SEVEN DAY LOAN

This book is to be returned on
or before the date stamped below

1 2 MAR 2003
2 3 MAR 2004
29 MAR 2004.

CARBON MONOXIDE
AND
CARDIOVASCULAR
FUNCTIONS

CARBON MONOXIDE
AND
CARDIOVASCULAR
FUNCTIONS

Edited by

Rui Wang, M.D., Ph.D.

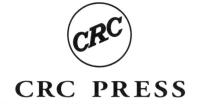

CRC PRESS

Boca Raton   London   New York   Washington, D.C.

Library of Congress Cataloging-in-Publication Data

Carbon monoxide and cardiovascular functions / Rui Wang, editor.
    p. ; cm.
    Includes bibliographical references and index.
    ISBN 0-8493-1041-5 (alk. paper) ✔
      1. Cardiovascular system--Physiology. 2. Carbon monoxide--Physiological effect. I.
Wang, Rui, M.D.
      [DNLM: 1. Cardiovascular Physiology--Congresses. 2. Carbon
Monoxide--metabolism--Congresses. WG 102 C264 2001]
    QP101 .C28 2001
    612.1--dc21

                                         2001037767

Visit the CRC Press Web site at www.crcpress.com

© 2002 by CRC Press LLC

No claim to original U.S. Government works
International Standard Book Number 0-8493-1041-5
Library of Congress Card Number 2001037767
Printed in the United States of America 1 2 3 4 5 6 7 8 9 0
Printed on acid-free paper

Dedications

To my parents, Chunmin Wang and Zhenyuan Li
   To my wife, Lingyun Wu, and my daughters, Jennifer Wang and Jessica Wang

Also to the Magnificent Five:
   Guangnan Wen, my supervisor of M.Sc. study, a Doctor of Never Give Up
      Peter K. Pang, my supervisor of Ph.D. study, a Doctor of Energy
         Ed Karpinski, my co-supervisor of Ph.D. study, a Doctor of Good Fellas
            Jacques de Champlain, my supervisor of post-doctoral study, a Doctor of
            Doctors
               Remy Sauvé, my co-supervisor of post-doctoral study, a Doctor of
               Finding the Needle in the Haystack

Preface

Carbon monoxide (CO) assumed its "silent killer" image as early as the 17th century and this image remains in the 21st century. For the most part, this conception arises because: (1) CO is produced by the incomplete combustion of organic materials including the most abundant air pollutants; (2) it is the most extensively studied and the best understood component of either mainstream or side-stream cigarette smoke; and (3) environmental exposure to CO is consistently associated with life-threatening hypoxic intoxication.

The first indication of a vascular effect of CO was provided by Duke and Killick (1952), who showed a decrease in pulmonary vascular resistance in the presence of CO. It was, however, not recognized until the early 1990s that CO-induced vasorelaxation might play a physiological role. The last ten years witnessed an astonishing surge of discoveries and re-discoveries of the physiological effects of CO. The cardiovascular effects of CO have been systematically mapped for the heart and the various vascular components. Heme oxygenases, which cleave the heme rings to form biliverdin and CO, have been located in the cardiovascular system and cloned. The endogenous production and induction of CO from the cardiovascular system have been documented. Advancements in the pharmacology of CO have provided an array of drugs that modulate CO metabolism. The altered functions and metabolism of CO have been related to many cardiovascular diseases. Thus, the status of CO has been transformed from a purely toxic gas to a dual-function compound involved in the homeostatic control of cardiovascular functions.

What makes the resurgence of interest in CO possible are the continuous advances in chemistry, biochemistry, biology, molecular biology, physiology, and electrophysiology. These advances demanded an arena to bring together the expertise of all these basic disciplines to enable practitioners to keep up with the explosive developments in this field. To meet the challenge, in December of 1998 an international symposium entitled "Carbon Monoxide and Cardiovascular Function" brought together a panel of distinguished scientists to exchange thoughts and generate new ideas about the cardiovascular effects of CO. Interestingly, this important event later took center stage at the Fifth Internet World Congress for Biomedical Sciences. The enthusiastic responses received from far and beyond after this virtual symposium encouraged me to take the mandate to use another medium to disseminate this important information. This book on the biological effects of CO on the cardiovascular system, the first of its kind, was thus produced. This idea was further encouraged by the First International Symposium on Heme Oxygenase held in July of 2000, which once again highlighted the physiological and pathophysiological importance of the cardiovascular effects of CO.

This book is the product of the collected wisdom of many respected scientists around the world. Concise up-to-date reviews of the fundamentals of the biological actions of CO on the cardiovascular system include all the most recent developments, scientific controversies, and future directions. The comprehensive coverage is maintained throughout the book without minimizing the complexity of the subject. To broaden our understanding of the biological roles of CO, a number of disorders in which the cardiovascular effects of CO are suspected to have been altered, including hypertension, diabetes, inflammation, and ischemic heart damage are addressed. This book also combines cutting-edge explanations of the mechanisms of CO actions with practical approaches to study the biological roles of CO under different conditions.

We may argue that earlier studies on the biological effects of CO were incomplete and oversimplified, but we cannot deny that today's understanding of the novel cardiovascular actions of CO has developed from the zigzag path of trial and error. Only time will tell whether what we know today about CO will still be valid or require modification. In this context, the progress reported in this book should be viewed as the beginning rather than the end of the exploration of the cardiovascular effects of CO.

Rui Wang, M.D., Ph.D.

Editor

Rui Wang, M.D., Ph.D., is a professor of physiology at the University of Saskatchewan, Canada. He graduated in 1982 from Weifang Medical College and completed his M.Sc. graduate study in 1984 at the Fourth Military Medical University, both in the People's Republic of China. In 1990, Dr. Wang obtained his Ph.D. with distinction from the University of Alberta, Canada. Thereafter, he pursued postdoctoral training at the Marine Biology Laboratory of the Woods Hole Oceanographic Institution in the U.S. and at the University of Montreal, Canada. He served as a faculty member at the University of Montreal from 1993 to 1997.

Dr. Wang is an expert on ion channel regulation of vascular smooth muscle functions. His research interests encompass hypertension and cardiovascular complications of diabetes. In recent years, Dr. Wang focused his investigations on the physiological roles of endogenous vasoactive gaseous molecules, including carbon monoxide, hydrogen sulfide, and nitric oxide. He organized the First International Internet Symposium entitled "Carbon Monoxide and Cardiovascular Function" in 1998. He has published more than 60 peer-reviewed articles, reviews, and book chapters covering many areas of health sciences and biology. Dr. Wang's academic achievements have been recognized internationally. Among the impressive honors and awards he has received is the Canadian Institutes of Health Research Scientist Award (2000–2005). He was named McDonald Scholar by the Heart and Stroke Foundation of Canada (1994–1999). He also received the Young Investigator Award of the Canadian Cardiovascular Society (1995) and the Stevenson Visiting Professorship of the Canadian Physiology Society (1996).

Contributors

Nader G. Abraham, Ph.D.
Department of Pharmacology
New York Medical College
Valhalla, New York

James F. Brien, Ph.D.
Department of Pharmacology and
 Toxicology
Queen's University
Kingston, Ontario, Canada

Kun Cao, M.D., Ph.D.
Department of Physiology
University of Saskatchewan,
Saskatoon, Saskatchewan, Canada

Dipak K. Das, Ph.D.
Cardiovascular Research Center
University of Connecticut School of
 Medicine
Farmington, Connecticut

Phyllis A. Dennery, M.D.
Division of Neonatal and Developmental
 Medicine
Stanford University School of Medicine
Palo Alto, California

William Durante, Ph.D.
Department of Medicine and
 Pharmacology
Houston VA Medical Center
Baylor College of Medicine
Houston, Texas

Roberta Foresti, Ph.D.
Department of Surgical Research
Northwich Park Institute for Medical
 Research
Harrow, Middlesex, England

Colin J. Green, M.D.
Department of Surgical Research
Northwich Park Institute for Medical
 Research
Harrow, Middlesex, England

Fruzsina K. Johnson, M.D.
Department of Physiology
Tulane University Medical Center
School of Medicine
New Orleans, Louisiana

Robert A. Johnson, Ph.D.
Department of Physiology
Tulane University Medical Center
School of Medicine
New Orleans, Louisiana

Attallah Kappas, Ph.D.
Department of Pharmacology
Gene Therapy Program
New York Medical College
Valhalla, New York

A. Kawashima, M.D.
Department of Pediatrics
Kanazawa University
Kanazawa, Japan

S. Koizumi, M.D.
Department of Pediatrics
Kanazawa University
Kanazawa, Japan

Pier Francesco Mannanoni, M.D.
Department of Preclinical and Clinical
  Pharmacology
University of Florence
Florence, Italy

Gerald S. Marks, Ph.D.
Department of Pharmacology and
  Toxicology
Queen's University
Kingston, Ontario, Canada

Emanuela Masini, M.D.
Department of Preclinical and Clinical
  Pharmacology
University of Florence
Florence Italy

Nilanjana Maulik, Ph.D.
Center for Cardiovascular Research
University of Connecticut School of
  Medicine
Farmington, Connecticut

Brian E. McLaughlin, Ph.D.
Department of Pharmacology and
  Toxicology
Queen's University
Kingston, Ontario, Canada

Roberto Motterlini, M.D.
Department of Surgical Research
Northwich Park Institute for Medical
  Research
Harrow, Middlesex, England

Kanji Nakatsu, Ph.D.
Department of Pharmacology and
  Toxicology
Queen's University
Kingston, Ontario, Canada

Joseph Fomusi Ndisang, Ph.D.
Department of Physiology
University of Saskatchewan
Saskatoon, Saskatchewan, Canada

K. Ohta, M.D.
Department of Pediatrics
Kanazawa University
Kanazawa, Japan

Shuo Quan, M.D., Ph.D.
Department of Pharmacology
New York Medical College
Valhalla, New York

Y. Saikawa, M.D.
Department of Pediatrics
Kanazawa University
Kanazawa, Japan

Sylvia Shenouda, Ph.D.
Department of Pharmacology
Gene Therapy Program
New York Medical College
Valhalla, New York

David K. Stevenson, M.D.
Department of Pediatrics
Neonatal and Developmental
  Medicine
Stanford University School
  of Medicine
Stanford, California

Hendrik J. Vreman, Ph.D.
Department of Pediatrics
Neonatal and Developmental Medicine
Stanford University School of Medicine
Stanford, California

Rui Wang, M.D., Ph.D.
Department of Physiology
College of Medicine
University of Saskatchewan
Saskatoon, Saskatchewan, Canada

Ronald J. Wong, M.Sc.
Department of Pediatrics
Neonatal and Developmental Medicine
Stanford University School of Medicine
Stanford, California

Lingyun Wu, M.D., Ph.D.
Department of Anatomy and Cell
  Biology
University of Saskatchewan
Saskatoon, Saskatchewan, Canada

Akihiro Yachie, M.D.
Department of Laboratory
  Sciences
Kanazawa University
Kanazawa, Japan

Weimin Zhao, M.D., Ph.D.
Department of Physiology
University of Saskatchewan
Saskatoon, Saskatchewan, Canada

Table of Contents

SECTION 2
Carbon Monoxide and Pathophysiology of the Cardiovascular System

SECTION 3
Techniques Used in Carbon Monoxide Research

Section 1

Carbon Monoxide and
Physiological Functions
of the Cardiovascular System

1 The Physiological Role of Carbon Monoxide Derived from Heme Oxidation Catalyzed by Heme Oxygenase

Gerald S. Marks, Brian E. McLaughlin, James F. Brien, and Kanji Nakatsu

CONTENTS

I. INTRODUCTION

A. GLYCERYL TRINITRATE AND NITRIC OXIDE

Our interest in the heme oxygenase (HO)–carbon monoxide (CO) system stems from our studies on the mechanism of action of nitroglycerin (GTN) which we have conducted for approximately 20 years.[1-5] In 1974, a prominent U.S. pharmacologist, Dr. John C. Krantz, who had worked for many years on the mechanism of action of GTN and other organic nitrates, wrote the following:[6]

> One who has watched this field of medicine change from empiricism to scientific exactness is still awed by the fact that GTN, the active ingredient in dynamite, dilates the coronary vessels. At present, this remains an enigma enveloped in an inscrutable puzzle. Perhaps some day the puzzle will yield to the researches of man.

In recent years this puzzle has been solved.[7-10] We have learned that nitric oxide (NO), a small gaseous molecule, is formed in the endothelial cells lining blood vessels by the action of an enzyme, nitric oxide synthase, on L-arginine. NO diffuses from the endothelial cells into the medial layer of blood vessels where it enhances soluble guanylyl cyclase (sGC) activity, elevates cyclic GMP (cGMP), and leads to vasorelaxation. Glyceryl trinitrate enters the medial layers of blood vessels where it is biotransformed to NO or an NO-adduct. sGC activity is enhanced, leading to vasorelaxation. Thus, GTN is biotransformed to NO or an NO-adduct,[5] thereby imitating a natural vasorelaxant process.

B. STUDIES OF GLYCERYL TRINITRATE BIOTRANSFORMATION USING CARBON MONOXIDE

We carried out studies to determine the mechanism by which GTN is biotransformed to NO or an NO-adduct. One hypothesis that we set out to test and which arose from an earlier study showing GTN biotransformation by deoxyhemoglobin[11] was that GTN was biotransformed to NO and/or an NO-adduct in vascular smooth muscle cells by a hemoprotein. In order to test this hypothesis, CO, a selective inhibitor of hemoprotein action, was bubbled into a tissue bath containing Krebs' solution in which a rabbit aortic smooth muscle, precontracted with phenylephrine, was mounted.[12,13] If a hemoprotein was responsible for biotransformation of GTN to NO and/or an NO-adduct, then it was anticipated that CO would inhibit biotransformation of GTN and inhibit GTN-induced vasorelaxation. However, CO was without effect on GTN biotransformation and GTN-induced relaxation, allowing us to conclude that in rabbit aortic strips, GTN biotransformation and GTN-induced relaxation were not dependent upon interaction with a hemoprotein.[12,13] During the above study, we observed, to our surprise, that CO relaxed rabbit aortic strips, although it was considerably less potent as a vasorelaxant than NO. Perusal of the literature revealed that other investigators had reported on the vasorelaxant effect of CO. CO was reported to relax rat coronary and aortic vascular smooth muscle,[14] lamb ductus venosus sphincter,[15] and dog femoral, carotid, and coronary arterial preparations.[16,17]

C. Formulation of Hypothesis — Does Carbon Monoxide Have a Physiological Function?

It has been proposed[16,17] that CO endogenously produced by lipid peroxidation[18] modulated blood vessel tone. Since CO shares the ability of NO to activate sGC,[19,20] it has been proposed that the modulation of blood vessel tone by CO occurs by activation of sGC.[16,17] Since lipid peroxidation is only a minor source of endogenous CO, we drew attention to the fact that the major source of endogenous CO was heme which would be metabolized by the HO enzyme to biliverdin, iron, and CO[20a] (Figure 1.1). CO is formed at the rate of 16.4 μmol/h in the human body. It has been customary to think of HO as the source of biliverdin and bilirubin (Figure 1.1) and as an enzyme whose activity results in the important clinical problem of hyperbilirubinemia. A paradigm shift occurred with regard to thinking about this enzyme when both biliverdin and bilirubin were shown to function as antioxidants and data supported the idea of a "beneficial" role for bilirubin as a physiological, chain-breaking antioxidant.[21]

As a result of these studies, we published a paper in 1991 entitled "Does carbon monoxide have a physiological function?"[22] We suggested that CO, which is formed endogenously from heme catabolism by HO and shares some of the chemical and biological roles of NO, may play a similar role. The L-arginine–NO pathway is accepted as a widespread signal transduction mechanism for the regulation of cell function and communication[23] and we suggested that the heme–CO pathway plays a similar role.

We envisaged that CO would bind to the iron atom of the heme moiety of sGC in a manner analogous to that of NO. This would result in activation of sGC and elevation of cGMP content, which would lead through a series of enzymic reactions to the physiological effect. The proposal that CO, regarded by medical science as a toxic agent, would have a widespread physiological role was difficult for some investigators to accept and the proposal initially met with disbelief. However, the proposal was easier to consider if one was familiar with a basic principle of toxicology put forward by Paracelsus in the 16th century:

> All substances are poisons, there is none which is not a poison; the right dose differentiates between a poison and a remedy.

Three forms of HO have been identified, namely HO-1 (inducible form), HO-2 (non-inducible form),[49] and a newly recognized form whose role is yet to be clarified.[49a] HO-1 has been identified as a 32-kDa mammalian stress protein. HO-1 participates in cellular defense mechanisms and its induction in mammalian cells is an indicator of oxidative stress.[49]

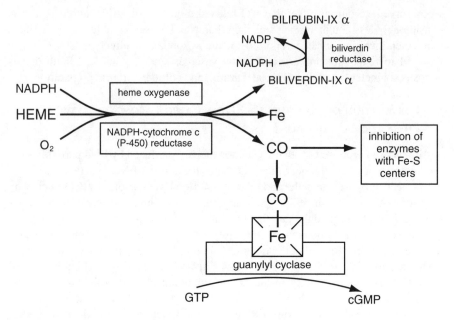

FIGURE 1.1 Schematic illustration of the formation of biliverdin-IXα, iron (Fe), and carbon monoxide (CO) following heme metabolism, catalyzed by heme oxygenase acting in concert with NADPH-cytochrome c (P-450) reductase. Biliverdin-IXα is subsequently converted to bilirubin-IXα by biliverdin reductase. It is proposed that CO binds to the iron atom of the heme moiety of cytosolic guanylyl cyclase in the cell in which CO is produced or in an adjacent cell. Activation of guanylyl cyclase results in elevated cGMP content, which leads via enzymatic reactions to the physiological effect, e.g., smooth muscle relaxation. It is also proposed that in macrophages, CO activates guanylyl cyclase and elevates cGMP, thereby changing metabolism and facilitating microbicidal and/or tumoricidal effects. CO produced by macrophages binds to Fe–S centers of enzymes, causing inhibition, and thereby facilitates microbicidal and/or tumoricidal effects. (Reproduced from Marks, G.S. et al., *Trends Pharmacol. Sci.*, 12, 185, 1991. With permission.)

II. EXPERIMENTAL INVESTIGATIONS DIRECTED TO DETERMINE WHETHER CARBON MONOXIDE HAS A PHYSIOLOGICAL ROLE

A. PRESENCE OF HEME OXYGENASE IN BLOOD VESSELS

In our original paper,[22] we outlined a series of experimental investigations that needed to be conducted in order to test the hypothesis that CO has a physiological function. Our first experiments were directed to determining whether HO was present in blood vessels since we were primarily interested in the vasorelaxant effects of CO. We utilized a sensitive gas chromatographic technique[24] for measurement of CO as an index of HO enzymatic activity. In our own laboratory[25] and in collaboration with other investigators,[26,27] we measured HO enzymatic activity in a wide variety of arteries and veins. These findings were confirmed by other investigators.[28]

The presence of HO protein and HO mRNA has been confirmed by studies in our laboratories[29] and those of others.[30,31]

B. ENDOGENOUS FORMATION OF CARBON MONOXIDE IN BLOOD VESSELS AND OTHER TISSUES

Our next studies were directed to measuring CO production by various tissues. In 1997, we reported for the first time that endogenous CO formation occurs in the hippocampus of the guinea pig and that the magnitude of CO formation rate was age-dependent.[32] The magnitude of CO formation rate was greater in the fetal than in the adult hippocampus. The maximum CO formation was found at gestational day 62 (term, about gestational day 68) and was 0.034 nmol/mg dry weight/hr. In recent studies in our laboratory,[33] preliminary data demonstrate time-dependent CO formation in the chorionic villi of human placenta. The results were obtained by direct analytical measurement of CO without the addition of exogenous heme to the experimental system. A CO production rate of 0.052 nmol/mg protein/h was measured by a radioactive (^{14}C) method in cultured cells from the rat olfactory bulb.[34] Kaide et al.[35] used gas chromatography–mass spectroscopy to measure CO formation from rat interlobar arteries and found CO formation of 0.095 nmol/mg protein/hr. The release of CO was inhibited by chromium mesoporphyrin.

Recently, Moromito et al.[36] carried out real-time measurements of endogenous CO production from rat aortic vascular smooth muscle cells using an ultrasensitive laser sensor and choosing a strong infrared absorption line of CO (4.67 μm) for CO detection without interference from other gases. The basal rate of CO production was found to be 0.072 nmol/mg protein/hr. Increases in CO production were demonstrated after addition of the HO substrate, hemin, followed by decreases after the addition of the HO inhibitor, tin protoporphyrin IX. The facts that the synthetic machinery for CO is present in blood vessels and that real-time endogenous CO production in vascular cells and vascular preparations is measurable satisfy important criteria for a physiological role of CO in blood vessels.

Hypoxia has been shown to be a strong stimulus for vascular smooth muscle cell (VSMC) proliferation. Under conditions of hypoxia, the expression of HO-1 is up-regulated, resulting in increased production of CO. Morita et al.[37] have shown that the enhanced production of CO leads to an elevation of cGMP levels and to diminished proliferation of VSMCs. Thus, the HO-1/CO system is thought to represent a "counter-proliferative" system which appears during hypoxic conditions. The authors[37] suggest that CO antagonizes the proliferative effects of hypoxia on VSMC growth, thus limiting blood vessel wall hyperplasia.

C. USE OF METALLOPORPHYRIN INHIBITORS TO STUDY POSSIBLE PHYSIOLOGICAL ROLE OF CARBON MONOXIDE

In our 1991 paper, we suggested that a possible physiological role of CO might be explored by the use of inhibitors of HO.[22] This suggestion was based on the fact that inhibitors of enzymatic activity served as useful chemical probes in establishing physiological roles for specific enzymes. Thus, N^ω-nitro-L-arginine methyl ester (L-NAME) has played an important role in elucidating the biological role of NO. We were also aware that a series of metalloporphyrins such as tin mesoporphyrin served as inhibitors of HO and were utilized therapeutically to reduce hyperbilirubinemia in the neonate.[38,39] The potency of metalloporphyrins as inhibitors of HO is dependent upon the metal cation associated with the porphyrin ring as well as upon different ring substituents.[40]

Many investigators used metalloporphyrins to test the hypothesis that CO has a physiological role. Zakhary et al.[41,42] used tin protoporphyrin (SnPP) to investigate a possible role for CO as a vasodilator. Zinc protoporphyrin (ZnPP) has also been used to demonstrate an apparent role for CO in long-term potentiation.[43-45] Several investigators have shown that metalloporphyrins are not selective inhibitors of HO; they also inhibit NOS, sGC, and possibly other enzymes and/or receptors.[46-48] For this reason, the conclusions reached by investigators who used metalloporphyrins to establish a physiological role for CO in biological systems, in which NOS and sGC are also active, have been criticized. In contrast, Zakhary et al.[41] reported that SnPP was ten times more potent in inhibiting HO-2 than NOS or sGC, and based on this finding, used SnPP to study CO-induced vasodilation.

Maines[49] points out that the heme pocket of HO is not occupied so that the substrate, heme, and metalloporphyrin inhibitors can gain ready access to the pocket. For this reason, HO activity can be inhibited by small concentrations of metalloporphyrins and a concentration of ZnPP as low as $2\ \mu M$ was found to inhibit HO-2 activity by 50%.[50] In contrast, heme is bound to NOS and sGC and higher concentrations of metalloporphyrin inhibitor would be required to displace heme bound to the protein. Maines therefore advocates using low concentrations of metalloporphyrins to test for the selective inhibition of HO.

We tested a series of metalloporphyrins previously shown to inhibit HO activity for their ability to inhibit HO without inhibition of NOS or sGC activities.[51] We measured the activities of HO in rat brain microsomes and NOS in rat brain cytosol in samples incubated with metalloporphyrins (0.15 to $50\ \mu M$) including ZnPP, zinc deuteroporphyrin IX 2,4-bis-ethylene glycol (ZnBG), chromium mesoporphyrin IX (CrMP), SnPP, and zinc N-methyl protoporphyrin IX (ZnNMePP). The results are shown in Figure 1.2. We were able to determine a maximum selective inhibitory (MSI) concentration at or below which inhibition of HO occurs with no effect on NOS. We concluded from our studies that CrMP and ZnBG, at concentrations at and below $5\ \mu M$, were selective inhibitors of HO activity relative to NOS activity in rat brain.

Meffert et al.,[47] who concluded that some metalloporphyrins are non-selective and would therefore not be useful in biological studies involving CO, employed metalloporphyrins in the concentration range of 10 to $100\ \mu M$. Grundemar et al.,[48] who arrived at a similar conclusion, utilized a concentration of ZnPP of $100\ \mu M$. The message that emerges is that, to achieve selectivity of metalloporphyrin-induced inhibition of HO vs. NOS, the concentration used is critically important and must be kept $\leq 5\ \mu M$.

To further characterize the selectivity of metalloporphyrins as inhibitors of HO, the effect of CrMP and ZnBG on basal and S-nitrosopenicillamine (SNAP)-induced

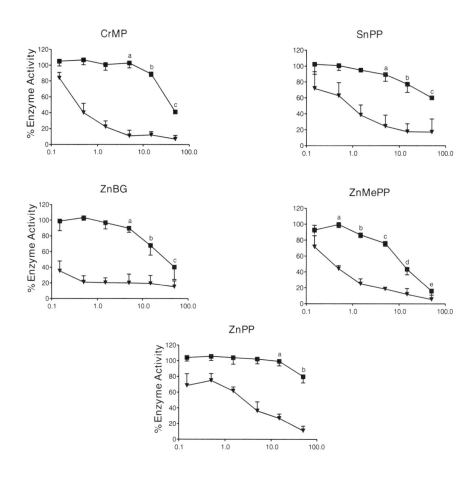

Log Metalloporphyrin Concentration (μM)

FIGURE 1.2 Inhibition of HO and NOS activity by CrMP, SnPP, ZnBG, ZnMePP, and ZnPP. Concentration–response curves for HO (▼) and NOS (■) activity in rat brain microsomes and cytosols, respectively, were obtained. The data are presented as group means ± S.D. ($n = 4$). The *a* represents the MSI concentration at or below which there is selective inhibition of HO activity with no effect on NOS activity. NOS activities for lower concentrations of metalloporphyrins were no different from the MSI concentration. Group means with different letters are statistically different from each other, $p < 0.05$. (Reproduced from Appleton, S.D. et al., *Drug Metab. Dispos.*, 27, 1214, 1999. With permission.)

sGC activity was determined using metalloporphyrin concentrations of 0.15 to 15 μ*M*. ZnBG did not affect basal sGC activity, but did potentiate SNAP-induced activity. CrMP did not affect basal or SNAP-induced activity. We conclude that careful exploration of concentration–response relationships with a variety of metalloporphyrins potentially can lead to the identification of an appropriate selective inhibitor for the biological model used.[51]

Confirmation of the selectivity of HO inhibition by metalloporphyrins comes from the work of Zakhary et al.,[42] who used HO-2 knockout mice and SnPP to demonstrate that CO plays a role in non-adrenergic, non-cholinergic (NANC) relaxation evoked by electrical field stimulation of mouse ileal segments. Thus, in mice in which the HO-2 gene had been deleted, SnPP did not affect NANC transmission, whereas in wild-type mice, SnPP partially inhibited NANC transmission. Zhuo et al.,[45] who studied the respective roles of NO and CO in long-term potentiation (LTP) in the rat hippocampus, carried out a careful study of the selectivity of the HO inhibitors, ZnPP, SnPP, ZnBG, and copper protoporphyrin (CuPP). Inhibitors of HO have been shown to inhibit the induction of LTP in the hippocampus by several groups of investigators, suggesting that CO in addition to NO was a retrograde messenger. This suggestion has been criticized because of evidence that HO inhibitors might also inhibit NOS and therefore NO production.[46-48] Zhuo et al.[45] were able to demonstrate that LTP induced by four trains of stimulation was significantly reduced by inhibitors of HO but only slightly reduced by inhibitors of NOS, suggesting that HO inhibitors do not act by inhibiting NOS.

Zhuo et al.[45] considered the possibility that the HO inhibitors might act by inhibiting sGC, which would then block induction of LTP. It was thought that if the HO inhibitors act by direct inhibition of sGC, they should block LTP produced by CO. The fact that in the presence of 10 μM ZnPP or 10 μM ZnBG, CO paired with weak stimulation still produced long-lasting LTP was in accord with the idea that metalloporphyrins inhibited HO rather than sGC. These investigators conclude that low doses of HO inhibitors have little effect on NOS or sGC.[45]

Thus, the studies of Zhuo et al.[45] and Zakhary et al.[42] are consistent with those of Appleton et al.,[51] that low doses of HO inhibitors have little effect on NOS or sGC. On a cautionary note, we suggest that, with different biological models, the concentration of metalloporphyrins that will selectively inhibit HO activity without inhibiting NOS and sGC activities should be determined and the most appropriate metalloporphyrin selected. Consideration will also be required of the facility with which metalloporphyrins distribute across multi-membrane systems such as the blood–brain barrier and the placenta.

D. EFFECT OF INHIBITION OF SOLUBLE GUANYLYL CYCLASE ON VASCULAR EFFECTS OF CARBON MONOXIDE

It has been proposed that the modulation of blood vessel tone by CO occurs by activation of sGC.[19,22] We were interested in determining whether this was the case, and in order to do so, sought to investigate the effects of inhibitors of sGC on CO-mediated relaxation of rabbit aortic rings. Methylene blue[52] and LY83583[53] have been widely used as sGC inhibitors. However, results have been inconclusive because of their demonstrated lack of selectivity. In 1995, ODQ (IH-[1,2,4]oxadiazolo[4,3-a]quinoxalin-1-one) was introduced by Garthwaite et al.[54] with the claim that it was a specific inhibitor of sGC, leading to its widespread use to detect involvement of cGMP in a pharmacological response. We investigated the role of sGC in the relaxation of rabbit aortic rings by CO.[55] CO relaxed rabbit aortic rings 47% and this relaxation was reduced to 26% by pretreatment with 0.1 μM ODQ

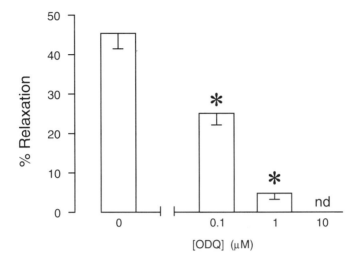

FIGURE 1.3 Effects of ODQ on relaxation by 30 μM CO gas. Inclusion of 0.1, 1, or 10 μM ODQ for 10 min prior to submaximal contraction resulted in an increasing attenuated relaxation to a single dose of CO compared with the control containing only DMSO vehicle. Each bar represents the mean ± S.D. of four determinations. Significant differences between ODQ-treated RARs and the DMSO control were determined by a one-way analysis of variance (ANOVA); *$p < 0.01$; nd, no detectable relaxation. (Reproduced from Hussain, A.S. et al., *Can. J. Physiol. Pharmacol.*, 75, 1034, 1997. With permission.)

(Figure 1.3). The relaxation was lowered to 7.4% by 1 μM ODQ and completely blocked by 10 μM ODQ. In a subsequent study, CO-induced relaxation of rat aortic strips was shown to be inhibited by 1 μM ODQ.[56] These studies supported the idea that CO-induced relaxation occurs by activation of sGC.

Supporting evidence for this idea comes from the studies of Morita et al.[57] and Christodoulides et al.,[58] who showed in cultured vascular myocytes that induction of HO to produce CO resulted in cGMP accumulation. Recent studies of Feelisch et al.[59] have shown that ODQ is not as selective as previously claimed[55] and that, in addition to the heme protein, sGC, it is capable of inhibiting other heme proteins such as cytochrome P-450 and NOS. These investigators suggest that particular care is required when ODQ is used to inhibit the action of endothelium-dependent vasodilators such as acetylcholine, where NOS is involved, or with NO donors requiring metabolic activation by cytochrome P-450. Since CO vasorelaxation is not dependent upon NOS nor upon metabolic activation by cytochrome P450, we conclude that ODQ is an appropriate inhibitor to use in probing the involvement of the heme protein, sGC, in CO-induced vasorelaxation.

E.   POTENTIATION OF CARBON MONOXIDE-INDUCED RELAXATION OF RAT AORTA BY YC-1 [3-(5′-HYDROXYMETHYL-2′-FURYL)-1-BENZYLINDAZOLE]

The proposal that CO plays an important role in vascular smooth muscle relaxation has been criticized because CO alone is a poor activator of sGC compared with

NO.[60,61] Moreover, CO has less than one thousandth of the potency of NO in the relaxation of rabbit aorta.[20] Studies by Friebe et al.[62] have muted that criticism. These investigators showed that YC-1, an NO-independent activator of sGC, potentiated CO stimulation of the activity of this enzyme to a magnitude similar to that achieved with NO. They proposed that CO may have a physiological role in the regulation of blood vessel tone should an endogenous analogue of YC-1 exist. This idea was also proposed by Stone and Marletta.[63]

We have recently shown that 1 μM YC-1, a concentration that did not cause vasodilation, potentiated CO-induced relaxation of rabbit aortic strips approximately 10-fold.[56] This is comparable in magnitude to an approximately 30-fold increase in CO-induced sGC activation produced by YC-1 in the study of Friebe et al.[62] We concluded that, should an endogenous compound exist with properties similar to those of YC-1, then the potency of CO as a vasorelaxant in the presence of this factor would be enhanced sufficiently that CO could play a role in the regulation of blood vessel tone comparable to that of NO.[56]

F. Kinetics of Carbon Monoxide in Tissue Bath Medium

We have noted that, upon adding CO solutions to a tissue bath containing vascular smooth muscle in an aerated Krebs' solution, the vasorelaxation is of very short duration.[56] The short duration of vasorelaxation might be due, at least in part, to rapid loss of CO from the medium and the concentration of CO in the medium was less than that derived from theoretical calculation. We used a gas chromatographic method[24] to obtain an accurate measurement of CO concentration in the tissue bath medium and showed that the time-dependent loss of CO from Krebs' solution was statistically significant after 1 min and complete after 10 min (Figure 1.4). For each volume of CO-containing solution added to the tissue bath, the actual concentration of CO measured 20 s later in the tissue bath was approximately one half of the calculated value (Table 1.1). It was concluded that CO has a vasorelaxant potency two times greater than previously estimated based on theoretical calculation of its concentration.

III. SITES OF ACTION OF CARBON MONOXIDE OTHER THAN SOLUBLE GUANYLYL CYCLASE

A. Calcium-Dependent Potassium Channels

Wang et al.[64] studied the vasorelaxant effects of CO in phenylephrine or U-46619 precontracted rat tail artery. The concentration-dependent relaxation of rat tail artery by CO was only partially inhibited by the sGC inhibitor, methylene blue, in contrast to complete inhibition observed of CO-dependent relaxation of rat aortic strip (RtAS) and rabbit aortic rings (RARs) using the sGC inhibitor, ODQ.[55,56] It was thus concluded that, in contrast to RARs and RtAS, an additional cGMP-independent mechanism was involved in CO-dependent relaxation in the rat tail artery.

Wang et al.[64] also explored the possibility that the cGMP-independent CO-induced relaxation involved K$^+$ channels. They showed that tetraethylammonium

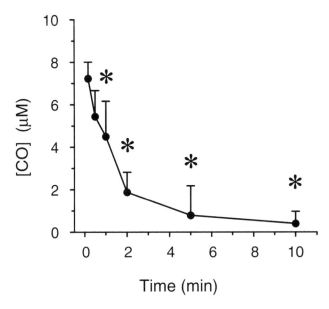

FIGURE 1.4 Relationship of CO concentration in Krebs' solution to time of incubation following the addition of 100 μL of CO-saturated solution to a tissue bath ($n = 4$ experiments). (Reproduced from McLaughlin, B.E. et al., *Can. J. Physiol. Pharmacol.*, 78, 343, 2000. With permission.)

cation (TEA), an inhibitor of K^+ channels, produced partial inhibition of CO-induced relaxation of rat tail artery (RTA). Using more selective inhibitors, these investigators were able to relate the CO effect to the opening of high conductance K_{Ca} channels in vascular smooth muscle.[64] The CO-induced relaxation was completely inhibited by a combination of TEA and methylene blue, showing that CO-induced vasorelaxation is mediated both by activation of sGC and the opening of high conductance K_{Ca} channels in RTA. Further studies were directed to determining the mechanism by which CO increases the opening of high conductance K_{Ca} channels.

Investigators are accustomed to thinking that CO interacts with the iron atom of heme. Wang and Wu[65] obtained a novel result indicating that the CO-induced increase in the open probability of K_{Ca} channels may rely on hydrogen bond formation of CO with a histidine residue in the K_{Ca} channels located on the external surfaces of the cell membranes. The involvement of K_{Ca} channels in CO-induced vasorelaxation has been confirmed by several other investigators. Nasjletti[66] studied the effects of CO on small arterial vessels: gracilis muscle arterioles (GMAs) and renal interlobar arteries (ILAs). CO-induced relaxation of PE-contracted GMAs and ILAs was prevented by the potassium channel inhibitor, TEA. Since both GMA and ILA contain K_{Ca} channels, it was concluded that endogenously produced CO inhibits constrictor stimuli in GMAs and ILAs by stimulation of K_{Ca} channels.

Brian et al.[67] reported that adult rabbit and dog cerebral arteries *in vitro* were unresponsive to CO even at very high concentrations. In contrast, Leffler et al.[68] showed that CO is a potent dilator of newborn pig cerebral microcirculation. The

TABLE 1.1

Concentration of CO in Krebs' solution following the addition of CO-saturated saline solution to tissue bath medium aerated with 95% O_2–5% CO_2, as demonstrated by (a) theoretical calculation, and (b) analytical measurement using a gas chromatographic method

Volume of CO-saturated saline solution (µl)	CO concentration (µM)	
	Theoretical[a]	Measured[b]
3	0.26	0.10 ± 0.26
10	0.87	0.31 ± 0.34
30	2.6	1.3 ± 0.4
100	8.7	5.3 ± 0.7
300	26	13 ± 1.2
1000	87	36 ± 5.7

[a] Theoretical calculation for CO concentration was made using the mole fraction solubility of CO in water at 1 atm and 35°C, reported by Gevantman (1998) to be 1.562×10^{-5}.
[b] Data for CO concentration measured using a gas chromatographic method, are presented as group means ± S.D. for five experiments. (Reproduced from McLaughlin, B.E. et al., *Can. J. Physiol. Pharmacol.*, 78, 343, 2000. With permission.)

possibility that CO functions physiologically as a vasodilator has been criticized because of its low potency compared to NO as a vasodilator and as a stimulant of sGC.[60,61] It is therefore of particular interest that in piglet pial arterioles (< 60 µm in diameter), significant vasodilation was reached at 10^{-11} M CO, and at 10^{-10} M in larger arterioles (> 60 µm in diameter). At 10^{-9} M CO, maximal dilation was observed in vessels of both sizes.[68] Thus, the potency of CO as a vasodilator in this system is comparable to the potency observed with NO as a vasodilator in other systems. Moreover, the CO-induced vasodilation is blocked by TEA and iberiotoxin, inhibitors of K_{Ca} channels, and appears to be unrelated to sGC activation. Leffler et al.[68] suggest the following reasons for the differences observed in their experiments and those previously reported by Brian et al.[67]: (1) the small diameters of the arterioles they employed vs. the large diameters of the arteries employed by Brian et al.[67]; (2) their use of an *in vivo* preparation vs. the *in vitro* preparation used by Brian et al.[67]; (3) their use of newborn vs. adult animals; and, finally, (4) species differences.

B. P38 MITOGEN-ACTIVATED PROTEIN (MAP) KINASE

Scientists have known for some time that HO-1, an inducible HO isozyme, is a 32-kDa mammalian stress protein that participates in cellular defense mechanisms.

Induction of HO-1 in mammalian cells is an indicator of oxidative stress.[68a] Since HO-1 has antiinflammatory properties,[69,70] it is thought that these properties may be the reason for cytoprotection.

Support for this idea was obtained by demonstrating diminished tumor necrosis factor-α (TNF-α) production in RAW264.7 macrophages overexpressing HO-1 after exposure to lipopolysaccharide (LPS). Otterbein et al.[70] showed *in vivo* in mice and *in vitro* in RAW264.7 cells that CO inhibited the expression of LPS-induced proinflammatory cytokines, tumor necrosis factor-α, interleukin 1-β, and macrophage inflammatory protein-1β. Moreover, CO enhanced the LPS-induced expression of the antiinflammatory cytokine interleukin-10. Of considerable interest is the fact that the concentrations of CO used in these studies were 10 to 500 ppm (0.001 to 0.05%). As pointed out by Otterbein et al.,[69,70] these concentrations of CO are comparable to concentrations used in humans (0.03%) in the measurement of CO lung diffusion capacity. Moreover, after exposure of rodents to 500 ppm CO for 2 years, no significant alterations were noted by either physiological or biochemical tests. The investigators were surprised to find that the CO-induced effects were not due to stimulation of sGC and elevated cGMP levels, nor could they be attributed to production of NO which is known to have antiinflammatory effects. The mechanism of CO antiinflammatory action was found to be attributable to CO selectively affecting the LPS-induced activation of p38 mitogen-activated protein (MAP) kinase while showing no effect on the extracellular signal-regulated kinase ERK1/ERK2 or c-*jun* N-terminal kinase (JNK) MAP kinases.

Brouard et al.[71] have shown that HO-1 exerts antiapoptotic effects in bovine aortic endothelial cells and in murine 2F-2B endothelial cell lines that is mediated by CO and involves activation of p38 MAP kinase. Moreover, low concentrations of CO (0.025%) were found to protect mice against oxidant-induced lung injury via the same pathway.[72] Finally, CO was found to substitute for HO-1 in suppressing the rejection of mouse to rat cardiac transplants.[73] The biochemical mechanism by which CO modulates MAP kinases is not known. Of interest is the fact that new protein synthesis is required in order for the protective effects of CO to be observed.[70] These studies led to the suggestion that CO may serve as a therapeutic agent for septic shock syndrome, lung disorders such as acute respiratory diseases (ARDs), and other inflammatory disease states.[70,71,74]

IV. SUMMARY

Galbraith[75] points out in a recent interesting review entitled "Heme oxygenase: Who needs it?" that since our group in 1991[22] posed the question, "Does carbon monoxide have a physiological role?," the literature in favor of a physiological role for CO continues to grow. Numerous studies now provide evidence that the heme–CO pathway serves as a widespread signal transduction mechanism for the regulation of cell function and communication in the cardiovascular system,[76,77] in the CNS,[78,79] in neuroendocrine systems,[80] in the gastrointestinal system,[81] in the placenta,[82] and in the myometrium.[83]

The most conclusive evidence for a physiological role for CO comes from studies employing mice with genomic deletions of HO-2 (HO2$^-$) or HO-1 (HO1$^-$). Such

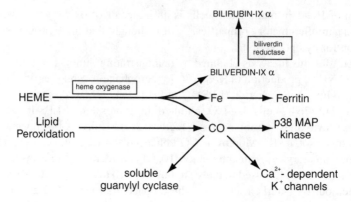

FIGURE 1.5 Schematic illustration of the formation of CO following heme metabolism catalyzed by heme oxygenase. Biliverdin is converted to bilirubin by biliverdin reductase. An additional source of CO is lipid peroxidation.[20a] The biological actions of CO are mediated by several pathways: soluble guanylyl cyclase (sGC), Ca^{2+}-dependent K^+ channels, and p38 MAP kinase. Fe^{2+} mediates the induction of the iron-storage protein, ferritin, which has antioxidant properties.

studies reveal that CO functions as a neurotransmitter in the myenteric plexus.[42] The most plausible product of HO-2 regulation of the neuromuscular reflex mechanisms involved in ejaculation is CO.[84] HO-1 is important for mammalian iron homeostasis, rapid protection of cells from stress-induced oxidative damage, and production of CO for participation in a variety of second messenger signaling systems.[85,86] The importance of HO-1 is illustrated by the first case of HO-1 deficiency reported from Japan.[87] A 2-year old patient exhibited relapsing fever, erythematous rash, and joint pain. When the patient reached 6 years of age, massive amyloid deposition was noted in the liver. The major target of HO-1 deficiency was endothelial cell and renal tubular epithelial cell injury. Liver parenchymal damage and monocyte dysfunction were present. These effects were attributed to the toxic effects of concentrated heme.

Our hypothesis put forward in 1991[22] is shown in Figure 1.1. Later developments led to a modified version of our hypothesis (Figure 1.5). Thus, while heme degradation catalyzed by HO is the major source of CO in the body, it has other sources such as lipid peroxidation.[20a] Moreover, it is now clear that sGC is not the sole target for CO, and that other targets such as Ca^{2+}-dependent K^+ channels[64] and p38 MAP kinase[70] exist. Coceani et al.[88] suggested in 1996 that, in the ductus arteriosus of the lamb, endogenous CO-induced relaxation occurs during endotoxin treatment and is attributable to inhibition of cytochrome P-450-mediated production of the vasoconstrictor endothelin-1 (ET-1). This operational linkage between CO and the cytochrome P-450/ET-1 system in the endotoxin-treated tissue could not be confirmed, at least to a significant degree, and the apparent inconsistency was ascribed to the overriding action of alternative agent(s), such as a cyclooxygenase product competing with CO in the curtailment of ET-1 synthesis.[89] Some investigators have queried the possible deleterious effects of the release of Fe^{2+} from heme by HO because of the possible generation of the hydroxyl radical following the Fenton reaction between

Fe^{2+} and the superoxide radical anion (O_2^-).[75] Other investigators suggest that iron is rapidly sequestered by the ferritin iron-storage protein, and that ferritin is up-regulated with an increase in cytoprotection.[69]

Tepperman suggests that CO may be considered for use in a number of clinical settings and stated in a recent editorial[90] that, because CO appears to participate in the regulation of host inflammatory responses, it may be the next "molecule of the year." Barinaga,[91] who wrote an article in 1993 entitled "Carbon monoxide: killer to brain messenger in one step," predicts that CO "was likely to provide fuel to run plenty of labs." The latter prediction certainly turned out to be true. Observing the last 10 years of research on the physiological role of CO has been enjoyable and gratifying. The next decade promises to yield even more exciting results.

ACKNOWLEDGMENT

This work was supported by the Heart and Stroke Foundation of Ontario, Canada (Grant No. NA-4438).

REFERENCES

1. Brien, J.F. et al., Biotransformation of glyceryl trinitrate occurs concurrently with relaxation of rabbit aorta, *J. Pharmacol. Exp. Ther.*, 237, 608, 1986.
2. Brien, J.F. et al., Mechanism of glyceryl trinitrate-induced vasodilation. I. Relationship between drug biotransformation, tissue cyclic GMP elevation and relaxation of rabbit aorta, *J. Pharmacol. Exp. Ther.*, 244, 322, 1988.
3. Marks, G.S. et al., Direct evidence for nitric oxide formation from glyceryl trinitrate during incubation with intact bovine pulmonary artery, *Can. J. Physiol. Pharmacol.*, 70, 308, 1992.
4. Marks, G.S. et al., Time-dependent increase in nitric oxide formation concurrent with vasodilation induced by sodium nitroprusside, 3-morpholinosydnonimine, and S-nitroso-N-acetylpenicillamine but not by glyceryl trinitrate, *Drug Metab. Dispos.*, 23, 1248, 1995.
5. Hussain, A.S. et al., Superoxide does not inhibit glyceryl trinitrate-rabbit aortic strip-mediated relaxation of rabbit taenia coli: evidence against a role for nitric oxide as the smooth muscle active drug metabolite? *Drug Metab. Dispos.*, 24, 780, 1996.
6. Krantz, J.C., Jr., *Historical Medical Classics Involving New Drugs*, Williams & Wilkins, Baltimore, 1974, Chap. 5.
7. Furchgott, R.F., Studies on relaxation of rabbit aorta by sodium nitrite: the basis for the proposal that the acid-activatable inhibitory factor from bovine retractor penis is inorganic nitrite and the endothelium-derived relaxing factor is nitric oxide, in *Vasodilation: Vascular Smooth Muscle, Peptides, Autonomic Nerves, and Endothelium*, Vanhoutte, P.M., Ed., Raven Press, New York, 1988, 401.
8. Ignarro, L.J., Byrns, R.E., and Wood, K.S., Biochemical and pharmacological properties of endothelium-derived relaxing factor and its similarity to nitric oxide radical, in *Vasodilation: Vascular Smooth Muscle, Peptides, Autonomic Nerves, and Endothelium*, Vanhoutte, P.M., Ed., Raven Press, New York, 1988, 427.
9. Palmer, R.M.J., Ferrige, A.G., and Moncada, S., Nitric oxide release accounts for the biological activity of endothelium-derived relaxing factor, *Nature*, 327, 524, 1987.

10. Palmer, R.M.J., Ashton, D.S., and Moncada, S., Vascular endothelial cells synthesize nitric oxide from L-arginine, *Nature*, 333, 664, 1988.
11. Bennett, B.M. et al., Biotransformation of glyceryl trinitrate to glyceryl dinitrate by human hemoglobin, *Can. J. Physiol. Pharmacol.*, 62, 704, 1984.
12. Liu, Z. et al., Carbon monoxide does not inhibit glyceryl trinitrate biotransformation by or relaxation of aorta, *Eur. J. Pharmacol.*, 211, 129, 1992.
13. Liu, Z. et al., Lack of evidence for the involvement of cytochrome P-450 or other hemoproteins in metabolic activation of glyceryl trinitrate (GTN) in rabbit aorta, *J. Pharmacol. Exp. Ther.*, 264, 1432, 1993.
14. Ramos, K.S., Lin, H., and McGrath, J.J., Modulation of cyclic guanosine monophosphate levels in cultured aortic smooth muscle cells by carbon monoxide, *Biochem. Pharmacol.*, 38, 1368, 1989.
15. Adeagbo, A.S.O. et al., Lamb ductus venosus: evidence of a cytochrome P-450 mechanism in its contractile tension, *J. Pharmacol. Exp. Ther.*, 252, 875, 1990.
16. Vedernikov, Y.P., Gräser, T., and Vanin, A.F., Similar endothelium-independent arterial relaxation by carbon monoxide and nitric oxide, *Biomed. Biochim. Acta*, 48, 601, 1989.
17. Gräser, T., Vedernikov, Y.P., and Li, D.S., Study on the mechanism of carbon monoxide induced endothelium-independent relaxation in porcine coronary artery and vein, *Biomed. Biochim. Acta*, 49, 293, 1990.
18. Wolff, D.G. and Bidlack, W.R., The formation of carbon monoxide during peroxidation of microsomal lipids, *Biochem. Biophys. Res. Commun.*, 73, 850, 1976.
19. Brune, B. and Ullrich, V., Inhibition of platelet aggregation by carbon monoxide is mediated by activation of guanylate cyclase, *Mol. Pharmacol.*, 32, 497, 1987.
20. Furchgott, R.F. and Jothianandan, D., Endothelium-dependent and -independent vasodilation involving cyclic GMP: relaxation induced by nitric oxide, carbon monoxide and light, *Blood Vessels*, 28, 52, 1991.
20a. Vreman, H.J., Wong, R.J., and Stevenson, D.K., Carbon monoxide in breath, blood and other tissues, in *Carbon Monoxide Toxicity*, Penney, D.G., Ed., CRC Press, Boca Raton, FL, 2000, Chap. 2.
21. Stocker, R. et al., Bilirubin is an antioxidant of possible physiological importance, *Science*, 235, 1043, 1987.
22. Marks, G.S. et al., Does carbon monoxide have a physiological function? *Trends Pharmacol. Sci.*, 12, 185, 1991.
23. Moncada, S., Palmer, R.M.J., and Higgs, E.A., Nitric oxide: physiology, pathophysiology and pharmacology, *Pharmacol. Rev.*, 43, 109, 1991.
24. Vreman, H.J. and Stevenson, D.K., Heme oxygenase activity as measured by carbon monoxide production, *Anal. Biochem.*, 168, 31, 1988.
25. Cook, M.N. et al., Heme oxygenase activity in the adult rat aorta and liver as measured by carbon monoxide formation, *Can. J. Physiol. Pharmacol.*, 73, 515, 1995.
26. Coceani, F. et al., Carbon monoxide formation in the ductus arteriosus in the lamb: implications for the regulation of muscle tone, *Br. J. Pharmacol.*, 120, 599, 1997.
27. Vreman, H.J. et al., Haem oxygenase activity in human umbilical cord and rat vascular tissues, *Placenta*, 21, 337, 2000.
28. Grundemar, L. et al., Haem oxygenase activity in blood vessel homogenates as measured by carbon monoxide production, *Acta Physiol. Scand.*, 153, 203, 1995.
29. Marks, G.S. et al., Heme oxygenase activity and immunohistochemical localization in bovine pulmonary artery and vein, *J. Cardiovasc. Pharmacol.*, 30, 1, 1997.
30. Ewing, J.F., Raju, V.S., and Maines, M.D., Induction of heart heme oxygenase-1 (HSP32) by hyperthermia: possible role in stress-mediated elevation of cyclic 3':5'-guanosine monophosphate, *J. Pharmacol. Exp. Ther.* 271, 408, 1994.

31. Zakhary, R. et al., Heme oxygenase 2: endothelial and neuronal localization and role in endothelium-dependent relaxation, *Proc. Natl. Acad. Sci. U.S.A.*, 93, 795, 1996.
32. Cook, M.N. et al., Carbon monoxide formation in the guinea pig hippocampus: ontogeny and effect of *in vitro* ethanol exposure, *Dev. Brain Res.*, 101, 283, 1997.
33. McLaughlin, B. et al., Formation of endogenous carbon monoxide by chorionic villi of term human placenta, *FASEB J.*, 15, A935, 2001.
34. Ingi, T., Cheng, J., and Ronnett, G.V., Carbon monoxide: an endogenous modulator of the nitric oxide–cyclic GMP signaling system, *Neuron*, 16, 835, 1996.
35. Kaide, J.-I. et al., Role of heme oxygenase-derived carbon monoxide on vascular reactivity to vasopressin, *Acta Haematol.*, 103 (Suppl. 1), 68, 2000.
36. Morimoto, Y. et al., Real-time measurements of endogenous CO production from vascular cells using an ultrasensitive laser sensor, *Am. J. Physiol.*, 280, H483, 2001.
37. Morita, T. et al., Carbon monoxide controls the proliferation of hypoxic vascular smooth muscle cells, *J. Biol. Chem.*, 272, 32804, 1997.
38. Valaes, T. et al., Control of jaundice in preterm newborns by an inhibitor of bilirubin production: studies with tin mesoporphyrin, *Pediatrics*, 93, 1, 1994.
39. Martinez, J.C. et al., Control of severe hyperbilirubinemia in full-term newborns with the inhibitor of bilirubin production Sn-mesoporphyrin, *Pediatrics*, 103, 1, 1999.
40. Vreman, H.J., Ekstrand, B.C., and Stevenson, D.K., Selection of metalloporphyrin heme oxygenase inhibitors based on potency and photoreactivity, *Pediatr. Res.*, 33, 195, 1993.
41. Zakhary, R. et al., Heme oxygenase 2: endothelial and neuronal localization in endothelium-dependent relaxation, *Proc. Natl. Acad. Sci. U.S.A.*, 93, 795, 1996.
42. Zakhary, R. et al., Targeted gene deletion of heme oxygenase 2 reveals neural role for carbon monoxide, *Proc. Natl. Acad. Sci. U.S.A.*, 94, 14848, 1997.
43. Stevens, C.F. and Wang, Y., Reversal of long-term potentiation by inhibitors of haem oxygenase, *Nature*, 364, 147, 1993.
44. Zhuo, M. et al., Nitric oxide and carbon monoxide produce activity-dependent long-term synaptic enhancement in hippocampus, *Science*, 260, 1946, 1993.
45. Zhuo, M. et al., On the respective roles of nitric oxide and carbon monoxide in long-term potentiation in the hippocampus, *Learn. Mem.*, 6, 63, 1999.
46. Luo, D. and Vincent, S.R., Metalloporphyrins inhibit nitric oxide-dependent cGMP formation *in vivo*, *Eur. J. Pharmacol.*, 267, 263, 1994.
47. Meffert, M.K. et al., Inhibition of hippocampal heme oxygenase, nitric oxide synthase, and long-term potentiation by metalloporphyrins, *Neuron*, 13, 1225, 1994.
48. Grundemar, L. and Ny, L., Pitfalls using metalloporphyrins in carbon monoxide research, *Trends Pharmacol. Sci.*, 18, 193, 1997.
49. Maines, M.D., The heme oxygenase system: a regulator of second messenger gases, *Annu. Rev. Pharmacol. Toxicol.*, 37, 517, 1997.
49a. McCoubrey, W.K., Jr., Huang, T.J., and Maines, M.D., Isolation and characterization of a cDNA from the rat brain that encodes hemoprotein heme oxygenase-3, *Eur. J. Biochem.*, 247, 725, 1997.
50. Rublevskaya, I.N. and Maines, M.D., Interaction of Fe-protoporphyrin IX and heme analogues with purified recombinant heme oxygenase-2, the constitutive isozyme of the brain and testes, *J. Biol. Chem.*, 269, 26390, 1994.
51. Appleton, S.D. et al., Selective inhibition of heme oxygenase without inhibition of nitric oxide synthase or soluble guanylyl cyclase by metalloporphyrins at low concentrations, *Drug Metab. Dispos.*, 27, 1214, 1999.
52. Mayer, B., Brunner, F., and Schmidt, K., Inhibition of nitric oxide synthesis by methylene blue, *Biochem. Pharmacol.*, 45, 367, 1993.

53. Wolin, M.S. et al., Methylene blue inhibits vasodilation of skeletal muscle arterioles to acetylcholine and nitric oxide via the extracellular generation of superoxide anion, *J. Pharmacol. Exp. Ther.*, 254, 872, 1990.

54. Garthwaite, J. et al., Potent and selective inhibition of nitric oxide sensitive guanylyl cyclase by 1H-[1,2,4]oxadiazolo[4,3-a]quinoxalin-1-one, *Mol. Pharmacol.*, 48, 184, 1995.

55. Hussain, A.S. et al., The soluble guanylyl cyclase inhibitor 1H-[1,2,4]oxadiazolo-[4,3-a]quinoxalin-1-one (ODQ) inhibits relaxation of rabbit aortic rings induced by carbon monoxide, nitric oxide, and glyceryl trinitrate, *Can. J. Physiol. Pharmacol.*, 75, 1034, 1997.

56. McLaughlin, B.E. et al., Potentiation of carbon monoxide-induced relaxation of rat aorta by YC-1 [3-(5′-hydroxymethyl-2′-furyl)-1-benzylindazole], *Can. J. Physiol. Pharmacol.*, 78, 343, 2000.

57. Morita, T. et al., Smooth muscle cell-derived carbon monoxide is a regulator of vascular cGMP, *Proc. Natl. Acad. Sci. U.S.A.*, 92, 1475, 1995.

58. Christodoulides, N. et al., Vascular smooth muscle cell heme oxygenases generate guanylyl cyclase-stimulatory carbon monoxide, *Circulation*, 91, 2306, 1995.

59. Feelisch, M. et al., The soluble guanylyl cyclase inhibitor 1H-[1,2,4]oxadiazolo[4,3-a]-quinoxalin-1-one is a nonselective heme protein inhibitor of nitric oxide synthase and other cytochrome P-450 enzymes involved in nitric oxide donor bioactivation, *Mol. Pharmacol.* 56, 243, 1999.

60. Stone, J.R. and Marletta, M.A., Soluble guanylate cyclase from bovine lung: activation with nitric oxide and carbon monoxide and spectral characterization of the ferrous and ferric states, *Biochemistry*, 33, 5636, 1994.

61. Burstyn, J.N. et al., Studies of the heme coordination and ligand binding properties of soluble guanylyl cyclase (sGC): characterization of Fe(II)sGC and Fe(II)sGC(CO) by electronic absorption and magnetic circular dichroism spectroscopies and failure of CO to activate the enzyme, *Biochemistry*, 34, 5896, 1995.

62. Friebe, A., Schultz, G., and Koesling, D., Sensitizing soluble guanylyl cyclase to become a highly CO-sensitive enzyme, *EMBO J.*, 15, 6863, 1996.

63. Stone, J.R. and Marletta, M.A., Synergistic activation of soluble guanylate cyclase by YC-1 and carbon monoxide: implications for the role of cleavage of the iron–histidine bond during activation by nitric oxide, *Chem. Biol.*, 5, 255, 1998.

63a. Gevantman, L.H., Solubility of selected gases in water in *CRC Handbook of Chemistry and Physics*, Lide, D.R., Ed., CRC Press, New York, 1998, 86.

64. Wang, R., Wang, Z., and Wu, L., Carbon monoxide-induced vasorelaxation and the underlying mechanisms, *Br. J. Pharmacol.*, 121, 927, 1997.

65. Wang, R. and Wu, L., The chemical modification of K_{Ca} channels by carbon monoxide in vascular smooth muscle cells, *J. Biol. Chem.*, 272, 8222, 1997.

66. Nasjletti, A., Carbon monoxide of vascular origin is an inhibitory regulator of vasoconstrictor responsiveness to myogenic and hormonal stimuli, *Acta Haematol.*, 103 (Suppl. 1), 68, 2000.

67. Brian, J.E., Jr., Heistad, D.D., and Faraci, F.M., Effect of carbon monoxide on rabbit cerebral arteries, *Stroke*, 25, 639, 1994.

68. Leffler, C.W. et al., Carbon monoxide and cerebral microvascular tone in newborn pigs, *Am. J. Physiol.*, 276, H1641, 1999.

68a. Ryter, S.W., Kvam, E., and Tyrrell, R.M., Heme oxygenase activity: current methods and applications, in *Methods in Molecular Biology*, Vol. 99, *Stress Response: Methods and Protocols*, Keyse, S.M., Ed., Humana Press Inc., Totowa, NJ, 2000, Chap. 23.

69. Otterbein, L.E. and Choi, A.M.K., Heme oxygenase: colors of defense against cellular stress, *Am. J. Physiol.*, 279, L1029, 2000.

70. Otterbein, L.E. et al., Carbon monoxide has antiinflammatory effects involving the mitogen-activated protein kinase pathway, *Nat. Med.*, 6, 422, 2000.

71. Brouard, S. et al., Carbon monoxide generated by heme oxygenase 1 suppresses endothelial cell apoptosis, *J. Exp. Med.*, 192, 1015, 2000.

72. Otterbein, L.E. et al., Carbon monoxide protects against oxidant-induced lung injury in mice via the p38 mitogen activated protein kinase pathway, *Acta Haematol.*, 103 (Suppl. 1), 83, 2000.

73. Sato, K. et al., Carbon monoxide can fully substitute heme oxygenase-1 in suppressing the rejection of mouse to rat cardiac transplants, *Acta Haematol.*, 103 (Suppl. 1), 87, 2000.

74. Otterbein, L.E., Mantell, L.L., and Choi, A.M.K., Carbon monoxide provides protection against hyperoxic lung injury, *Am. J. Physiol.*, 276, L688, 1999.

75. Galbraith, R., Heme oxygenase: who needs it? *Proc. Soc. Exp. Biol. Med.*, 222, 2999, 1999.

76. Johnson, R.A. and Johnson, F.K., The effects of carbon monoxide as a neurotransmitter, *Curr. Opin. Neurol.*, 13, 709, 2000.

77. Maines, M.D., The heme oxygenase system and its functions in the brain, *Cell. Mol. Biol.*, 46, 5, 2000.

78. Durante, W. and Schafer, A.I., Carbon monoxide and vascular cell function (review), *Int. J. Mol. Med.*, 2, 255, 1998.

79. Johnson, R.A., Kozma, F., and Colombari, E., Carbon monoxide: from toxin to endogenous modulator of cardiovascular functions, *Braz. J. Med. Biol. Res.*, 32, 1, 1999.

80. Grossman, A. et al., Gaseous neurotransmitters in the hypothalamus. The roles of nitric oxide and carbon monoxide in neuroendocrinology, *Horm. Metab. Res.*, 29, 477, 1977.

81. Hu, Y. et al., Contribution of carbon monoxide-producing cells in the gastric mucosa of rat and monkey, *Histochem. Cell Biol.*, 109, 369, 1998.

82. Yoshiki, N., Kubota, T., and Aso, T., Expression and localization of heme oxygenase in human placental villi, *Biochem. Biophys. Res. Commun.*, 276, 1136, 2000.

83. Acevedo, C.H. and Ahmed, A., Heme oxygenase-1 inhibits human myometrial contractility via carbon monoxide and is up-regulated by progesterone during pregnancy, *J. Clin. Invest.*, 101, 949, 1998.

84. Burnett, A.L. et al., Ejaculatory abnormalities in mice with targeted disruption of the gene for heme oxygenase-2, *Nat. Med.*, 4, 84, 1998.

85. Poss, K.D. and Tonegawa, S., Heme oxygenase 1 is required for mammalian iron reutilization. *Proc. Natl. Acad. Sci. U.S.A.*, 94, 10919, 1997.

86. Poss, K.D. and Tonegawa, S., Reduced stress defense in heme oxygenase 1-deficient cells, *Proc. Natl. Acad. Sci. U.S.A.*, 94, 10925, 1997.

87. Yachie, A. et al., What did we learn from the first case of human heme oxygenase-1 deficiency? *Acta Haematol.*, 103 (Suppl. 1), 82, 2000.

88. Coceani, F., Kelsey, L., and Seidlitz, E., Carbon monoxide-induced relaxation of the ductus arteriosus in the lamb: evidence against the prime role of guanylyl cyclase, *Br. J. Pharmacol.*, 118, 1689, 1996.

89. Coceani, F. and Kelsey, L., Endothelin-1 release from the lamb ductus arteriosus: are carbon monoxide and nitric oxide regulatory agents? *Life Sci.*, 66, 2613, 2000.

90. Tepperman, B., The next molecule of the year? Carbon monoxide as a regulator of host inflammatory responses, *J. Pediatr. Gastroenterol. Nutr.*, 31, 2, 2000.

91. Barinaga, M., Carbon monoxide: killer to brain messenger in one step, *Science*, 259, 309, 1993.

2 Carbon Monoxide-Induced Vasorelaxation and the Underlying Mechanisms

Weimin Zhao and Rui Wang

CONTENTS

0-8493-1041-5/02/$0.00+$1.50
© 2002 by CRC Press LLC

I. OVERVIEW OF THE VASCULAR EFFECTS OF CO

The vascular production of carbon monoxide (CO) and the vascular effects of this gas have been known for more than half a century. Soon after the discovery in the late 1940s of the endogenous production of CO in humans during heme catabolism,[1] the vascular effect of CO was detected by Duke and Killick[2] who showed that CO decreased pulmonary vascular resistance. In the following 40 years, the reputation of CO as a toxic hypoxic gas was widely known. Neither the endogenous production nor the physiological effect of CO was further investigated. The resurgent interest in the vascular production and effects of CO started to emerge in the mid 1980s. Early studies of the ductus arteriosus,[3] femoral arterial rings,[4] and rat thoracic aorta[5,6] demonstrated the vasorelaxant effects of CO. The endogenous production of CO from the vascular wall, including smooth muscle,[7,8] endothelium, and neurons,[8,9] was later documented.

It is now well known that CO can induce relaxation of vascular tissues with different diameters and from various species (Table 2.1). The affected vascular tissues include aorta,[10] tail artery,[11] pulmonary artery and vein,[12] mesenteric artery,[12] renal arteries,[13] hepatic arteries,[14] ductus arteriosus,[3] and femoral arteries.[4] Exogenously applied CO induced a concentration-dependent relaxation of rat tail artery tissues precontracted with phenylephrine.[11] The CO-induced vasorelaxation was not due to antagonism of α-adrenoreceptors since CO also relaxed the vascular tissue precontracted with U-46619 (9,11-dideoxy-11α, 9α-epoxymethano-prostaglandin F2α), which induces vasoconstriction mainly by releasing intracellular calcium. The CO-induced vasorelaxation was sustained, but reversible upon the withdrawal of CO, and independent of the presence of an intact endothelium. The vasorelaxant effects of CO are further exemplified in several specific vascular beds below.

Pulmonary circulation is under the influence of CO. Steinhorn et al.[15] showed that the contraction force of rabbit pulmonary artery was decreased by exogenously applied CO in an endothelium-independent way. Furthermore, the presence of heme oxygenase (HO) in bovine pulmonary artery and pulmonary vein has been demonstrated, indicating a multifaceted role for the enzyme in the regulation of heme content in vascular tissues and in the formation of CO with consequent regulation of vascular tone.[16]

Coronary circulation is not an exception regarding the vasorelaxant effects of CO. Coronary flow was reversibly increased by exogenously applied CO in perfused rat heart.[17] The vasodilatation effect of CO on coronary blood flow was not due to carboxyhemoglobin formation or changes of heart rate and was independent of α-adrenergic activities, release of adenosine, or prostaglandins.[18] Thus, CO likely exerts

TABLE 2.1
The Effects of CO on Vascular Tissues from Different Species

Tissue Type	Species	CO Source	Vascular Effect	Ref.
Pial arterioles	Piglet[a]	Exogenous and endogenous	Relaxation	27
Mesenteric artery	Piglet[a]	Exogenous	Relaxation	12
Pulmonary artery, vein	Piglet[a]	Exogenous	Relaxation	12
Extramural arteries of the bladder	Pig	Exogenous	No effect	28
Coronary artery and vein	Pig	Exogenous	Relaxation	19
Femoral artery, carotid artery, coronary artery	Dog	Exogenous	Relaxation	4
Basilar and middle cerebral arteries	Dog, Rabbit	Exogenous	No effect	29
Gracilis muscle arterioles	Rat	Endogenous	Relaxation	30
Renal artery	Rat	Exogenous	Relaxation	13
Tail artery	Rat	Exogenous	Relaxation	10, 11
Coronary artery	Rat	Exogenous	Relaxation	17
Aorta	Rat	Exogenous	Relaxation	10
Hepatic vein	Rat	Endogenous	Relaxation	26
Hepatic artery	Rat	Endogenous	No effect	26
Pulmonary artery	Rabbit	Exogenous	Relaxation	15
Aorta	Rabbit	Exogenous	Relaxation	29, 31

[a] Unless otherwise specified, adult animals were used.

a direct effect on coronary vascular smooth muscle. In superfusion experiments on isolated porcine coronary arterial and venous ring preparations precontracted with prostaglandin F2α, repeated bolus applications of CO induced a reproducible relaxation. The endothelium had been removed from these preparations. Therefore, a direct interaction of CO and smooth muscle cells was evidenced.[19]

Hepatic circulation is also significantly affected by CO in a unique way. Liver tissues exhibit specific expression patterns of HO isoforms and generate detectable endogenous CO under basal conditions.[20,21] The roles of CO in the regulation of the contractility of bile canaliculus in hepatocytes[22] and biliary transport[23] have also been shown. The inhibition of endogenous CO production increased the perfusion pressure under the constant flow conditions of the isolated perfused rat liver. This phenomenon was reversed by the application of exogenous CO to the perfusate.[24,25] In the hepatic circulation, CO mainly exerts vasodilatory effects in the hepatic portal vein and within sinusoids. Pannen and Bauer[26] surgically investigated anesthetized SD rats to monitor the changes in hepatic arterial and portal venous vascular resistance in response to intravenous bolus administration of HO inhibitor. The inhibition of endogenous production of CO significantly increased the hepatic vein resistance, but not the artery resistance. Thus, CO seems to exert a selective effect on vascular resistance in the two inflows to the liver. While it has no relaxant effect on the hepatic artery, CO actively participates in the modulation of portal venous vascular tone.

The sensitivities of different vascular beds to CO are variable. CO-induced vasorelaxation was more marked in pulmonary veins than in pulmonary or mesenteric arteries.[12] Additionally, CO has been found ineffective on cerebral vasculature. One study showed that exogenously applied CO at concentrations between 1 and 300 μM failed to induce vasorelaxation in isolated rabbit and dog basilar and rabbit middle cerebral arteries.[29]

In contrast to CO, nitric oxide (NO) produced rapid relaxation in all examined cerebral vessels with similar ED_{50} values. A distinct intracellular mechanism between NO and CO may explain their different effects on cerebral vessels. The effect of NO is due to the activation of the soluble guanylyl cyclase (sGC)–cGMP pathway that mediates target cell responses such as in vascular smooth muscle.[32] However, CO may relax vascular smooth muscle through several pathways other than cGMP, e.g., by inhibiting the cytochrome P450–endothelin-1 system[33] or by stimulating the calcium-activated K (K_{Ca}) channels,[11] depending on the tissue types.

In most vascular tissues, CO may stimulate cGMP formation.[31,34] This stimulating effect becomes less pronounced or even absent in some vascular beds such as the ductus arteriosus in which CO can still induce relaxation, but the relaxation develops virtually unabated in the presence of sGC inhibitors; the magnitude of this relaxation was not correlated with tissue levels of cGMP.[33]

At different developmental stages, certain types of vascular tissues may be equipped with different signaling mechanisms and the expression of cellular targets of CO in these tissues may have different profiles. This might well be the case for the effect of CO on porcine vascular tissues. Leffler et al.[27] showed that CO relaxed pial mesenteric artery tissues from piglets, but Werkstrom et al.[28] did not observe any vascular effect of CO on the extramural arteries of bladders from adult pigs. The interaction between CO and NO in different vascular tissues should also be taken into account when the differential vascular responses to CO are considered. At concentrations between 0.1 and 10 μM, CO released NO from a large intracellular pool in rat renal artery, leading to vasorelaxation.[13] The vasorelaxant potency of NO is much greater than that of CO. Conceivably, in vascular tissues with large CO-releasable NO pools, the CO-induced vasorelaxation could be largely due to secondarily released NO. To extrapolate this hypothesis, in other vascular tissues with small CO-releasable pools of NO, the vascular effects of CO would be significantly reduced or even absent. It should be pointed out, however, that this NO-mediated model of CO action cannot fully explain the vascular effect of CO since in many cases the blockade of the NO pathway did not interfere with the CO effect.

II. THE EFFECTS OF CO ON DIFFERENT CELLULAR COMPONENTS OF VASCULAR WALLS

A. EFFECT OF CO ON CULTURED VASCULAR SMOOTH MUSCLE CELLS

Numerous studies have demonstrated that the CO-induced vasorelaxation does not depend on the functional integrity of the endothelium. Further evidence supporting the direct effect of CO on smooth muscle cells (SMCs) has been obtained by studying cultured vascular SMCs *in vitro*. Direct bubbling of the culture medium with 5%

CO gas induced a time-dependent increase in intracellular cGMP level in cultured rat aortic SMCs,[35] which could consequently decrease intracellular free calcium levels and reduce the contraction force.

CO also exerts a profound effect in either a paracrine or autocrine fashion on the proliferation of SMCs. Morita et al.[36] demonstrated that increased endogenous CO production or exposing cells to exogenous CO led to markedly attenuated cell growth. Conversely, inhibiting CO formation or scavenging CO with hemoglobin increased vascular SMC proliferation induced by serum or endothelin stimulation. Many chronic cardiovascular disorders, including atherosclerosis, intimal hyperplasia, and pulmonary hypertension are characterized by increased proliferation of vascular SMCs. Increased CO production in cultured vascular SMCs facing a hypoxic challenge provides a protective mechanism for blood vessel walls from hyperplasia. More detailed discussion of the influence of CO on vascular SMC proliferation can be found in Chapter 3.

B. The Role of Endothelium in the Metabolism and Function of CO

1. Expression of HO Isoforms and Production of CO in Endothelial Cells

Endothelium constitutes a monolayer covering the inner surface of the entire circulatory system. Several vasoconstricting factors and vasorelaxing factors are secreted from the endothelium to finely tune vascular tones. For example, endothelium-derived relaxant factor (NO) and hyperpolarizing factor (EDHF) as well as prostacyclin are responsible for the relaxation of vascular smooth muscles, whereas endothelin induces vasoconstriction by acting on endothelin receptors on SMCs. Whether different isoforms of HO are expressed in vascular endothelial cells and whether CO can be generated from endothelium in a meaningful amount are unclear. Early studies supported the idea that CO production in vascular walls was mainly from vascular SMCs. To a large extent, this still holds true.

The expression of HO isoforms in vascular endothelial cells is indeed demonstrated in several recent studies. The vascular endothelia of the intramural vessels of the urethra, bladder, and oesophagogastric junction, and the extramural vessels of the bladders of piglets, displayed HO-2 immunoreactivity, but not HO-1 reactivity.[28] HO-2 reactivity was also demonstrated in the endothelial lining of porcine aorta.[8] Based on current knowledge, CO generated from endothelial HO-2 is not likely to play an important role in the acute regulation of vascular tone since HO-2 is not inducible except in response to adrenal glucocorticoids.[37]

Interestingly, the acutely regulated release of CO from endothelium was reported in one case. Inhibition of HO activity by tin protoporphyrin IX (SnPPIX) reversed the ACh-induced and NO-independent relaxation of porcine distal pulmonary arteries.[8] In the absence of endothelium, ACh failed to relax vascular tissue. Therefore, this study was presented to support the idea that ACh released CO from endothelium in addition to NO release. This extremely important discovery reveals an acute mechanism controlling the endogenous release of CO for the phasic modulation of vascular tone. To substantiate this mechanism, a few key experiments are needed. The expression of HO isoforms should be confirmed in the endothelium layers of these vessels. The CO levels from these endothelial cells need to be determined.

The direct stimulation of HO isoforms by ACh should be directly documented. Similar phenomena should be confirmed in more vascular preparations.

The chronically regulated CO release from endothelium was reported in pathophysiological situations. Using immunocytochemical methods, a marginally increased expression of HO-1 in endothelial layer of aorta and adventitial arterioles was observed 9 hours after lipopolysaccharide (LPS) injection in rats.[38] This increase in HO-1 expression was much weaker in the endothelial layer than in the smooth muscle layer. In the absence of LPS stimulation, HO-1 staining in endothelial layers of these vascular tissues was hardly detectable.

In another study, aortic tissues from chronically hypoxic rats exhibited greater contractile response after inhibition of NO synthase (NOS) and HO than tissues treated only with the NOS inhibitor.[9] Removal of endothelium from these aortic tissues abolished the HO-mediated vascular contractile response. This result could be explained if hypoxia up-regulated the expression of HO-1 or increased the activity of existing HO-2 in the vascular endothelium. Inhibition of HO activity with zinc protoporphyrin-9 (ZnPPIX) did not alter the contractile property of these vascular tissues from normal control rats independent of the presence of endothelium,[9] suggesting that, under physiological conditions, endothelium-derived CO is not essential for the regulation of vascular tone. In short, there is no evidence for the production of CO from vascular endothelial cells under physiological conditions and limited study has not firmly demonstrated the regulated production of CO from endothelial cells. Therefore, one should be very cautious in evaluating the importance of endothelium-derived CO.

2.   Mediation of Vascular Effect of CO by Endothelial Cells

Generally speaking, the vasorelaxant effect of CO is not endothelium-dependent. This conclusion does not come as a surprise. NO is another gaseous vasoactive factor that acts directly on vascular SMCs independent of the presence of endothelium once it is generated from endothelium. However, possible modulation of the vascular action of CO by endothelium should be considered. For CO in the circulation to act on SMCs, thus affecting vascular contractility, it must pass though the endothelium layer of vessel walls. Endothelial cells and their cellular contents may function as physical barriers or traps to limit the access of CO to SMCs. For CO generated in SMCs or endothelial cells to exert an autocrine or paracrine vasoactive effect, it may stimulate endothelium to modulate the release of endothelium-derived vasoactive factors. CO-induced vasorelaxation can thus be indirectly regulated by endothelium.

Gene expression of many endothelium-derived factors is under the influence of CO. A case in point is hypoxia, which suppresses both the transcriptional rate of the endothelial NOS gene and the stability of its mRNA in pulmonary artery endothelial cells. In contrast, hypoxia increases the expression of a number of genes encoding vascular cell mitogens produced by endothelial cells, including platelet-derived growth factor B (PDGF-B) and endothelin-1 (ET-1).[39] In acute hypoxia, the expression of HO-1 in vascular SMCs is greatly induced and CO production escalates.

Besides its autocrine effect of inhibiting the proliferation of SMCs, the released CO suppresses the production of ET-1 and PDGE-B from endothelial cells in a paracrine fashion.[40] The inhibition by CO of the binding activity of a hypoxia-inducible factor-1 (HIF-1) to the 5′ region of the concerned vascular mitogen genes may be critical for this effect of CO. Excluding the input of SMC-derived CO, acute hypoxia causes pulmonary vasoconstriction and chronic hypoxia causes smooth muscle cell replication and extracellular matrix accumulation, resulting in vessel wall remodeling. To take into account the hypoxia-stimulated CO production from SMCs, pulmonary vasoconstriction would be reduced and SMCs proliferation regressed. The endothelium-derived CO may inhibit eNOS activity and suppress NO release from the endothelium. Consequently, the vasorelaxant effect of CO would be compensated by the reduced NO release.[9,41] Again, this hypothesis assumes that a large part of CO effect is actually due to the vascular effect of NO, which needs to be further investigated.

3. Regulation of Non-Contractile Functions of Vascular Tissues by Endothelium-Derived CO

The presence of HO in vascular endothelial cells suggests that CO may also serve as an endothelium-derived factor that may not necessarily be a vasorelaxant factor. For instance, in certain pig vascular tissues, HO-2 was detected in the endothelium layer but no relaxations of these vascular tissues can be elicited by exogenous CO.[28] The endothelium-derived CO probably participates in the regulation of non-contractile activities of vascular tissues, including cell–cell interaction, proliferation, apoptosis, and inflammation.

C. Effect of CO on Nerve Terminals and Neurotransmitters within Vascular Walls

The interaction of CO and the peripheral nerve system may influence vascular contractility in at least two ways. First, chronic CO exposure may affect the development and function of the nerve system.[42,43] Tetrodotoxin (TTX) inhibited the contraction of rat mesenteric vascular beds evoked by electrical perivascular nervous stimulation. This inhibitory effect of TTX was significantly increased in vascular tissues from prenatal pups after exposing the pregnant mother rats to 150 ppm CO for 5 to 7 days.[44] TTX blocks voltage-gated Na^+ channels in the nerve endings and inhibits the neurotransmitter release upon the electrical depolarizing stimulation. A reduced TTX effect indicates that chronic CO treatment somehow altered the electrophysiological properties of pre-synaptic membranes and facilitated the neurotransmitter release. Moreover, in the chronic CO-treated prenatal pups, the ACh-induced relaxation of the mesenteric arterial beds with intact endothelium appeared about 4 days earlier than in non-CO-treated control pups,[44] indicating an accelerated maturation of the muscarinic receptor–eNOS system.

Second, CO may serve as a neurotransmitter, possibly released by non-adrenergic, non-cholinergic (NANC) nerve endings.[45] ZnPPIX antagonized the NANC relaxation induced by electrical field stimulation in opossum and sphincter muscles.[45] Furthermore, a recent study shows that the relaxation of small intestinal smooth muscles and the release of inhibitory neurotransmission are reduced in HO-2/nNOS double-knockout mice. The electrical field stimulation-induced contraction of small intestinal muscles was almost abolished in HO-2 knockout mice although nNOS expression was intact. The NANC inhibitory transmission was restored by exogenously applied CO in HO-2 knockout mice. Thus, CO appears essential for NANC neurotransmission in these tissues.[46] Whether CO plays a similar role in NANC neurotransmission in vascular tissues is unknown.

The vascular effect of CO released from perivascular neurons has gained support from histological and anatomical studies on the location of HO. HO-2 has been localized by immunohistochemistry to adventitial nerves of blood vessels. HO-2 is also localized to neurons in autonomic ganglia, including the petrosal, superior cervical, and nodose ganglia, as well as ganglia in the myenteric plexus of the intestine.[8] In non-vascular smooth muscle tissues, HO-2 immunoreactivity, but not HO-1 immunoreactivity, was also found in nerve cell bodies and nerve fibers in feline lower oesophageal sphincters.[47] Whether HO-1 is expressed or can be up-regulated in perivascular nerve tissues is unclear.

The proposed role of endogenous CO generated from SMCs, endothelial cells, and perivascular neurons in the regulation of vascular tone is summarized in Figure 2.1. Our opinion is that SMC-generated CO is most important for the regulation of vascular tone; that endothelium-generated CO may mainly act on endothelial cells in an autocrine manner; and that CO with a neuronal origin may facilitate the neuronal regulation of vascular contractility. In terms of the production of CO, the expression and up-regulation of HO-1 in endothelial cells and perivascular neurons are still issues for debate.

III. THE VASORELAXANT EFFECTS
OF ENDOGENOUS CO

A. CHANGES IN VASCULAR CONTRACTILITY INDUCED BY HEMIN AND OTHER HO INDUCERS

Endogenously formed CO is mainly derived from degeneration of monometric free heme. Heme forms a 1:1 complex with HO, an enzyme catalyzing the reaction result in CO formation, and serves as the substrate and cofactor of the enzyme.[48] During the reaction, heme is degraded into equimolar iron, biliverdin, and CO. The HO-catalyzed metabolism of heme is the predominant source of endogenously formed CO. To date, at least three isoforms of HO have been identified.[49,50] HO-1 is substrate-inducible and its levels in many cellular systems are regulated to match the load of heme.[51] HO-2 is constitutive and appears to be regulated solely by steroids.[52] Both HO-1 and HO-2 can be inhibited by certain heme analogues, such as SnPPIX and ZnPPIX. HO-3 is a newly identified HO isoform. Its predicted amino acid structure differs from those of HO-1 and HO-2 but is closely related to HO-2. The expression of HO-3 has been found in brain, heart, kidney, liver, testis, and spleen but not in the vasculature. Very little is known about its function and regulation.[50]

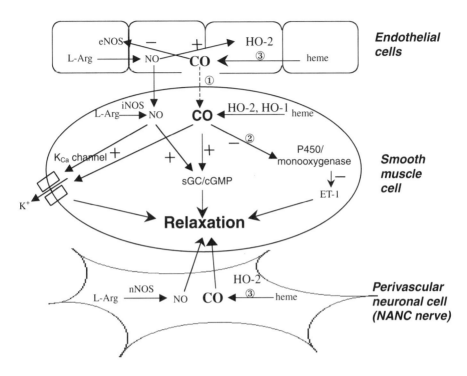

FIGURE 2.1 Mechanism of CO-induced vascular smooth muscle relaxation. Three major hypotheses for CO-induced SMCs relaxation: cGMP accumulation, large conductance potassium channel activation, and inhibition of the cytochrome P450–monooxygenase system are illustrated. ① Whether the endothelium-produced CO can diffuse into the underlying SMCs is unclear. ② Whether this pathway is applicable to adult vascular beds is unclear. ③ The expression and the presence of functional HO-1 are unclear.

The vascular effect of endogenous CO has been studied by using the HO substrate and/or inducers such as hemin, heme arginate, or heme-L-lysinate.[27] A good HO inducer should not alone affect vascular tone and its direct effects on blood vessels should be distinguished from the effects mediated by the increased HO activity. Results from *in vivo* studies showed that HO inducers can decrease blood pressure in spontaneously hypertensive rats (SHRs) and increase coronary blood flow in isolated perfused hearts.[53,54] Moreover, the development of hypertension in SHRs was chronically retarded by HO inducers such as $SnCl_2$.[55] Heme-induced decreases in blood pressure can be prevented by pre-treating the animals with HO inhibitors, suggesting that the vasodilating action of heme is consequent to the formation of HO products.[56] These results suggest that endogenous HO products may be responsible for the relaxation of vascular smooth muscle *in vivo*. As biliverdin did not induce vasodilatation and chelation of free iron had no effect on the heme-L-lysinate-induced vasorelaxation, CO was the only vasoactive molecule resulting from HO induction.[30,54]

After intraperitoneal injection of hemin for 18 hours, HO-1 expression in hepatocytes increased in a time-dependent fashion. Concurrently, the vascular resistance in perfused rat liver was reduced by 13% and the CO level in venous effluent was markedly increased.[57] The application of oxyhemoglobin that scavenges both NO and CO abolished the hemin treatment-induced reduction of vascular resistance. The specific involvement of CO was further demonstrated by the failure of methemoglobin, which traps NO but not CO, to modulate the hemin effect. Clearly, hepatic circulation is significantly modulated by overproduced CO from extrasinusoidal liver tissues. The vascular effect of CO is also demonstrated in other vascular tissues. For example, the vascular tone of isolated lamb ductus arteriosus was significantly decreased after hemin was added to the bath solution.[58]

S-nitroso-N-acetyl penicillamine (SNAP), an NO donor, was also effective in increasing HO-1 mRNA and protein expression in aorta.[7] Consequently, the endogenous levels of CO and intracellular cGMP were elevated, and aortic contractile response to phenylephrine was reduced. NO and cAMP were also found to enhance the expression of HO-1 at mRNA and protein levels.[59,60] However, it is difficult to separate the vasorelaxant effects of NO and cAMP from the increased CO production due to the induced HO expression.

B. Changes in Vascular Contractility Induced by Zinc-Protoporphyrin-IX and Other HO Inhibitors

It may be argued that the change in vascular contractility after the application of HO inducers represents the effect of over-produced endogenous CO. It is still physiologically relevant but does not reflect what can happen under basal conditions. Application of HO inhibitors will help to determine the vascular effect of endogenous CO under basal or resting conditions. The most often used HO inhibitors belong to the family of metalloporphyrins, including ZnPPIX, SnPPIX, cobalt protoporphyrin IX (CoPPIX), and chromium mesoporphyrin (CrMP).[61] Intraperitoneal injection of HO inhibitors such as ZnPPIX increased blood pressure and peripheral resistance in normal SD rats.[62] The application of HO inhibitors also abolished the anti-hypertensive effect of HO inducers in vivo[53,55] and the vasorelaxant effect of HO inducers in vitro.[7,58,59]

To elucidate whether endogenously generated CO is a vasorelaxant in the hepatic microcirculation, Suematsu et al.[25] applied ZnPPIX to isolated perfused rat liver. This treatment eliminated the CO flux in the venous effluent, which is otherwise at the level of 0.7 nmol/min/gram of liver. The vascular resistance was increased by 30% and sinusoidal constriction occurred. These effects of ZnPPIX were attenuated significantly by the application of exogenous CO to the perfusate. These results support the physiological effects of endogenous CO on the hepatic microcirculation at basal conditions. Similar observations were made using other HO inhibitors in other types of vascular beds. CrMP induced a marked increase in the contraction forces of small branches of isolated femoral artery in vitro.[61] In contrast, the contraction forces of large arteries like the aorta and femoral artery were not significantly affected. Thus, endogenously produced CO appears to play a more important vasorelaxant role in small resistance vessels than in large capacity arteries.

TABLE 2.2
The Effects of HO Modulators on Vascular Tissues from Different Species

Tissue Type	Species	Treatment	Vascular Effect	Ref.
Hepatic vein	Wistar rat	Hemin–HO inducer	Relaxation	57
Ductus arteriosus	Lamb	Hemin	Relaxation	58
Aorta	Lewis rat	SNAP–HO inducer	Relaxation	7
Hepatic vein	SD rat	SnPPIX–HO inhibitor	Contraction	26
Aorta	Lewis rat	SnPPIX	Contraction	7
Ductus arteriosus	Lamb	ZnPPIX–HO inhibitor	Contraction	58
Aorta	SD rat	ZnPPIX	Contraction	9
Gracilis muscle arterioles	SD rat	CrMP–HO inhibitor	Contraction	61

Metalloporphyrins are membrane permeable and potent in blocking HO activity. However, their photosensitivity may lead to non-specific biological effects not related to HO inhibition.[63] Metalloporphyrins may also inhibit other heme-dependent enzymes, such as NOS and sGC.[63,64] ZnPPIX is more potent in blocking purified sGC ($K_i =$ 50 nM) than in suppressing HO activities ($K_i = 212$ nM).[65] Recent studies also showed that ZnPPIX inhibited voltage-gated calcium channels in pituitary cells[66] and suppressed G protein-mediated vascular smooth muscle relaxation via mechanisms other than HO inhibition.[47,67] Finally, the inhibitory effects of metalloporphyrins on HO activity are not isoform-specific. Thus, whether the activities of HO-1 or HO-2 are inhibited cannot be distinguished by using these inhibitors.[68] Despite these pitfalls, metalloporphyrins are useful and irreplaceable tools for investigating the role of endogenously produced CO. Independent lines of evidence, such as production of the same effects by using CO scavengers (e.g., oxidized hemoglobin) and other types of HO inhibitors and the reversed effects of exogenously applied CO or HO inducers, will help support the conclusions derived from the experiments employing metalloporphyrins.

The modulation of endogenous production of CO and the consequent vascular contractility changes are summarized in Table 2.2.

IV. THE MECHANISMS FOR
CO-INDUCED VASORELAXATION

Three major mechanisms have been proposed to explain the vascular effects of CO: (1) the vascular effect of CO may be mostly mediated by the sGC pathway; (2) the vasodilatory effect of CO may be related to the modulation of K^+ channel activities[11,69,70–73]; and (3) the inhibition of the cytochrome P450 pathway may also be involved in the vascular effect of CO.[3] Taking into account the diversity of the responsiveness of different vascular beds from different species to CO, none of these three mechanisms alone can fully explain the vascular effect of CO. Most likely, all three mechanisms coexist with additional mechanisms, with one predominant in certain vascular beds and others in different vascular beds.

A. Stimulation of cGMP Pathway

Like NO, CO is a potent stimulator of sGC.[19,31] CO binds to the heme regulatory subunit of sGC and activates the enzyme.[74] The activation of sGC results in an increase in cGMP level. In vascular smooth muscle, increased cGMP production subsequently induces relaxation by lowering intracellular calcium concentration and/or decreasing the sensitivity of the contractile system to free calcium. The mechanism producing the stimulating effect of CO on the sGC system is discussed in detail in Chapter 4.

B. Modulation of K$^+$ Channels by CO

The activities of the potassium channel have a great impact on smooth muscle contractility. Smooth muscle cell membrane is characterized by high input resistance. A small amount of K$^+$ channel activation is sufficient to hyperpolarize the cell membrane.[48] This membrane hyperpolarization results in vasorelaxation by inactivating voltage-dependent calcium channels, inhibiting the agonist-induced increase in inositol triphosphate (IP$_3$), and reducing contractile system Ca^{2+} sensitivity.[75]

Earlier studies at the vascular tissue level indicated the involvement of K$^+$ channel activation in the CO effect. The muscle-relaxing effect of CO was relatively weaker in high concentrations of KCl-precontracted than in agonist-precontracted tissues.[76] The CO-induced relaxation of rat tail artery was also significantly reduced by tetraethylammonium (TEA, 30 mM), a K$^+$ channel blocker.[73] Charybdotoxin (ChTX), a large conductance K$_{Ca}$ channel blocker, inhibited the vascular effect of CO as TEA did, whereas apamin, a small conductance K$_{Ca}$ inhibitor, had no effect.

These results clearly indicate that the activation of large conductance K$_{Ca}$ channels constitutes an important mechanism for CO-induced vasorelaxation. Furthermore, CO-induced vasorelaxation was completely abolished by co-application of either TEA and methylene blue (MB) or ChTX and Rp-8-Br-cGMPS.[73] Leffler et al.[27] showed that topically applied CO dose-dependently dilated piglet pial arterioles *in vivo* over the range 10^{-11} to 10^{-9} M. The channel inhibitors TEA and iberiotoxin K$_{Ca}$ abolished CO-induced cerebrovascular dilation. TEA also inhibited the relaxation of piglet pial arterioles induced by endogenous CO generated from the HO substrate heme-L-lysinate. These functional studies support the idea that CO-induced vascular relaxation is partially mediated by the opening of high conductance K$_{Ca}$ channels in vascular SMCs.

In rabbit corneal epithelial cells, Rich et al.[77] found that 1% CO increased delayed rectifier K$^+$ channel currents by 84% and hyperpolarized the membrane from –42 to –51 mV. In the same study, CO increased open probability of single K$^+$ channels without changing the single channel conductance. K$^+$ channels are widely distributed in different tissues and the modulation of different types of K$^+$ channels by CO is also tissue-type specific. In a whole cell patch-clamp study, CO transiently increased a TEA-insensitive K$^+$ channel current and induced membrane potential oscillation in human jejunal circular muscle cells.[78] However, that study could not distinguish whether a delayed rectifier or a K$_{Ca}$ channel was activated.

In the thick ascending limb of kidney, an apical 70-pS K^+ channel was inhibited by chromium mesoporphyrin, an inhibitor of HO.[79] Moreover, heme-L-lysinate (the HO substrate) significantly stimulated the channel activity in cell-attached patches. The excitation of this 70-pS channel was finally ascribed to the effect of CO because a CO-bubbled bath solution increased channel activity, whereas biliverdin, another HO-dependent metabolite of heme, had no effect. The modulation of K^+ channel activity by CO was also demonstrated in vascular SMCs. Wang et al.[11] showed that CO hyperpolarized single SMCs isolated from rat tail artery by approximately 20 mV, and reversibly enhanced whole-cell outward K^+ channel currents. Wang and colleagues[72] further reported that CO, applied both extracellularly and intra-cellularly, increased the open probability of single large conductance K_{Ca} channels in a concentration-dependent fashion without affecting single channel conductance. This effect of CO was antagonized by bath-applied ChTX.

It has been suggested that a chemical interaction between CO and certain amino acid residues may be responsible for the CO-induced reversible activation of K_{Ca} channels.[48] The detailed experimental observations and putative mechanisms are discussed in Chapter 5.

C. INHIBITION OF CYTOCHROME P450 BY CO

Cytochrome P450-linked mono-oxygenase is responsible for the generation of vas-oconstricting substances, such as an arachidonic metabolite[3,80] or ET-1.[81] A decreased formation of these vasoconstrictors would lead to vascular relaxation.[48] CO and cytochrome P450 function are closely related. CO is an inhibitor of cytochrome P450[82] and the levels of cytochrome P450 are controlled by the availability of cellular heme[53] which can be catalyzed to CO and biliverdin. Therefore, it has been hypoth-esized that the vascular effect of CO may result from the inhibition of a cytochrome P450-dependent mono-oxygenase.

In rat thymocytes, capacitance-induced calcium entry was prevented by some known cytochrome P450 inhibitors as well as a 3-min treatment with CO, whereas elevation of cGMP or cAMP level had little or no effect.[83] These results suggest that a cytochrome P450-based mechanism may be involved in the effect of CO. In the lamb ductus arteriosus, exogenously applied CO and most of the known cytochrome P450 inhibitors relaxed the tissue precontracted with either indomethacin or KCl.[3,82] The CO-induced relaxation was maximally reversed by light illumination at 450 nm, indicating the involvement of cytochrome P450 in the process.[82] Since the contractile mechanism for the lamb ductus arteriosus may be ascribed to a cytochrome P450-based mono-oxygenase reaction controlling the synthesis of ET-1, Coceani et al.[58,81] proposed that the CO-induced relaxation of the lamb ductus arteriosus may result from the reduced synthesis of ET-1.

Utz and Ullrich[76] had a different view on the involvement of cytochrome P450 in the relaxing effect of CO. They observed a maximal photoreversibility of the relaxant effect of CO on ileal smooth muscles at 422 nm. This wavelength corresponds exactly to the maximum absorption of a reduced heme–CO complex, i.e., guanylate cyclase.[84] Obviously, further experiments are needed to examine the wavelength spectrum of the photoreversibility of the relaxing effects of CO on different types of blood vessels as well as the interactions of CO and other cytochrome P450 inhibitors.

Wang and colleagues[48,70,71] reported that the CO-induced relaxation of tail artery tissues from adult rats was not affected by the presence or absence of 4-phenylimidazole (4-PD), an antagonist of cytochrome P450. Indeed, 4-PD alone relaxed the precontracted endothelium-free rat tail artery. After the 4-PD induced relaxation reached the maximum, however, additional relaxation could be induced by CO. The CO-relaxed vascular tissues could also be further relaxed by 4-PD. These results, together with the observation that the simultaneous inhibition of both cGMP pathway and K_{Ca} channels completely eliminated the CO-induced relaxation, do not support the involvement of a cytochrome P450 system in the CO-induced relaxation of rat tail artery tissues. Tail arteries from adult rats are different from the lamb ductus arteriosus/venosus in many ways. For instance, indomethacin contracts the lamb ductus arteriosus/venosus but not the rat tail artery. The discrepancy in the importance of a cytochrome P450 system in the CO effect between adult rat tail artery and the lamb ductus arteriosus/venosus may shed light on our understanding of the developmental regulation of the vascular effect of CO.

D. OTHER MECHANISMS POSSIBLY LINKED TO CO-INDUCED VASCULAR RELAXATION

1. Calcium Channels and Intracellular Free Calcium Concentration

It was reported previously that CO reduced the KCl-induced increase in $[Ca^{2+}]_i$ by 29% in rat aortic segments, detected by the Ca^{45} uptake technique. This effect of CO was mimicked by verapamil, a blocker for voltage-gated calcium channels, that reduced the KCl-induced increase in intracellular Ca^{2+} concentration by 40%.[5,6] The suggestion was that CO might relax vascular tissue directly by blocking calcium entry to SMCs and consequently lowering the intracellular calcium concentration or indirectly by activating the sGC–cGMP pathway.[85] Direct measurement of intracellular free calcium concentration in cultured vascular SMCs in the presence of CO was reported recently.[48] The relative resting level of $[Ca^{2+}]_i$ in acutely isolated rat tail artery SMCs was not altered by CO (10 μM). CO also had no effect on the KCl-induced increase in $[Ca^{2+}]_i$ in vascular SMCs.

Studies of the effect of CO on calcium mobilization in non-vascular SMCs also yielded controversial results. In GH_3 (a clonal line derived from a rat anterior pituitary tumor with the properties of somatomammotrophs) and chromaffin cells, voltage-dependent Ca^{2+} entry was not affected by CO.[86] Bile canaliculus associated with the couplet cells in cultured rat hepatocyte suspension exhibited periodic contractions. The addition of ZnPPIX to the culture medium increased both the contraction frequency and intracellular calcium concentrations observed with time-lapse video microscopy. Concurrently, the endogenous production of CO was diminished. Exogenous CO antagonized the ZnPPIX-elicited increases in contractile frequency and intracellular calcium concentrations.[22]

Carotid body provides another example of tissue in which opposite observations of the CO effect on cellular calcium levels were made. In one study, the binding of

CO to membrane heme-containing proteins in rat carotid body appeared to stimulate calcium influx through voltage-gated Ca^{2+} channels and depolarize cell membranes since the stimulatory effect of CO on the carotid body was blocked by Cd^{2+}, a voltage-gated Ca^{2+} channel blocker.[87] In another study, the inhibitory effect of CO on carotid body was argued since CO inhibited sensory discharge by inhibiting calcium channels and lowering intracellular calcium in glomus cells.[88]

2. Voltage-Gated Na⁺ Channels

Carratu et al.[43] showed that low level CO exposures (75 and 150 ppm) to rats from day 0 to day 20 of pregnancy produced modifications of Na^+ channel current properties of sciatic nerve fibers of pups. In particular, the inactivation kinetics of transient Na^+ current was significantly slowed. The percentage of the maximum number of available Na^+ channels at the normal resting potential (–80 mV) was increased to approximately 85% in the CO-exposed pups. The equilibrium potential for Na^+ ions also exhibited a negative shift in the CO-treated animals. It appears that mild prenatal exposure to CO produces reversible changes in Na^+ channel inactivation kinetics and irreversible changes in Na^+ equilibrium potential. These alterations may reflect the role of CO in the development and structural changes of Na^+ channels. As voltage-gated Na^+ channels are not generally expressed in vascular SMCs or endothelial cells, at least in adult subjects, the likelihood that Na^+ channels mediate the vascular effects of CO is remote.

3. Ion Channels without Voltage Dependence

Pineda et al.[89] examined the effects of NO and CO on locus coeruleus (LC) neurons with electrophysiological techniques on rat brain slices. Bath application of various NO donors increased the firing rates of most LC neurons. The NO effect was associated with a voltage-independent TTX-insensitive non-selective inward current, which was not an Na^+–Ca^{2+} exchanger or Cl^- channel. Within 3 to 10 min of the application of CO-saturated saline to the brain slices, the firing rates of LC neurons increased, then gradually returned to the previous level. This effect of CO was partially mediated by cGMP-dependent protein kinase. However, the ionic basis of this effect of CO is unknown. Whether CO also induced non-selective ion channels, as NO did in these neurons, was not further explored.

Leinders–Zufall et al.[90] showed that CO at submicromolar concentrations induced a significant inward current in isolated olfactory receptor neurons (ORNs) of the tiger salamander. This inward current was conducted through cyclic nucle-otide-gated (CNG) channels previously thought to mediate odor transduction. Like-wise, CO effectively depolarized the membrane potentials of ORNs through tonic activation of CNG channels. Similar to the results with LC neurons,[89] the effect of CO on CNG channels in ORNs was also mediated by the cGMP pathway rather than directly acting on CNG channels.

4. Cyclic AMP (cAMP) Pathway in Vascular SMCs

Whether CO can modify the activity of the cAMP pathway is questionable.[48] A study of rat tail artery showed that forskolin, an adenylate cyclase inhibitor, inhibited phenylephrine-induced vasoconstriction. This effect was not affected by the administration of MB, TEA, or MB plus TEA. The latter treatment may have completely inhibited the CO-induced vasorelaxation in the same preparation.[48] These results indirectly suggest that the cAMP pathway is not involved in CO-induced vasorelaxation.

5. Na^+/K^+ ATPase as the Target of CO

CO has been shown to stimulate ouabain-sensitive Na^+/K^+ ATPase in rat Purkinje neurons.[91] Changes in intracellular Na^+ concentrations or free radical levels did not affect this action of CO. Evidence also showed that the effect of CO on Na^+/K^+ ATPase was mediated by the activation of both membrane and soluble GC, the subsequently increased cGMP level, and the activity of cGMP-dependent protein kinase. The activation of Na^+/K^+ ATPase in Purkinje neurons may lead to membrane hyperpolarization and the inhibition of neuronal excitability. Does CO also affect the activity of Na^+/K^+ ATPase in vascular SMCs? The answer is not yet available.

One pertinent clue is the differential distribution of isoforms of Na^+/K^+ ATPase among tissues. The Na^+/K^+ ATPase in Purkinje neurons, which is sensitive to CO modulation, appears to be the $\alpha 3$ isoform.[91] The $\alpha 1$ isoform of Na^+/K^+ ATPase in rat kidney, on the other hand, is inhibited by the increased cGMP level.[92] Although all three α subunit isoforms have been identified in cardiac and skeletal muscles, a structurally distinct isoform, the truncated $\alpha 1$ subunit ($\alpha 1$-T Na^+/K^+ ATPase) is exclusively expressed in vascular SMCs.[93] The sensitivity of this evolutionarily conserved, truncated Na^+/K^+ ATPase isoform to CO is not yet known.

V. CONCLUSIONS

Investigations started several decades ago and intensified in the last 10 years demonstrated that CO is an important endogenous gaseous vasoactive factor. CO acts on vascular SMCs to induce relaxation and shares many similar mechanisms with NO. However, depending on the types of vascular tissues and species, vascular responses to CO vary for still unknown reasons. The up-regulation of the CO-generating enzyme HO-1 is achieved by the surge of many endogenous factors, and the down-regulation of HO becomes successful with the use of pharmacological agents, such as metalloporphyrin compounds or steroids.[94] Among the mechanisms underlying the vascular effects of CO, the activation of cGMP, the opening of K_{Ca} channels, and the modulation of cytochrome P450 have attracted the most attention. Whether CO also acts on other cellular and molecular targets is still being investigated.

We still face many challenges on the road to establishing the role of CO as a physiological and endogenous vasoactive factor. Whether CO has a regulatory role in modulating vascular tone cannot be ascertained before an endogenous substance or substances releasing CO in response to internal environmental changes can be identified. On a chronic scale, heme, free radical, hypoxia, and many other stimuli can stimulate HO-1 expression. In an acute scenario, ACh may directly stimulate existing HO (HO-1 and HO-2) to release CO.[8] These reports are promising but more research is needed.

Another long standing question that puzzled and frustrated us from the beginning of the journey is the endogenous level of CO which can be further divided into circulating levels and local levels in vascular walls.

Allow us to consider the case of NO. Do we know the circulating level of NO? Do we know the local level of NO in the interstitial fluid of vascular walls? The answers are uncertain now but definitive answers should be sought.

Returning to CO, its circulating level has been traditionally evaluated based on the level of carboxyhemoglobin. Does carboxyhemoglobin fully represent the CO level in circulation, considering the different affinities of hemoglobin to CO under varying conditions? The question becomes even more problematic where the tissue level of CO is concerned. Although the generation of CO from vascular SMCs of rats,[95] lambs,[58] and humans[96] has been determined *in vitro*, the physiological concentration of CO in the adjacent neighborhoods of vascular SMCs *in vivo* is still unknown. Knowing the interstitial concentrations of CO in vascular walls will facilitate the interpretation of the physiological relevance of the concentrations of CO tested in various reports. Nevertheless, studies of brain tissues[91] have indicated that the concentrations of CO produced *in vivo* are higher than those of NO, and are at least as high as those of CO used *in vitro* to stimulate guanylyl cyclase in cerebellar slices (1 to 200 μM). More studies on vascular tissues and the development of novel techniques in detecting CO concentrations in the interstitial spaces will justify our endeavors and advance our knowledge of this specific aspect of CO activity.

ACKNOWLEDGMENTS

This work was supported by research grants from the Canadian Institutes of Health Research (CIHR), the Natural Science and Engineering Research Council of Canada, and the Heart and Stroke Foundation of Canada. W. Zhao was supported by a post-doctoral fellowship award from University of Saskatchewan. R. Wang was supported by a scientist award from CIHR.

REFERENCES

1. Sjostrand, T., Endogenous formation of carbon monoxide in man under normal and pathological conditions, *Scand. J. Clin. Lab. Invest.*, 1, 201, 1949.
2. Duke, H.N. and Killick, E.M., Pulmonary vasomotor responses of isolated perfused cat lungs to anoxia, *J. Physiol.*, 117, 303, 1952.
3. Coceani, F. et al., Cytochrome P450-linked monooxygenase: involvement in the lamb ductus arteriosus, *Am. J. Physiol.*, 246, H640, 1984.
4. Vedernikov, Y.P., Graser, T., and Vanin, A.F., Similar endothelium-independent arterial relaxation by carbon monoxide and nitric oxide, *Biomed. Biochim. Acta*, 48, 601, 1989.
5. Lin, H. and McGrath, J.J., Carbon monoxide effects on calcium levels in vascular smooth muscle, *Life Sci.*, 43, 1813, 1988.
6. Lin, H. and McGrath, J.J., Vasodilating effects of carbon monoxide, *Drug Chem. Toxicol.*, 11, 371, 1988.

7. Sammut, I.A. et al., Carbon monoxide is a major contributor to the regulation of vascular tone in aortas expressing high levels of haeme oxygenase-1, *Br. J. Pharmacol.*, 125, 1437, 1998.

8. Zakhary, R. et al., Heme oxygenase 2: endothelial and neuronal localization and role in endothelium-dependent relaxation, *Proc. Natl. Acad. Sci. U.S.A.*, 93, 795, 1996.

9. Caudill, T.K. et al., Role of endothelial carbon monoxide in attenuated vasoreactivity following chronic hypoxia, *Am. J. Physiol.*, 275, R1025, 1998.

10. Longo, M. et al., Effect of nitric oxide and carbon monoxide on uterine contractility during human and rat pregnancy, *Am. J. Obstet. Gynecol.*, 181, 981, 1999.

11. Wang, R., Wang, Z.Z., and Wu, L., Carbon monoxide-induced vasorelaxation and the underlying mechanisms, *Br. J. Pharmacol.*, 121, 927, 1997.

12. Villamor, E. et al., Relaxant effect of carbon monoxide compared with nitric oxide in pulmonary and systemic vessels of newborn piglets, *Pediatric Res.*, 48, 546, 2000.

13. Thorup, C. et al., Carbon monoxide induces vasodilatation and nitric oxide release but suppresses endothelial NOS, *Am. J. Physiol.*, 277, F882, 1999.

14. Zygmunt, P.M., Hogestatt, E.D., and Grundemar, L., Light-dependent effects of zinc protoporphyrin IX on endothelium-dependent relaxation resistant to N-L-arginine, *Acta Physiol. Scand.*, 152, 137, 1994.

15. Steinhorn, R.H., Morin, F.C., III, and Russell, J.A., The adventitia may be a barrier specific to nitric oxide in rabbit pulmonary artery, *J. Clin. Invest.*, 94, 1883, 1994.

16. Marks, G.S. et al., Heme oxygenase activity and immunohistochemical localization in bovine pulmonary artery and vein, *J. Cardiovasc. Pharmacol.*, 30, 1, 1997.

17. McGrath, J.J. and Smith, D.L., Response of rat coronary circulation to carbon monoxide and nitrogen hypoxia, *Proc. Soc. Exp. Biol. Med.*, 177, 132, 1984.

18. McFaul, S.J. and McGrath, J.J., Studies on the mechanism of carbon monoxide-induced vasodilatation in the isolated perfused rat heart, *Toxicol. Appl. Pharmacol.*, 87, 464, 1987.

19. Graser, T., Vedemikov, Y.P., and Li, D.S., Study on the mechanism of carbon monoxide induced endothelium-independent relaxation in porcine coronary artery and vein, *Biomed. Biochim. Acta*, 4, 293, 1990.

20. Makino, N. et al., Altered expression of heme oxygenase-1 in the livers of patients with portal hypertensive diseases, *Hepatology*, 33, 32, 2001.

21. Goda, N. et al., Distribution of heme oxygenase isoforms in rat liver. Topographic basis for carbon monoxide-mediated microvascular relaxation, *J. Clin. Invest.*, 101, 604, 1998.

22. Shinoda, Y. et al., Carbon monoxide as a regulator of bile canalicular contractility in cultured rat hepatocytes, *Hepatology*, 28, 286, 1998.

23. Sano, T. et al., Endogenous carbon monoxide suppression stimulates bile acid-dependent biliary transport in perfused rat liver, *Am. J. Physiol.*, 272, G1268, 1997.

24. Suematsu, M. et al., Carbon monoxide as an endogenous modulator of hepatic vascular perfusion, *Biochem. Biophys. Res. Commun.*, 205, 1333, 1994.

25. Suematsu, M. et al., Carbon monoxide: an endogenous modulator of sinusoidal tone in the perfused rat liver, *J. Clin. Invest.*, 96, 2431, 1995.

26. Pannen, B.H.J. and Bauer, M., Differential regulation of hepatic arterial and portal venous vascular resistance by nitric oxide and carbon monoxide in rats, *Life Sci.*, 62, 2025, 1998.

27. Leffler, C.W. et al., Carbon monoxide and cerebral microvascular tone in newborn pigs, *Am. J. Physiol.*, 276, H1641, 1999.

28. Werkstrom, V. et al., Carbon monoxide-induced relaxation and distribution of haem oxygenase isoenzymes in the pig urethra and lower oesophagogastric junction, *Br. J. Pharmacol.*, 120, 312, 1997.

29. Brian, J.E., Jr., Heistad, D.D., and Faraci, F.M., Effect of carbon monoxide on rabbit cerebral arteries, *Stroke*, 25, 639, 1994.
30. Kozma, F., Johnson, R.A., and Nasjletti, A., Role of carbon monoxide in heme-induced vasodilatation, *Eur. J. Pharmacol.*, 323, R1, 1997.
31. Furchgott, R.F. and Jothianandan, D., Endothelium-dependent and -independent vasodilatation involving cyclic GMP: relaxation induced by nitric oxide, carbon monoxide and light, *Blood Vessels*, 28, 52, 1991.
32. Ignarro, L.J., Endothelium-derived nitric oxide: actions and properties, *FASEB J.*, 3, 31, 1989.
33. Coceani, F., Kelsey, L., and Seidlitz, E., Carbon monoxide-induced relaxation of the ductus arteriosus in the lamb: evidence against the prime role of guanylyl cyclase, *Br. J. Pharmacol.*, 118, 1689, 1996.
34. Ewing, J.F., Vulapalli, S.P., and Maines, M.D., Induction of heart heme oxygenase-1 (HSP32) by hyperthermia: possible role in stress-mediated elevation of cyclic 3′:5′-guanosine monophosphate, *J. Pharmacol. Exp. Ther.*, 271, 408, 1994.
35. Ramos, K.S., Lin, H., and McGrath, J.J., Modulation of cyclic guanosine monophosphate levels in cultured aortic smooth muscle cells by carbon monoxide, *Biochem. Pharmacol.*, 38, 1368, 1989.
36. Morita, T. et al., Carbon monoxide controls the proliferation of hypoxic vascular smooth muscle cells, *J. Biol. Chem.*, 272, 32804, 1997.
37. Maines, M.D., Eke, B.C., and Zhao, X., Corticosterone promotes increased heme oxygenase–2 protein and transcript expression in the newborn rat brain, *Brain Res.*, 722, 83, 1996.
38. Yet, S.F. et al., Induction of heme oxygenase-1 expression in vascular smooth muscle cells, *J. Biol. Chem.*, 272, 4295, 1997.
39. Kourembanas, S. et al., Mechanisms by which oxygen regulates gene expression and cell–cell interaction in the vasculature, *Kidney Int.*, 51, 438, 1997.
40. Kourembanas, S. et al., Hypoxic responses of vascular cells, *Chest*, 114 (1 Suppl. 1), 25S, 1998.
41. Johnson, R.A. and Kozma, F., Endothelial-dependent and -independent actions of heme and carbon monoxide on vascular tone, *INABIS*, 1998.
42. Storm, J.E. and Fechter, L.D., Prenatal carbon monoxide exposure differentially affects postnatal weight and monoamine concentration of rat brain regions, *Toxicol. Appl. Pharmacol.*, 81, 139, 1985.
43. Carratu, M.R. et al., Changes in peripheral nervous system activity produced in rats by prenatal exposure to carbon monoxide, *Arch. Toxicol.*, 67, 297, 1993.
44. Montagnani, M. et al., Prenatal exposure to carbon monoxide and vascular responsiveness of rat resistance vessels, *Life Sci.*, 59, 1553, 1996.
45. Rattan, S., and Chakder, S., Inhibitory effect of CO on internal anal sphincter: heme oxygenase inhibitor inhibits NANC relaxation, *Am. J. Physiol.*, 265, G799, 1993.
46. Xue, L. et al., Carbon monoxide and nitric oxide as coneurotransmitters in the enteric nervous system: evidence from genomic deletion of biosynthetic enzymes, *Proc. Natl. Acad. Sci. U.S.A.*, 97, 1851, 2000.
47. Ny, L. et al., Carbon monoxide as a putative messenger molecule in the feline lower oesophageal sphincter of the cat, *Neuroreport*, 6, 1389, 1995.
48. Wang, R., Resurgence of carbon monoxide: an endogenous gaseous vasorelaxing factor, *Can. J. Physiol. Pharmacol.*, 76, 1, 1998.
49. Takahashi, S., Wang, J., and Rousseau, D.L., Heme-hemeoxygenase complex: structure and properties of the catalytic site from resonance Raman scattering, *Biochemistry*, 33, 5531, 1994.

50. McCoubrey, W.K., Jr., Huang, T.J., and Maines, M.D., Isolation and characterization of a cDNA from the rat brain that encodes heme protein heme oxygenase-3, *Eur. J. Biochem.*, 274, 725, 1997.
51. Jandl, J.H., Physiology of red cells, in *Blood: Textbook of Hematology*, Jandl, J.H., Ed., Little, Brown, Boston, 1987, 89.
52. Maines, M.D., The heme oxygenase system: a regulator of second messenger classes, *Annu. Rev. Pharmacol. Toxicol.*, 37, 517, 1997.
53. Levere, R.D. et al., Effect of heme arginate administration on blood pressure in spontaneously hypertensive rats, *J. Clin. Invest.*, 86, 213, 1990.
54. Johnson, R.A. et al., Heme oxygenase substrates acutely lower blood pressure in hypertensive rats, *Am. J. Physiol.*, 271, H1132, 1996.
55. Sacerdoti, D. et al., Treatment with tin prevents the development of hypertension in spontaneously hypertensive rats, *Science*, 243, 388, 1989.
56. Johnson, R.A., Kozma, F., and Colombari, E., Carbon monoxide — from toxin to endogenous modulator of cardiovascular functions, *Braz. J. Med. Biol. Res.*, 32, 1, 1999.
57. Wakabayashi, Y. et al., Carbon monoxide overproduced by heme oxygenase-1 causes a reduction of vascular resistance in perfused rat liver, *Am. J. Physiol.*, 277, G1088, 1999.
58. Coceani, F. et al., Carbon monoxide formation in the ductus arteriosus in the lamb: implications for the regulation of muscle tone, *Br. J. Pharmacol.*, 120, 599, 1997.
59. Durante, W. et al., cAMP induces heme oxygenase-1 gene expression and carbon monoxide production in vascular smooth muscle, *Am. J. Physiol.*, 273, H317, 1997.
60. Durante, W. et al., Nitric oxide induces heme oxygenase-1 gene expression and carbon monoxide production in vascular smooth muscle cells, *Circ. Res.*, 80, 557, 1997.
61. Kozma, F. et al., Contribution of endogenous carbon monoxide to regulation of diameter in resistance vessels, *Am. J. Physiol.*, 276, R1087, 1999.
62. Johnson, R.A. et al., A heme oxygenase product, presumably carbon monoxide, mediates a vasodepressor function in rats, *Hypertension*, 25, 166, 1995.
63. Grundemar, L. and Ny, L., Pitfalls using metalloporphyrins in carbon monoxide research, *Trends Pharmacol. Sci.*, 18, 193, 1997.
64. Luo, D. and Vincent, S.R., Metalloporphyrins inhibit nitric oxide — dependent cGMP formation *in vivo*, *Eur. J. Pharmacol.*, 267, 263, 1994.
65. Drummond, G.S. and Kappas, A., Prevention of neonatal hyperbilirubinaemia by tin protoporphyrin IX, a potent competitive inhibitor of heme oxidation, *Proc. Natl. Acad. Sci. U.S.A.*, 78, 6466, 1981.
66. Linden, D.J., Narasimhan, K., and Gurfel, D., Protoporphyrins modulate voltage-gated Ca current in AtT-20 pituitary cells, *J. Neurophysiol.*, 70, 2673, 1993.
67. Ny, L., Anderson, K.E., and Grundemar, L., Inhibition by zinc protoporphyrin-IX of receptor-mediated relaxation of the rat aorta in a manner distinct from inhibition of haem oxygenase, *Br. J. Pharmacol.*, 115, 186, 1995.
68. Maines, M.D. and Trakshel, G.M., Differential regulation of heme oxygenase isozymes by Sn- and Zn-protoporphyrins: possible relevance to suppression of hyper-bilirubinemia, *Biochim. Biophys. Acta*, 1131, 166, 1992.
69. Wang, R., Le monoxyde de carbone: un facteur vasoactif endogene chez les rats normaux et diabétiques? *Med. Sci.*, (Suppl. 2), 9, 1995.
70. Wang, R., Carbon monoxide may act as an endogenous gaseous vasorelaxing factor: studies in normal and diabetic rats, *Jpn. Circ. J.*, 60 (Suppl. 1), 543, 1996.
71. Wang, R., Vasorelaxation induced by carbon monoxide and underlying mechanisms. *Physiol. Can.*, 27, 37, 1996.

72. Wang, R. and Wu, L., The chemical modification of K_{Ca} channels by carbon monoxide in vascular smooth muscle cells, *J. Biol. Chem.*, 272, 8222, 1997.

73. Wang, R., Wu, L., and Wang, Z.Z., The direct effect of carbon monoxide on K_{Ca} channels in vascular smooth muscle cells, *Pflügers Arch.*, 434, 285, 1997.

74. Brüne, B. and Ullrich, V., Inhibition of platelet aggregation by carbon monoxide is mediated by activation of guanylyl cyclase, *Mol. Pharmacol.*, 32, 497, 1987.

75. Quast, U., Do the K^+ channel openers relax smooth muscle by opening K^+ channels? *Trends Pharmacol. Sci.*, 14, 332, 1993.

76. Utz J. and Ullrich, V., Carbon monoxide relaxes ileal smooth muscle through activation of guanylyl cyclase, *Biochem. Pharmacol.*, 41, 1195, 1991.

77. Rich, A., Farrugia, G., and Rae, J.L., Carbon monoxide stimulates a potassium-selective current in rabbit corneal epithelial cells, *Am. J. Physiol.*, 267, C435, 1994.

78. Farrugia, G. et al., Activation of whole cell currents in isolated human jejunal circular smooth muscle cells by carbon monoxide, *Am. J. Physiol.* 264, G1184, 1993.

79. Liu, H. et al., Carbon monoxide stimulates the apical 70-pS K^+ channel of the rat thick ascending limb, *J. Clin. Invest.*, 103, 963, 1999.

80. Harder, D.R. et al., Identification of a putative microvascular oxygen sensor, *Circ. Res.*, 79, 54, 1996.

81. Coceani, F. et al., Inhibition of the contraction of the ductus arteriosus to oxygen by 1-aminobenzotriazole, a mechanism-based inactivation of cytochrome P450, *Br. J. Pharmacol.*, 117, 1586, 1996.

82. Coceani, F. et al., Further evidence implicating a cytochrome P450-mediated reaction in the contractile tension of the lamb ductus arteriosus, *Circ. Res.*, 62, 471, 1988.

83. Alvarez, J., Montero, M., and Garcia-Sancho, J., Cytochrome P450 may regulate plasma membrane Ca^{2+} permeability according to the filling state of the intracellular Ca^{2+} stores, *FASEB J.*, 6, 786, 1992.

84. Gerzer, R. et al., Soluble guanylate cyclase purified from bovine lung contains heme and copper, *FEBS Lett.* 132, 71, 1981.

85. Carvajal, J.A. et al., Molecular mechanism of cGMP-mediated smooth muscle relaxation, *J. Cell. Physiol.*, 184, 409, 2000.

86. Villalobos, C. et al., Inhibition of voltage-gated Ca^{2+} entry into GH_3 and chromaffin cells by imidazole antimyocotics and other cytochrome P450 blockers, *FASEB J.*, 6, 2742, 1992.

87. Rozanov, C. et al., Chemosensory response to high pCO is blocked by cadmium, a voltage-sensitive calcium channel blocker, *Brain Res.* 833, 101, 1999.

88. Prabhakar, N.R., NO and CO as second messengers in oxygen sensing in the carotid body, *Respir. Physiol.*, 115, 161, 1999.

89. Pineda, J., Kogan, J.H., and Aghajanian, G.K., Nitric oxide and carbon monoxide activate locus coeruleus neurons through a cGMP-dependent protein kinase: involvement of a nonselective cationic channel, *J. Neurosci.*, 16, 1389, 1996.

90. Leinders–Zufall, T., Shepherd, G.M., and Zufall, F., Regulation of cyclic nucleotide-gated channels and membrane excitability in olfactory receptor cells by carbon monoxide, *J. Neurophysiol.*, 74, 1498, 1995.

91. Nathanson, J.A. et al., The cellular Na^+ pump as a site of action of carbon monoxide and glutamate: a mechanism for long-term modulation of cellular activity, *Neuron*, 14, 781, 1995.

92. McKee, M., Scavone, C., and Nathanson, J.A., Nitric oxide, cyclic GMP and hormone regulation of active sodium transport, *Proc. Natl. Acad. Sci. U.S.A.*, 91, 12056, 1994.

93. Medford, R.M. et al., Vascular smooth muscle expresses a truncated Na^+, K^+-ATPase alpha-1 subunit isoform, *J. Biol. Chem.*, 266, 18308, 1991.

94. Lutton, J.D. et al., Differential induction of heme oxygenase in the hepatocarcinoma cell line (Hep3B) by environmental agents, *J. Cell Biochem.*, 49, 259, 1992.
95. Cook, M.N. et al., Heme oxygenase activity in the adult rat aorta and liver as measured by carbon monoxide formation, *Can. J. Physiol. Pharmacol.,* 73, 515, 1995.
96. Grundemar, L. et al., Haem oxygenase activity in blood vessel homogenates as measured by carbon monoxide production, *Acta Physiol. Scand.*, 153, 203, 1995.

3 Carbon Monoxide and Vascular Smooth Muscle Cell Growth

William Durante

CONTENTS

I. INTRODUCTION

The blood vessel wall is an active, integrated organ composed of different cell types that are coupled to each other in a complex set of autocrine–paracrine interactions. The vessel wall is organized in three distinct layers. The innermost layer, the intima, consists of a single layer of endothelial cells (ECs) seated on a specialized extracellular matrix known as the basement membrane. The underlying media contain vascular smooth muscle cells (SMCs) that are densely packed into an interstitial matrix containing collagen, fibronectin, and proteoglycans. The outer adventitia consists of fibroblasts in a loose connective tissue, which also contains small blood vessels and nerves.

The fully differentiated medial SMC is a highly specialized cell whose principal function is contraction. It expresses a unique constellation of contractile proteins, ion channels, and signaling molecules that are required for its contractile function. These SMCs exhibit extremely low rates of proliferation and synthesize minimal extracellular matrix. However, in response to vascular injury, SMCs can switch to a synthetic phenotype and begin to proliferate, migrate, and secrete large amounts of extracellular matrix. Although this remarkable plasticity of vascular SMC function is essential for the development of the vascular system and for tissue repair following vascular trauma, it is also a characteristic feature of arterial lesions found in athero-sclerosis, postangioplasty restenosis, and hypertension.[1-4] Although most studies have focused on aberrant SMC growth as the fundamental process of vascular lesion formation, emerging evidence suggests that the balance between cell growth and programmed cell death or apoptosis governs the development of vascular lesions.

In this chapter we will examine the regulation of CO synthesis by vascular cells and review recent studies indicating that endogenously generated CO is a critical regulator of vascular SMC growth and apoptosis. In addition, we will investigate the role of CO in regulating vascular remodeling.

II. REGULATION OF VASCULAR CARBON MONOXIDE BIOSYNTHESIS

The predominant endogenous source of CO is the degradation of heme by the enzyme heme oxygenase (HO).[5] HO cleaves and oxidizes the α-methene bridge of the heme molecule yielding equimolar amounts of biliverdin, iron, and CO.[6] The catalytic activity of HO requires the concerted action of microsomal NADPH–cytochrome P450 reductase to transfer electrons to the HO–heme complex.[7] At least three different isoforms of HO (HO-1, HO-2, and HO-3) have been identified and cloned.[8-10] These isozymes are products of different genes and differ markedly in their tissue expression and their molecular properties. The HO-2 isoform is consti-tutively expressed and is present in high levels in both the brain and testes.[11] In contrast, the HO-1 isoform is rapidly induced by its own substrate and by several oxidants, including superoxide anion, hydrogen peroxide, and nitric oxide (NO).[12-15] The recently discovered HO-3 isoform is closely related to HO-2, is nearly devoid of HO activity, and may function as a heme-sensing or heme-binding protein.[10]

Several studies demonstrated the presence of HO in various blood vessels. Both HO-1 mRNA and protein have been detected in arterial and venous blood vessels.[16-19] Inducible HO-1 and constitutive HO-2 have been found in both cultured vascular endothelium and SMCs.[17,20-22] To date, however, there is no evidence that the HO-3 isoform is expressed in the vasculature. HO-catalyzed CO production has also been recorded by gas chromatography in tissue homogenates of animal and human blood vessels.[19,23,24] In addition, a recent study from our laboratory directly measured the synthesis of CO from intact cultured vascular SMCs using laser absorption spectroscopy.[25] Interestingly, this study found that vascular CO synthesis is not only dependent on HO expression, but also on cellular heme levels.

HO-1 can be induced in vascular SMCs and ECs by physiologically relevant stimuli. In an early study, Morita et al.[20] found that hypoxia induces HO-1 gene expression and CO synthesis in vascular SMCs. Similarly, we demonstrated that hemin, sodium arsenite, and other heavy metals also stimulate vascular SMC HO-1 expression and CO release.[21] More recent studies indicate that inflammatory cytok-ines,[14,15,22,26] endotoxin,[26] NO,[14,15,27] cyclic nucleotides,[28] and oxidized low density lipoproteins[29,30] are all capable of inducing HO-1 gene expression. In addition to humoral stimuli, specific hemodynamic forces such as fluid shear stress and cyclic strain stimulate vascular cell HO-1 expression and CO synthesis.[31,32]

More recently, our laboratory found that growth factors are also potent inducers of HO-1. Treatment of vascular SMCs with platelet-derived growth factor (PDGF) results in a marked increase in the expression of HO-1 mRNA and protein and the release of CO.[33] Other growth factors, including angiotensin II, transforming growth factor-β1, and serum have also been demonstrated to regulate HO-1 expression.[18,34-38] The up-regulation of HO-1 gene expression by growth factors is dependent on *de novo* RNA synthesis and probably involves transcriptional activation of the HO-1 gene.[33] In addition, growth factor-mediated HO-1 expression is dependent on the production of reactive oxygen species. We observed that PDGF stimulates a marked increase in the intracellular synthesis of reactive oxygen intermediates. Moreover, we found that the antioxidant N-acetyl-L-cysteine suppresses both the PDGF-mediated synthesis of reactive oxygen species and the expression of HO-1 in vascular SMCs. These findings indicate that reactive oxygen intermediates, which are well-established inducers of HO-1,[12,13] mediate the induction of HO-1 by PDGF. Interestingly, promoter studies have identified functionally responsive elements for the redox-sensitive transcription factors, activator protein-1 (AP-1) and nuclear factor-κB (NFκB), in the 5′-flanking region of the HO-1 gene, suggesting a possible role for these transcription factors in the induction of HO-1 by growth factors.[22,27,39,40]

In summary, these studies demonstrate that vascular cells generate CO by the action of HO on heme. Furthermore, they show that physiologically relevant biochemical and hemodynamic stimuli induce CO synthesis in vascular cells by specifically inducing HO-1 gene expression.

III. CARBON MONOXIDE AND VASCULAR SMOOTH MUSCLE CELL PROLIFERATION

In recent years, rapid progress has been made in identifying and understanding the molecular mechanisms regulating vascular cell proliferation. Cellular growth can be divided into five distinct phases (Figure 3.1). Quiescent cells are found in the G_0 phase of the cell cycle and exhibit minimal protein synthesis. When appropriately stimulated, a cell enters the cycle at the first gap (G_1) phase and begins to synthesize proteins necessary for DNA synthesis (S phase), after which the cell enters a second gap (G_2) phase. During G_2 the cell synthesizes additional proteins in preparation for cell division or mitosis (M phase) when the cell divides into two daughter cells. Several checkpoints exist within the cell cycle to ensure that cell division proceeds normally.[41] In the late G_1 phase, cells reach the primary checkpoint, known as the restriction point (R); cells are then committed to DNA replication and cell cycle progression.

The progression of vascular cells through the cell cycle is orchestrated by a family of cyclin-dependent kinases (cdk), whose activity depends upon cyclin binding and positive and negative phosphorylation. In particular, transition through the early G_1 phase of the cell cycle is controlled by three D-type cyclins (D1, D2, and D3) that assemble with their catalytic partners, cdk4 and cdk6.[42] The protein level of proliferating cell nuclear antigen (PCNA), a factor that increases the processing ability of DNA-polymerase-δ and increases and associates with cyclin D/cdk4 complexes.[43]

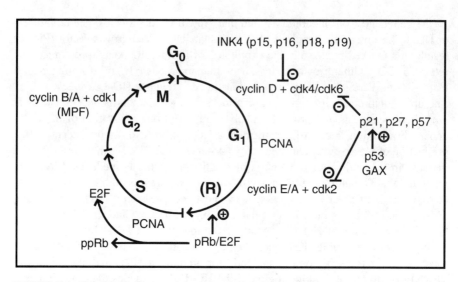

FIGURE 3.1 Simplified scheme of the cell cycle. Cell cycle progression is dependent on the expression and activation of cyclin-dependent kinases (cdk) which form holoenzymes with their regulatory subunits, the cyclins. Cdk inhibitors (the INK 4 and p21[cip1/waf1], p27[Kip1], and p57[Kip2] family of proteins) bind to and inhibit the activation of cdk/cyclin complexes. Activation of the complexes results in the phosphorylation of retinoblastoma protein (pRb) and the release of E2F, which is essential for DNA synthesis and cell division.

Free cyclin D/cdk4/PCNA complexes are subsequently activated through phosphorylation by a cdk-activating kinase (CAK). In the late G_1 phase, cyclins E and A are expressed, and they bind and activate their catalytic partner, cdk2.[42]

    The activation of G_1 phase cdk results in the phosphorylation of retinoblastoma protein (pRB) at the R point.[44] pRb acts as a timer of transcriptional events during the cell cycle. The hypophosphorylated form of pRb binds to and inhibits the transcription factor E2F. Hyperphosphorylation of pRb (ppRb) in late G_1 liberates E2F, which subsequently up-regulates the expression of several genes (dihydrofolate reductase, PCNA, cyclin E, and cyclin A) required for progression through S phase and DNA synthesis.[45] After DNA replication is complete, the cell enters the G_2 phase and cyclin B levels increase. This protein then binds with cdk1 to form mitosis-promoting factor (MPF). Activation of MPF requires the specific phosphorylation and dephosphorylation of cdk1 by CAK and cdc25 phosphatase, respectively.[46] Activated MPF initiates prophase and induces the destruction of cyclin B by stimulating the ubiquitin proteasome pathway.[47] This results in the inactivation of cdk1 and resets the cell cycle clock.

    Multiple redundant mechanisms have been developed to prevent inappropriate cell cycle entry. One important class of regulators is the cdk inhibitors. These proteins bind directly to cyclin/cdk complexes and block their ability to phosphorylate pRb. These cdk inhibitors consist of the INK 4 (p15, p16, p18, and p19), p21[cip1/waf1], p27[Kip1], and p57[Kip2] family of proteins. While the INK 4 proteins have selective inhibitory activity for cdk4 and cdk6, p21[cip1/waf1], p27[Kip1], and p57[Kip2] bind and inhibit a broad range of cdk as well as other proteins involved in cellular proliferation, such as PCNA.[48]

A role for the tumor suppressor protein, p53, in cell cycle regulation has also been suggested. p53 arrests cells in the G_1 phase in response to DNA damage and may provide the primary mechanism for the antiproliferative effect of radiation. This protective effect has been linked to the p53-mediated induction of p21[cip1/waf1 49,50] However, p53 can also stimulate cell death, providing another important defense against the propagation of cells with damaged DNA.[51] Finally, homeobox gene products are also important modulators of cell cycle entry. In particular, the arrest-specific homeobox, GAX, has been demonstrated to arrest cells in the G_0/G_1 phase of the cell cycle by stimulating the expression of p21[cip1/waf1 52].

Numerous positive and negative regulators of vascular SMC growth have been identified and are listed in Table 3.1. A detailed description of the biology of these growth regulators is beyond the scope of this chapter and is described else-where.[1,3,53-55] Most growth factors stimulate the entry of SMCs into the cell cycle by up-regulating the transcription of the protooncogenes c-*fos*, c-*myc*, c-*myb*, B-*myb*, and *ras*. Their gene products act as transcription factors that increase the expression of specific cell cycle regulatory genes. In contrast, many antiproliferative agents inhibit the expression of the protooncogenes by activating adenylate cyclase or guanylate cyclase, thereby elevating the intracellular levels of cAMP or cGMP, respectively. Interestingly, some regulators, such as transforming growth factor-β1 and cyclic strain, exhibit growth-inhibitory or growth-stimulatory properties depending on the type of SMCs and the local cellular milieu.

The observation that growth factors induce HO-1 gene expression raises the possibility that HO-1 may affect vascular SMC growth. Indeed, in a preliminary study,[38] we found that the HO inhibitors, tin protoporphyrin-IX (SnPP) and zinc protoporphyrin-IX (ZnPP), potentiate PDGF-mediated DNA synthesis in SMCs (Figure 3.2). In addition, the CO scavenger, hemoglobin, further increases PDGF-stimulated DNA synthesis (Figure 3.2). Interestingly, the mitogenic actions of angiotensin II, endothelin-1, and hypoxia are also potentiated by both HO inhibition and CO scavenging.[56,57] These results suggest that the HO-1-catalyzed release of CO may function in an autocrine manner to limit SMC proliferation. Consistent with these findings, the induction of HO-1 by hemin administration or by gene transfer has also been reported to inhibit the proliferation of vascular SMCs.[56-59]

In more recent studies, our laboratory found that exogenous administration of CO blocks vascular SMC proliferation. In these experiments, SMCs are exposed to CO via a specially constructed environmental chamber[60] (Figure 3.3). Air containing 1% CO is mixed with air containing 5% CO_2 in a stainless steel mixing cylinder prior to delivery into the exposure chamber. Flow into the humidified chamber is at 1 L/min and the temperature is maintained at 37°C. A CO analyzer (Interscan, Chatsworth, CA) is used to continuously measure CO levels in the chamber by electrochemical detection. Using this apparatus, exposure of SMCs to CO at a concentration of 100 parts per million (ppm) markedly attenuates PDGF-mediated SMC DNA synthesis (Figure 3.4). This concentration of exogenous CO was estimated to be comparable to that produced by HO-1 activity in cultured vascular

TABLE 3.1
Regulators of Vascular Smooth Muscle Cell Growth

Growth promoters	Growth inhibitors
Platelet-derived growth factor	Heparin sulfate
Fibroblast growth factor	Nitric oxide
Epidermal growth factor	Atrial natriuretic peptide
Heparin-binding epidermal growth factor	Type C natriuretic peptide
Insulin-like growth factor I	Prostaglandins
Insulin	Fibronectin
Transforming growth factor-β[a]	Transforming growth factor-β[a]
Thrombin	Collagen
Angiotensin II	Shear stress
Serotonin	Cyclic stretch[a]
Endothelin	
Norepinephrine	
Vasopressin	
Substance P	
Leukotrienes	
Thromboxane	
Interleukin-1	
Interleukin-6	
Cyclic stretch[a]	

[a] These regulators have bifunctional growth properties depending on the type of smooth muscle cell and the local cellular milieu.

cells.[61] Thus, physiologically relevant levels of CO are able to inhibit vascular SMC growth.

To date, little is known regarding the actions of CO on the cell cycle machinery. Recent reports indicate that inhibition of vascular SMC growth following HO-1 expression is due to G_1 arrest.[58,59] Consistent with this finding, Morita et al.[56] observed that induction of HO-1 suppresses the expression of the transcription factor E2F-1. These inhibitory effects on the cell cycle likely result from the CO-mediated activation of soluble guanylate cyclase and the consequent rise in the cGMP levels.[62-64] In support of this proposal, inhibition of soluble guanylate cyclase with methylene blue or 1H-[1,2,4]oxadiazolo-[4,3-α]quinoxaline-1-one (ODQ) reverses the inhibition of cell cycle progression and SMC growth by HO-1.[53,56] Moreover, lipophilic analogues of cGMP mimic the antiproliferative action of CO on vascular SMCs.[56] Interestingly, cGMP regulates the expression of numerous cell cycle regulatory proteins, including cyclin D, cyclin A, p27[Kip1], and p53.[65-68] This raises the possibility that CO interacts at multiple sites to block S phase entry and SMC growth.

In addition to directly inhibiting cell proliferation, CO may regulate SMC growth by modulating the release of vascular mitogens. Using a co-culture system of ECs and SMCs, it was found that SMC-derived CO inhibits the synthesis of endothelin-1 and PDGF from hypoxic EC.[68] The CO-mediated inhibition of endothelin-1 and

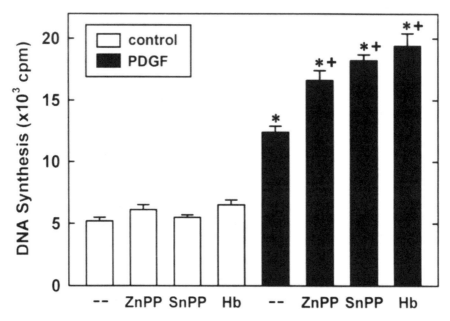

FIGURE 3.2 Effect of platelet-derived growth factor (PDGF) on vascular smooth muscle cell (SMC) DNA synthesis. SMCs were treated with PDGF (30 ng/ml) for 24 hours in the presence or absence of zinc protoporphyrin-IX (ZnPP; 20 μM), tin protoporphyrin-IX (SnPP; 20 μM), or hemoglobin (Hb; 50 μM). Results are means ± SEM of four separate experiments. Asterisks indicate statistically significant effects of PDGF. Plus signs indicate statistically significant effects of HO inhibition and CO scavenging.

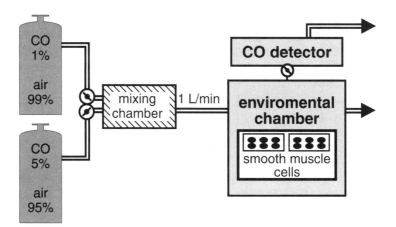

FIGURE 3.3 Schematic diagram of the CO environmental chamber. CO at 1% concentration in air was mixed with air containing 5% CO_2 in a stainless steel mixing cylinder prior to delivery into a humidified 37°C environmental chamber. Flow into the chamber was at 1 L/min and CO levels were continuously monitored by electrochemical detection using a CO analyzer (Interscan, Chatsworth, CA).

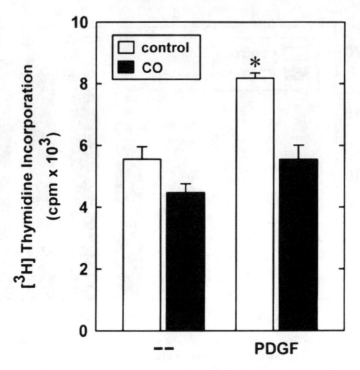

FIGURE 3.4 Effect of CO on vascular smooth muscle cell (SMC) DNA synthesis. SMCs were treated with platelet-derived growth factor (PDGF; 10 ng/ml) for 24 hours in the presence or absence of 100 parts per million of CO. Results are means ± SEM of four separate experiments. Asterisk indicates a statistically significant increase in DNA synthesis.

PDGF production is paralleled by a decrease in both endothelin-1 and PDGF mRNA, suggesting that CO suppresses endothelin-1 and PDGF gene expression. However, these actions of CO are not mediated by cGMP since inhibition of soluble guanylate cyclase or the administration of lipophilic analogues of cGMP does not affect the expression of endothelin-1 and PDGF.[69]

Platelets are another important source of vascular mitogens. The recruitment and aggregation of circulating platelets to sites of vascular injury and the subsequent release of growth factors from platelet alpha granules stimulate SMC proliferation and contribute to the formation of a neointima.[1,70,71] Utilizing a platelet/SMC coincubation system, our laboratory demonstrated that SMC-derived CO is capable of inhibiting platelet aggregation. Co-incubation of platelets with SMC treated with an HO-1 inducer (shear stress or Na arsenite) inhibits ADP-stimulated platelet aggregation.[31] In contrast, co-incubation of platelets with untreated control SMCs has no significant effect on platelet aggregation.[31] The inhibition of platelet aggregation by SMCs following HO-1 induction is associated with a marked rise in platelet cGMP concentration that is reversed by treating SMCs with SnPP.[31] These results are consistent with earlier studies demonstrating that the exogenous administration of CO inhibits platelet aggregation via a cGMP-mediated pathway.[72,73] Thus, SMC-derived CO is able to function in a paracrine fashion to block the release of growth factors from vascular cells and circulating blood cells in both cGMP-dependent and -independent manners.

In contrast to its effect on vascular SMCs, HO-1 appears to stimulate EC growth. Transfection of the HO-1 gene stimulates the proliferation of coronary ECs and promotes the formation of capillary-like tube structures when the cells are embedded within a matrigel matrix.[74] These findings suggest that HO-1 may play an important role in angiogenesis. In addition, since ECs exert an inhibitory effect on SMC growth by releasing various antiproliferative factors, the ability of HO-1 to induce EC growth may represent another mechanism by which HO-1 down-regulates SMC growth.[75]

IV. CARBON MONOXIDE AND VASCULAR SMOOTH MUSCLE CELL APOPTOSIS

Vascular pathologists have long been intrigued by the observation of cell death within the arterial wall in the absence of overt necrosis.[76,77] In the early 1970s, Kerr and colleagues termed this novel form of cell death *apoptosis*.[78] Apoptosis or programmed cell death was initially described in cells on the basis of characteristic morphology. In contrast to the classic cellular swelling and membrane rupture associated with necrosis, apoptotic cells shrink and maintain their membrane integrity. Other hallmarks of apoptosis include chromatin margination and condensation, internucleosomal DNA fragmentation, redistribution of membrane phospholipids, and cell budding.[79] Recent studies suggest that apoptosis plays a pivotal role in both normal development and pathology of the vascular system. Indeed, programmed cell death is a prominent feature of the remodeling process that occurs in atherosclerosis, hypertension, and restenosis following angioplasty.[80-83]

Apoptosis is regulated by a complex interplay between cell surface signals and the expression of specific intracellular proteins (Figure 3.5). Apoptosis may be triggered via ligand binding to specific death receptors, such as the tumor necrosis factor and Fas family of receptors. These receptors consist of an extracellular domain, a hydrophobic transmembrane domain, and a cytoplasmic domain. Ligand binding to these receptors recruits adapter molecules (FADD, TRADD, and RIP) to the receptors, leading to the activation of caspase-8, which initiates the lethal caspase cascade.[84] Caspases are present as inactive proenzymes that are activated by proteolytic cleavage. They are responsible for the deliberate disassembly of the cell into apoptotic bodies.

Apoptosis is also modulated via the expression of specific intracellular proteins. In particular, the Bcl-2 family of proteins plays a crucial role in regulating apoptosis. While some Bcl-2 proteins, such as Bax, Bad, Bid, and Bak, promote apoptosis, others including Bcl-2 and Bcl-x_L, suppress it.[85] The Bcl-2 family of proteins regulates apoptosis in several ways. The apoptosis promoters, such as Bax and Bid, play an important role in the release of cytochrome c, a potent pro-apoptotic stimulus, from the mitochondria. In the cytoplasm, cytochrome c binds to apoptosis activating factor-1 (Apaf-1), resulting in the activation of caspase-9 and the subsequent caspase cascade.[86] In contrast, the Bcl-2 family members that suppress apoptosis, such as Bcl-2 and Bcl-x_L, prevent the activation of the caspase cascade by binding to Apaf-

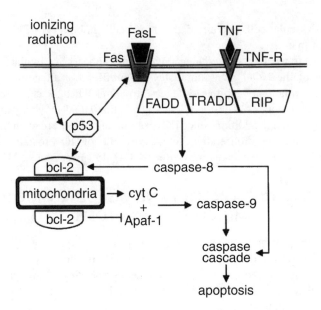

FIGURE 3.5 Schematic diagram of the main apoptotic pathways. Ligand binding to death receptors (TNF-R and Fas) results in the activation of caspase-8 and the subsequent activation of the caspase cascade. Caspase-9 is activated in response to the release of cytochrome c and its binding to Apaf-1. Activation of the caspase cascade is responsible for the disassembly of the cell into apoptotic bodies.

l protein and/or inhibiting the release of cytochrome c from the mitochondria.[87] Overall, the ratio of Bcl-2 suppressors to promoters helps determine a cell's susceptibility to apoptosis.

The activity of Bcl-2 family of proteins is regulated by changes in the expression of the genes that encode them or by modifications of the proteins through enzymatic cleavage. The transcription factor, p53, promotes apoptosis by inducing the expression of Bax while inhibiting the expression of Bcl-2.[87,88] In addition, activation of p53 increases cell surface expression of Fas by stimulating the transport of the receptor from the Golgi apparatus.[89] Alternatively, caspase-8 promotes apoptosis by cleaving Bid, which then translocates to the mitochondrial membrane, inducing cytochrome c release and caspase-9 activation.[90]

Vascular SMC apoptosis is induced by a wide variety of agents, including inflammatory mediators, vasoactive substances, oxidized lipids, viruses, protooncogenes, and biomechanical forces.[91-95] In contrast, growth factors exert potent antiapoptotic effects on vascular SMCs. In fact, many known growth factors have been shown to act as survival factors rather than true mitogens.[91,96,97] Interestingly, some factors, such as NO, exert opposite effects on SMC apoptosis depending on their concentration.[98]

Recent evidence indicates that CO may also be an important regulator of apoptosis. In a preliminary report,[99] Juan and Chau found that adenovirus-mediated HO-1 overexpression in cultured vascular SMCs induces apoptotic cell death as revealed by DNA fragmentation and the activation of the caspase cascade. Incubation of cells with the HO inhibitor, SnPP, or the CO scavenger, hemoglobin, markedly reduces cell death, suggesting that CO mediates the apoptotic effect of HO-1. Further experiments revealed that HO-1-induced SMC apoptosis is associated with the release of cytochrome c into the cytosol and increased expression of the proapoptotic proteins, p53 and Bax. In addition, the level of the antiapoptotic protein, Bcl-2, is down-regulated. In contrast, in a preliminary study,[100] our laboratory found that exposure of vascular SMCs to CO (100 ppm) markedly attenuated cytokine-mediated apoptosis. Clearly, additional studies are required to reconcile these important preliminary findings and to further define the molecular mechanisms by which CO regulates the apoptotic pathway in vascular SMCs.

Interestingly, Brouard et al.[61] recently found that overexpression of HO-1 protects ECs from apoptosis induced by various stimuli, including serum deprivation, etoposide, and the combination of tumor necrosis factor-α and actinomycin D (Figure 3.6). The induction of HO-1 also inhibits EC apoptosis during antibody-induced transplant arteriosclerosis, indicating an important role for HO-1 in promoting EC survival *in vivo*.[101] The ability of HO-1 to enhance EC survival may, in part, contribute to the growth-promoting activity of HO-1 in these cells.

The antiapoptotic effect of HO-1 in the vascular endothelium appears to be mediated by CO since hemoglobin is able to prevent this response.[61] However, both apoptotic and antiapoptotic effects have been reported following the exogenous administration of CO to cultured ECs.[61,102] The reasons for these divergent results are not known but may reflect differences in the dose and duration of CO exposure and/or in the vascular source of ECs.

The molecular mechanism by which HO-1 inhibits EC apoptosis appears to involve the p38 mitogen-activated protein kinase (MAPK) pathway. Recombinant adenovirus-mediated overexpression of HO-1 promotes the activation of p38 MAPK.[61] Moreover, the antiapoptotic action of HO-1 is prevented when p38 MAPK activation is blocked by the specific inhibitor of p38 MAPK, SB203580.[61] In addition, overexpression of a dominant-negative mutant of p38 MAPK inhibits the ability of HO-1 to suppress EC apoptosis.[61] Although activation of p38 MAPK regulates apoptosis in numerous cell types, the molecular mechanism by which this kinase modulates the apoptotic pathway remains unclear.[103]

V. CARBON MONOXIDE AND VASCULAR REMODELING

The process of vascular remodeling involves the intrinsic capacity of the vessel wall to alter its geometry as an adaptive response to its environment. It is an active process that involves changes in vascular cell growth and death. Although vascular remodeling is a critical biological process during the ontogeny of the circulatory system, it is also involved in the pathogenesis of a variety of vascular disorders, including postangioplasty restenosis, atherosclerosis, and hypertension.[3]

Considerable evidence indicates that HO-1 regulates the arterial remodeling response following balloon angioplasty.[57,104,105] This remodeling response is characterized by the loss of vascular ECs, the formation of an SMC-rich neointima, and

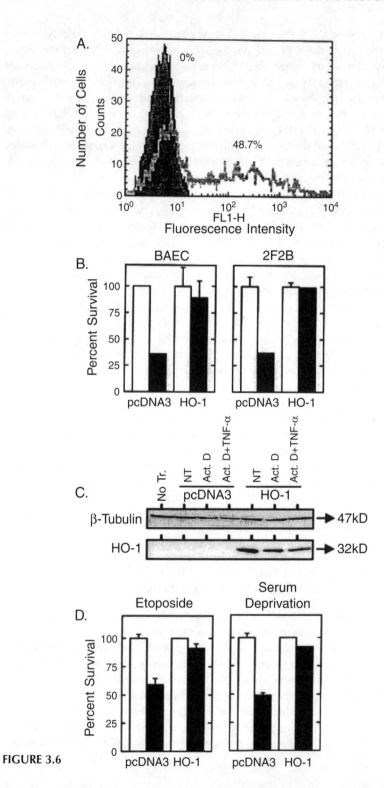

FIGURE 3.6

a collagen-enriched adventitia with a major diminution in luminal patency.[53,54] Figure 3.7A shows a Verhoff's elastic tissue-stained cross-section of a balloon-injured left carotid artery 14 days post-injury from a control rat. A significant and concentric elastin-rich neointima is evident with elastin fibers stained black. Collagen is highly expressed in the adventitia. However, treatment of rats with the HO-1 inducer, hemin, markedly reduced intimal thickening following balloon injury. Animals treated with daily injections of hemin starting 2 days prior to injury and continuing throughout the duration of the experiment demonstrated a significantly reduced neointima appearing as a thin cellular layer adjacent to the internal elastic lamina. Also evident is a decreased adventitia and reduced collagen staining (Figure 3.7B). The reduction in both neointima and adventitia formation by hemin are dependent on HO-1 activity since the HO inhibitor SnPP restores them to control levels (Figure 3.7C). Consistent with these findings, a recent study found that adenoviral-mediated overexpression of HO-1 significantly reduces intimal hyperplasia following vascular injury.[59]

There are several potential mechanisms by which HO-1 inhibits intimal thickening following vascular injury. However, the HO-1-mediated production of CO may be of paramount importance since it promotes the loss of vascular SMCs from the vessel wall by directly inhibiting SMC growth and stimulating SMC apoptosis.[56,57,99] CO may also exert an indirect effect on SMC proliferation by blocking the release of growth factors from the vessel wall and from platelets recruited to the site of vascular injury.[31,67] In addition, the ability of CO to block the synthesis of proinflammatory cytokines from activated vascular cells may also be important,[106] since these inflammatory mediators promote SMC growth.[107]

Consistent with a role for CO in mediating the inhibitory effects of HO-1 on vascular remodeling, the reduction in neointima formation is associated with a pronounced increase in vessel wall cGMP, a known target of CO.[57] Moreover, in a

---

FIGURE 3.6 (opposite) HO-1 inhibits endothelial cell (EC) apoptosis. (A) 2F-2B ECs were transfected with a GFP-expressing plasmid and monitored for green fluorescent protein expression by flow cytometry. The percentage of transfected ECs was assessed by fluorescence intensity in ECs transfected with control (pcDNA3; filled histogram) vs. GFP (open histogram) expression plasmids. (B) ECs were cotransfected with β-galactosidase plus control (pcDNA3) or HO-1 (β-actin/HO-1) expression vectors. EC apoptosis was induced by tumor necrosis factor-α (TNF-α) plus actinomycin D (Act.D) and apoptosis of β-galactosidase-transfected cells was quantified. Open bars represent ECs treated with Act.D and black bars represent ECs treated with TNF-α plus Act.D. Results shown are the means ± SD from duplicate wells taken from one representative experiment out of ten. (C) HO-1 expression detected in bovine aortic endothelial cells (BAECs) by Western blot. No Tr = non-transfected; NT = non-treated. (D) 2F-2B ECs cotransfected with β-galactosidase plus control (pcDNA3) or HO-1 (β-actin/HO-1) expression vectors. Open bars represent untreated ECs and black bars represent ECs treated with etoposide (200 μM, 8 h) or subjected to serum-deprivation (0.1% FCS, 24 h). Results shown are the means ± SD from duplicate wells taken from one representative experiment out of three independent experiments. Similar results were obtained with BAECs. (Reproduced from Brouard, S. et al., *J. Exp. Med.*, 192, 1015, 2000 with copyright permission of the Rockefeller University Press.)

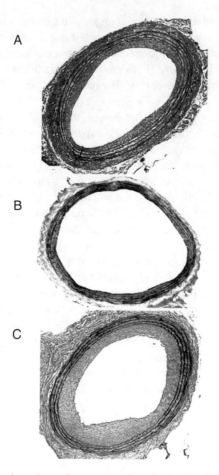

FIGURE 3.7 Representative photomicrographs of perfusion-fixed rat left carotid arteries (LCAs) 14 days after balloon injury. (A) Cross-section of a Verhoff's elastic tissue stained LCA from a control animal. (B) Effect of hemin treatment (50 mg/kg/day) starting 2 days prior to injury and continuing through sacrifice. (C) Simultaneous treatment with hemin (50 mg/kg/day) and tin protoporphyrin-IX (50 μM/kg/day). Magnification × 100.

recently published study,[108] we found that 3-(5'-hydroxymethyl-2'-furyl)-1-benzyl indazole (YC-1), a compound known to potentiate the stimulatory effects of CO on soluble guanylate cyclase,[109] elevates vessel wall cGMP levels and attenuates intimal thickening following balloon angioplasty.

Since the generation of reactive oxygen species contributes to the vascular response to injury,[110] HO-1 may also prevent intimal thickening by virtue of its antioxidant effects. HO-1 converts the prooxidant heme to biliverdin, which is subsequently metabolized to bilirubin by biliverdin reductase.[111] Moreover, both of these bile pigments are potent antioxidants that efficiently scavenge reactive oxygen species and inhibit lipid peroxidation.[112,113] Bilirubin also inhibits the migration of leukocytes, which is postulated to be a critical event in postangioplasty restenosis.[29]

Thus, the ability of HO-1 to generate both CO and bilirubin may provide a potent adaptive mechanism to maintain homeostasis at sites of vascular injury.

HO-1 may also play a critical role in regulating vascular remodeling in other pathophysiological settings. The induction of HO-1 protects against the development of antibody-induced arteriosclerosis in cardiac allografts.[101] In addition, preliminary studies indicate that HO-1 inhibits the formation of atherosclerotic plaques in both apoE and LDL receptor knockout mice.[114,115] Recent reports also indicate that vascular HO-1 expression is elevated in aortas of spontaneously hypertensive rats and angiotensin II-induced hypertensive rats, suggesting the possibility that CO may regulate the structural changes in hypertensive vessels.[18,116] Finally, a preliminary report indicates that CO also prevents pulmonary vascular remodeling during hypoxia.[117]

VI. CONCLUSIONS

Recent studies indicate that CO is not simply an irrelevant byproduct of heme metabolism and may assume physiologically important functions in the vasculature. In particular, the release of CO by the vessel wall serves as an endogenous regulator of vascular cell growth and survival. Emerging evidence indicates that CO is a potent inhibitor of vascular SMC growth. Although the antiproliferative effect of CO appears to be mediated via G_1 arrest, additional studies are required to precisely define the actions of CO on the cell cycle. In contrast, CO appears to promote the growth and survival of ECs. The capacity of CO to induce EC proliferation may also indirectly inhibit SMC growth, since ECs release various humoral factors that block SMC growth.

Finally, the HO-1/CO system may play an important role in regulating vascular remodeling. HO-1 markedly attenuates the arterial remodeling response following balloon angioplasty. Moreover, preliminary results suggest that HO-1 may inhibit vascular remodeling in a wide spectrum of vascular disorders. Thus, the ability of the HO-1/CO system to differentially regulate the growth of vascular cells may serve to maintain homeostasis at sites of vascular injury and prevent the development of occlusive vascular disease.

ACKNOWLEDGMENTS

I would like to thank Drs. Andrew I. Schafer, David A. Tulis, Xiao-ming Liu, and Gary B. Chapman for their many helpful contributions. This work was supported by National Heart, Lung, and Blood Institute Grant HL-59976. The author is an established investigator of the American Heart Association.

REFERENCES

1. Ross, R., The pathogenesis of atherosclerosis: a perspective for the 1990s, *Nature*, 362, 801, 1993.
2. Schwartz, S.M., Campbell, G.R., and Campbell, J.H., Replication of vascular smooth muscle cells in vascular disease, *Circ. Res.*, 58, 427, 1986.

3. Gibbons, G.H. and Dzau, V.J., The emerging concept of vascular remodeling, *New Engl. J. Med.*, 330, 1431, 1994.

4. Owens, G.K., Regulation of differentiation of vascular smooth muscle cells, *Physiol. Rev.*, 75, 487, 1995.

5. Rodgers, P.A. et al., Sources of carbon monoxide (CO) in biological systems and applications of CO detecting technologies, *Semin. Perinatol.*, 18, 2, 1994.

6. Tenhunen, R., Marver, H.S., and Schmidt, R., The enzymatic conversion of heme to bilirubin by microsomal heme oxygenase, *Proc. Natl. Acad. Sci. U.S.A.*, 244, 6388, 1968.

7. Trakshel, G.M., Kutty, R.K., and Maines, M.D., Cadmium-mediated inhibition of testicular heme oxygenase activity: the role of cytochrome-c (P-450) reductase, *Arch. Biochem. Biophys.*, 251, 175, 1986.

8. Maines, M.D., Trakshel, G.M., and Kutty, R.K., Characterization of two constitutive forms of rat liver microsomal heme oxygenase: only one molecular species of the enzyme is inducible, *J. Biol. Chem.*, 261, 411, 1986.

9. Trakshel, G.M. and Maines, M.D., Multiplicity of heme oxygenase isozymes: HO-1 and HO-2 are different molecular species in rat and rabbit, *J. Biol. Chem.*, 264, 1323, 1989.

10. McCoubrey, W.K. Jr., Huang, T.J., and Maines, M.D., Isolation and characterization of a cDNA from the rat brain that encodes hemoprotein heme oxygenase-3, *Eur. J. Biochem.*, 247, 725, 1997.

11. Maines, M.D., Heme oxygenase: function, multiplicity, regulatory mechanisms, and clinical applications, *FASEB J.*, 2, 2557, 1988.

12. Keyse, S.M. et al., Oxidative stress leads to the transcriptional activation of the human heme oxygenase gene in cultured skin fibroblasts, *Mol. Cell Biol.*, 10, 4967, 1990.

13. Vile, G.F. et al., Heme oxygenase 1 mediates an adaptive response to oxidative stress in human skin fibroblasts, *Proc. Natl. Acad. Sci. U.S.A.*, 91, 2607, 1994.

14. Motterlini, R. et al., NO-mediated activation of heme oxygenase: endogenous cytoprotection against oxidative stress to endothelium, *Am. J. Physiol.*, 270, H107, 1996.

15. Durante, W. et al., Nitric oxide induces heme oxygenase expression and carbon monoxide production in vascular smooth muscle cells, *Circ. Res.*, 80, 557, 1997.

16. Ewing, J.F., Raju, V.S., and Maines, M.D., Induction of heart heme oxygenase-1 (HSP-32) by hyperthermia: possible role in stress-mediated elevation of cyclic $3':5'$-guanosine monophosphate, *J. Pharmacol. Exp. Ther.*, 271, 408, 1994.

17. Zakhary, R. et al., Heme oxygenase-2: endothelial and neuronal localization and role in endothelium-dependent relaxation, *Proc. Natl. Acad. Sci. U.S.A.*, 93, 795, 1996.

18. Ishizaka, N. et al., Angiotensin II-induced hypertension increases heme oxygenase-1 expression in rat aorta, *Circulation*, 96, 1923, 1997.

19. Marks, G.S. et al., Heme oxygenase activity and immunohistochemical localization in bovine pulmonary artery and vein, *J. Cardiovasc. Res.*, 30, 1, 1997.

20. Morita, T. et al., Smooth muscle cell-derived carbon monoxide is a regulator of vascular cGMP, *Proc. Natl. Acad. Sci. U.S.A.*, 92, 1475, 1995.

21. Christodoulides, N. et al., Vascular smooth muscle cell heme oxygenases generate guanylyl cyclase-stimulatory carbon monoxide, *Circulation*, 91, 2306, 1995.

22. Terry, C.M. et al., Effect of tumor necrosis factor-α and interleukin-1α on heme oxygenase-1 expression in human endothelial cells, *Am. J. Physiol.* 274, H883, 1998.

23. Cook, M.N. et al., Heme oxygenase activity in the adult rat aorta and liver as measured by carbon monoxide formation, *Can. J. Physiol. Pharmacol.*, 73, 515, 1995.

24. Grundemar, L. et al., Haem oxygenase activity in blood vessel homogenates as measured by carbon monoxide production, *Acta Physiol. Scand.*, 153, 203, 1995.

25. Morimoto, Y. et al., Real-time measurements of endogenous CO production from vascular cells using an ultrasensitive laser sensor, *Am. J. Physiol.*, 280, H483, 2001.

26. Yet, S.F. et al., Induction of heme oxygenase-1 expression in vascular smooth muscle cells: a link to endotoxic shock, *J. Biol. Chem.*, 272, 4295, 1997.

27. Hartsfield, C.L. et al., Regulation of heme oxygenase-1 gene expression in vascular smooth muscle cells by nitric oxide, *Am. J. Physiol.*, 273, L980, 1997.

28. Durante, W. et al., cAMP induces heme oxygenase-1 gene expression and carbon monoxide production in vascular smooth muscle cells, *Am. J. Physiol.*, 273, H317, 1997.

29. Ishikawa, K. et al., Induction of heme oxygenase-1 inhibits the monocyte transmigration induced by mildly oxidized LDL, *J. Clin. Invest.*, 100, 1209, 1997.

30. Siow, R.C. et al., Induction of the antioxidant stress proteins heme oxygenase-1 and MSP23 by stress agents and oxidised LDL in cultured vascular smooth muscle cells, *FEBS Lett.*, 368, 239, 1995.

31. Wagner, C.T. et al., Hemodynamic forces induce the expression of heme oxygenase in cultured vascular smooth muscle cells, *J. Clin. Invest.* 100, 589, 1997.

32. De Keulenaer, G.W. et al., Oscillatory and steady laminar shear stress differentially affect human endothelial redox state: role of superoxide-producing NADH oxidase, *Circ. Res.*, 82, 1094, 1998.

33. Durante, W., Peyton, K.J., and Schafer, A.I., Platelet-derived growth factor stimulates heme oxygenase-1 gene expression and carbon monoxide production in vascular smooth muscle cells, *Arterioscler. Thromb. Vasc. Biol.*, 19, 2666, 1999.

34. Ishizaka, N. et al., Heme oxygenase-1 is regulated in the rat heart in response to chronic administration of angiotensin II, *Am. J. Physiol.*, 279, H672, 2000.

35. Ishizaka, N. and Griendling, K.K., Heme oxygenase-1 is regulated by angiotensin II in rat vascular smooth muscle cells, *Hypertension*, 29, 790, 1997.

36. Kutty, R.K. et al., Increased expression of heme oxygenase-1 in human retinal pigment epithelial cells by transforming growth factor-beta, *J. Cell. Physiol.* 159, 371, 1994.

37. Hill–Kapturczak, N. et al., Smad7-dependent regulation of heme oxygenase-1 by transforming growth factor-β in human epithelial cells, *J. Biol. Chem.*, 275, 40904, 2000.

38. Durante, W., Peyton, K.J., and Schafer, A.I., Heme oxygenase-1 is an autocrine inhibitor of vascular smooth muscle cell growth, *Circulation*, 102, II-298, 2000.

39. Lavrovsky, Y. et al., Identification of binding-sites for transcription factors NF-κB and AP-2 in the promoter region of the human heme oxygenase-1 gene, *Proc. Natl. Acad. Sci. U.S.A.*, 91, 5987, 1994.

40. Sen, C.K. and Packer, L., Antioxidant and redox regulation of gene transcription, *FASEB J.*, 10, 709, 1996.

41. Elledge, S.J., Cell cycle checkpoints: preventing an identity crisis, *Science*, 274, 1664, 1996.

42. Sherr, C.J., G_1 phase progression: cycling on cue, *Cell*, 79, 551, 1994.

43. Stillman, B., Smart machines and the DNA replication fork, *Cell*, 78, 725, 1994.

44. Weinberg, R.A., The retinoblastoma protein and cell cycle control, *Cell*, 81, 323, 1995.

45. DeGregori, J., Kowalik, T., and Nevins, J.R., Cellular targets for activation by E2F1 transcription factor include DNA synthesis- and G1/S-regulatory genes, *Mol. Cell Biol.*, 15, 4215, 1995.

46. King, R.W., Jackson, P.K., and Kirschner, M.W., Mitosis in transition, *Cell*, 79, 563, 1994.

47. King, R.W. et al., How proteolysis drives the cell cycle, *Science*, 274, 1652, 1996.

48. Pines, J., Cyclin-dependent kinase inhibitors: the age of crystals, *Biochem, Biophys. Acta*, 1332, M39, 1997.
49. el-Diery, W.S. et al., WAF1, a potential mediator of p53 tumor suppression, *Cell*, 75, 817, 1993.
50. Levine, A.J., p53, the cellular gatekeeper for growth and division, *Cell*, 88, 323, 1997.
51. Lowe, S.M. et al., p53 is required for radiation-induced apoptosis in mouse thymocytes, *Nature*, 362, 847, 1993.
52. Smith, R.C. et al., p21CIP-mediated inhibition of cell proliferation by overexpression of the GAX homeodomain gene, *Gene Dev.*, 11, 1674, 1997.
53. Schwartz, S.M., Heimark, R.L., and Majesky, M.W., Developmental mechanisms underlying pathology of arteries, *Physiol. Rev.*, 70, 1177, 1990.
54. Ferns, G.A.A. and Avades, T.J., The mechanisms of coronary stenosis: insights from experimental models, *Int. J. Exp. Pathol.* 81, 63, 2000.
55. Chapman, G.B. et al., Physiological cyclic stretch causes cell cycle arrest in cultured vascular smooth muscle cells, *Am. J. Physiol.*, 278, H748, 2000.
56. Morita, T. et al., Carbon monoxide controls the proliferation of hypoxic vascular smooth muscle cells, *J. Biol. Chem.*, 272, 32804, 1997.
57. Togane, Y. et al., Protective roles of endogenous carbon monoxide in neointimal development elicited by arterial injury, *Am. J. Physiol.*, 278, H623, 2000.
58. Duckers, H.J. et al., Protective properties of recombinant heme oxygenase 1 *in vitro* and *in vivo* in the balloon injured porcine artery, *Circulation*, 98, I-739, 1998.
59. Duckers, H.J. et al., Heme oxygenase 1 protects against vascular constriction and proliferation, *Nat. Med.*, 7, 693, 2001.
60. Petrache, I. et al., Heme oxygenase-1 inhibits TNF-α-induced apoptosis in cultured fibroblasts, *Am. J. Physiol.*, 278, L312, 2000.
61. Brouard, S. et al., Carbon monoxide generated by heme oxygenase 1 suppresses endothelial apoptosis, *J. Exp. Med.*, 192, 1015, 2000.
62. Brune, B., Schmidt, K.-U., and Ullrich, V., Activation of soluble guanylate cyclase by carbon monoxide and inhibition by superoxide anion, *Eur. J. Biochem.*, 192, 683, 1990.
63. Stone, J.R. and Marletta, M.A., Soluble guanylate cyclase from bovine lung: activation with nitric oxide and carbon monoxide and spectral characterization of the ferrous and ferric states, *Biochemistry*, 33, 5635, 1994.
64. Ramos, K.S., Lin, H., and McGrath, J.J., Modulation of cyclic guanosine monophosphate levels in cultured aortic smooth muscle cells by carbon monoxide, *Biochem. Pharmacol.*, 38, 1368, 1989.
65. Fukumoto, S. et al., Distinct role of cAMP and cGMP in the cell cycle control of vascular smooth muscle cells: cGMP delays cell cycle transition through suppression of cyclin D1 and cyclin-dependent kinase 4 activation, *Circ. Res.*, 85, 985, 1999.
66. Kronemann, N. et al., Growth-inhibitory effect of cyclic GMP- and cyclic AMP-dependent vasodilators on rat vascular smooth muscle cells: effect on cell cycle and cyclin expression, *Br. J. Pharmacol.*, 126, 349, 1999.
67. Suenobu, N. et al., Natriuretic peptides and nitric oxide induce endothelial apoptosis via a cGMP-dependent mechanism, *Arterioscler. Thromb. Vasc. Biol.*, 19, 140, 1999.
68. Morita, T. and Kourembanas, S., Endothelial cell expression of vasoconstrictors and growth factors is regulated by smooth muscle cell-derived carbon monoxide, *J. Clin. Invest.*, 96, 2676, 1995.
69. Kourembanas, S. et al., Nitric oxide regulates the expression of vasoconstrictors and growth factors by vascular endothelium under both normoxia and hypoxia, *J. Clin. Invest.*, 92, 99, 1993.

70. Ross, R., Raines, E.W., and Bowen–Pope, D.F., The biology of platelet-derived growth factor, *Cell*, 46, 155, 1986.
71. Assoian, R.K. et al., Cellular transformation by coordinate action of three peptide growth factors from human platelets, *Nature*, 309, 804, 1984.
72. Brune, B. and Ullrich, V., Inhibition of platelet aggregation by carbon monoxide is mediated by the activation of guanylate cyclase, *Mol. Pharmacol.*, 32, 497, 1987.
73. Mansouri, A. and Perry, C.A., Alteration of platelet aggregation by cigarrette smoke and carbon monoxide, *Thromb. Haemost.* 48, 286, 1982.
74. Deramaudt, B.M.J.M. et al., Gene transfer of human heme oxygenase into coronary endothelial cells potentially promotes angiogenesis, *J. Cell. Biochem.*, 68, 121, 1998.
75. Belle, E.V. et al., Endothelial regrowth after arterial injury: from vascular repair to therapeutics, *Cardiovasc. Res.*, 38, 54, 1998.
76. Cliff, W.J., The aortic tunica media in aging rats, *Exp. Mol. Pathol.*, 13, 172, 1970.
77. Thomas, W.A. et al., Population dynamics of arterial smooth muscle cells. V. Cell proliferation and cell death during initial three months in atherosclerotic lesions induced in swine by hypercholestrolemic diet and intimal trauma, *Exp. Mol. Pathol.*, 24, 360, 1976.
78. Kerr, J.F., Wyllie, A.H., and Currie, A.R., Apoptosis, a basic biological phenomenon with wide-ranging implications in tissue kinetics, *Br. J. Cancer*, 26, 239, 1972.
79. Allen, R.T., Hunter, W.J., III, and Agrawal, D.K., Morphological and biochemical characterization and analysis of apoptosis, *J. Pharmacol. Toxicol. Methods*, 37, 215, 1997.
80. Bennett, M.R., Evan, G.I., and Schwartz, S.M., Apoptosis of human vascular smooth muscle cells derived from normal vessels and coronary atherosclerotic plaques, *J. Clin. Invest.*, 95, 2266, 1995.
81. Geng, J.Y. and Libby, P., Evidence for apoptosis in advanced human atheroma: colocalization with interleukin-1β converting enzyme, *Am. J. Pathol.*, 147, 251, 1995.
82. Isner, J.M. et al., Apoptosis in human atherosclerosis and restenosis, *Circulation*, 91, 2703, 1995.
83. DeBlois, D. et al., Smooth muscle apoptosis during vascular regression in spontaneously hypertensive rats, *Hypertension*, 29, 340, 1997.
84. Ashkenazi, A. and Dixit, V.M., Death receptors: signaling and modulation, *Science*, 281, 1305, 1998.
85. Kroemer, G., The protooncogene Bcl-2 and its role in regulating apoptosis, *Nat. Med.*, 3, 614, 1997.
86. Zou, H. et al., Apaf-1, a human protein homologous to C-elegans CED-4, participates in cytochrome c-dependent activation of caspase-3, *Cell*, 90, 405, 1997.
87. Miyashita, T. and Reed, J.C., Tumor suppressor p53 is a direct transcriptional regulator of the human BAX gene, *Cell*, 80, 293, 1995.
88. Haldar, S. et al., Downregulation of bcl-2 by p53 in breast cancer cells, *Cancer Res.*, 54, 2095, 1994.
89. Bennett, M. et al., Cell surface trafficking of Fas: a rapid mechanism of p53-mediated apoptosis, *Science*, 282, 290, 1998.
90. Li, H. et al., Cleavage of BID by caspase-8 mediates the mitochondrial damage in the Fas pathway of apoptosis, *Cell*, 94, 491, 1998.
91. Mallat, Z. and Tedgui, A., Apoptosis in the vasculature: mechanisms and functional importance, *Br. J. Pharmacol.*, 130, 947, 2000.
92. Geng, Y.J. et al., Apoptosis of vascular smooth muscle cells induced by *in vitro* stimulation with interferon-γ, tumor necrosis factor-α, and interleukin-1β, *Arterioscler. Thromb. Vasc. Biol.*, 16, 19, 1996.

93. Joringe, S. et al., DNA fragmentation and ultrastructural changes of degenerating cells in atherosclerotic lesions and smooth muscle cells exposed to oxidized LDL, *Arterioscler. Thromb. Vasc. Biol.*, 17, 2225, 1997.

94. Bennett, M.R., Evan, G.I., and Newby, A.C., Deregulated expression of the c-*myc* oncogene abolishes inhibition of proliferation of rat vascular smooth muscle cells by serum reduction, interferon-γ, heparin, and cyclic nucleotide analogues and induces apoptosis, *Circ. Res.*, 74, 525, 1994.

95. Pollman, M.J., Hall, J.L., and Gibbons, G.H., Determinants of vascular smooth muscle cell apoptosis after balloon angioplasty injury, influence of redox state and cell phenotype, *Circ. Res.*, 84, 113, 1999.

96. Fox, J.C. and Shanley, J.R., Antisense inhibition of basic fibroblast growth factor induces apoptosis in vascular smooth muscle cells, *J. Biol. Chem.*, 271, 12578, 1996.

97. Pollman, M. et al., Vasoactive substances regulate vascular smooth muscle cell responses: countervailing influences of nitric oxide and angiotensin II, *Circ. Res.*, 79, 748, 1996.

98. Kim, Y.-M., Bombeck, C.A., and Billiar, T.R., Nitric oxide as a bifunctional regulator of apoptosis, *Circ. Res.*, 84, 253, 1999.

99. Juan, S.-H. and Chau, L.-Y., Induction of apoptosis in vascular smooth muscle cells by heme oxygenase-1-derived carbon monoxide, *Acta Haematol.*, 103 (Suppl. 1), 70, 2000.

100. Liu, X.-M., Chapman, G.B., and Durante, W., Carbon monoxide inhibits apoptosis in vascular smooth muscle and endothelium, *FASEB J.*, 15, 773a, 2001.

101. Hancock, W.W. et al., Antibody-induced transplant arteriosclerosis is prevented by graft expression of antioxidant and anti-apoptotic genes, *Nat. Med.*, 4, 1392, 1998.

102. Thom, S.R. et al., Adaptive responses and apoptosis in endothelial cells exposed to carbon monoxide, *Proc. Natl. Acad. Sci. U.S.A.*, 97, 1305, 2000.

103. Nemoto, S. et al., Induction of apoptosis by SB202190 through inhibition of p38-beta mitogen-activated protein kinase, *J. Biol. Chem.*, 273, 16415, 1998.

104. Aizawa, T. et al., Balloon injury does not induce heme oxygenase-1 expression, but administration of hemin inhibits neointima formation in balloon-injured rat carotid artery, *Biochem, Biophys. Res. Commun.*, 261, 302, 1999.

105. Tulis, D.A. et al., Heme oxygenase-1 attenuates vascular remodeling following balloon injury in rat carotid arteries, *Atherosclerosis*, 155, 113, 2001.

106. Otterbein, L.E. et al., Carbon monoxide has antiinflammatory effects involving the mitogen-activated protein kinase pathway, *Nat. Med.*, 6, 422, 2000.

107. Sasu, S. and Beasley, D., Essential roles of I-kappa-B kinases alpha and beta in serum and IL-1-induced human VSMCs proliferation, *Am. J. Physiol.*, 27, H1823, 2000.

108. Tulis, D.A. et al., YC-1, a benzyl indazole derivative, stimulates vascular cGMP and inhibits neointima formation, *Biochem. Biophys. Res. Commun.*, 279, 646, 2000.

109. Friebe, A., Schultz, G., and Koesling, D., Sensitizing soluble guanylate cyclase to become a highly CO-sensitive enzyme, *EMBO J.*, 15, 6863, 1996.

110. Gong, K.-W. et al., Effect of reactive oxygen species on intimal proliferation in rat aorta after arterial injury, *J. Vasc. Res.*, 33, 42, 1996.

111. Llesuy, S.F. and Tomaro, M.L., Heme oxygenase and oxidative stress: evidence of involvement of bilirubin as a physiologic protector against oxidative damage, *Biochim. Biophys. Acta*, 1223, 9, 1994.

112. Stocker, R.Y. et al., Bilirubin is an antioxidant of possible physiological importance, *Science*, 235, 1043, 1987.

113. Neuzil, J. and Stocker, R., Free and albumin-bound bilirubin are efficient co-antioxidants for alpha-tocopherol, inhibiting plasma and low density lipoprotein lipid peroxidation, *J. Biol. Chem.*, 269, 16712, 1994.

114. Ishikawa, K. et al., Heme oxygenase-1 inhibits atherosclerotic lesion formation in LDL receptor knockout mice, *Circulation*, 96, I-111, 1997.

115. Juan, S.-H. et al., Overexpression of HO-1 reduces iron overload in vascular smooth muscle cells *in vitro* and lesion formation in apoE-deficient mice, *Acta Haematol.*, 103 (Suppl. 1), 70, 2000.

116. Seki, T. et al., Roles of heme oxygenase carbon monoxide system in genetically hypertensive rats, *Biochem. Biophys. Res. Commun.*, 241, 574, 1997.

117. Carraway, M.S. et al., CO remodels pulmonary vessels in hypoxia, *Acta Haematol.*, 103 (Suppl. 1), 66, 2000.

4 Signal Transduction Pathways Involved in CO-Induced Vasodilation: The Role of Cyclic GMP/Soluble Guanylyl Cyclase

Kanji Nakatsu, James F. Brien,
Brian E. McLaughlin, and Gerald S. Marks

CONTENTS

0-8493-1041-5/02/$0.00+$1.50
© 2002 by CRC Press LLC

I. INTRODUCTION

It would be an understatement to say that the concept that CO derived from heme via heme oxygenase plays a physiological role in regulating vascular resistance, by virtue of its ability to inhibit the mechanical activities of various blood vessels, has been contentious since its articulation a decade ago.[1] Nevertheless, this mechanical inhibitory action has been documented in many different blood vessels in several species. The purpose of this chapter is to address the potential mechanisms by which CO brings about relaxation in vascular smooth muscle. It should come as no surprise that the actions of CO have been proposed to parallel those of NO; our initial report emphasized the many similarities between CO and NO: small molecular size, volatility, effect on blood vessels, and activation of soluble guanylyl cyclase (sGC).

The mechanisms underlying this vasorelaxant effect of CO may involve one or a combination of synthesis of cyclic nucleotides, extrusion of Ca^{++}, and activation of K^+ channels. As the effects of CO on K^+ channels are the topic of Chapter 5, the focus here will be on the sGC/cGMP axis with a brief comment on Ca^{++} disposition. The hypothesis addressed in this chapter may be stated as: *CO-induced relaxation of blood vessels is mediated by enhanced production of cGMP content.* It should be noted that some of the papers reviewed in this chapter refer to experiments on CO conducted in the context of issues other than its use as a physiological vasoregulator.

Sutherland, Robison, and Butcher,[2] in their elegant work on establishing a second messenger role for cAMP in hormone action, articulated a number of criteria to be fulfilled. These were adapted in a review considering the role of cGMP in smooth muscle relaxation[3] and can be restated as follows:

1. CO must be capable of stimulating the activity of sGC (or inhibiting the activity of cGMP phosphodiesterase) in broken cell preparations of appropriate blood vessels.
2. CO-induced relaxation of the blood vessels should be accompanied by increased tissue content of cGMP in an appropriate temporal and dose- (or concentration-) related basis.
3. Drugs that alter the activity of sGC in response to CO should also alter CO-induced blood vessel relaxation in a similar manner.

One of the earliest reports suggesting a role for sGC/cGMP as a mediator of the effects of CO was performed in platelets rather than vascular tissue. Brune and Ullrich[4] tested the functional effect of CO on platelets as well as its effect on cyclic nucleotides. Blood obtained from human volunteers was used to prepare platelet rich plasma (PRP). CO bubbled through the PRP for 15 to 30 sec completely inhibited serotonin-induced platelet aggregation. In the presence of a phosphodiesterase inhibitor, isobutylmethyl xanthine (IBMX), CO gassing of PRP induced an increase in cGMP to $143 \pm 10\%$ of control values, whereas no change was noted in the content of cAMP. These investigators also tested the effect of CO gassing on sGC activity of the $10,000 \times g$ platelet supernatant. In comparison to gassing with nitrogen, CO resulted in an increase in activity of sGC to 402%. These observations are consistent with the view that inhibition of platelet aggregation induced by CO is mediated via an elevation of intracellular cGMP content.

II. EFFECT OF CO ON CGMP CONTENT

A. ISOLATED BLOOD VESSEL PREPARATIONS

Several laboratories conducted experiments using isolated vascular preparations to examine the effect of CO on mechanical activity and cGMP. For example, Graser, Vedernikov, and Li[5] examined the relaxation of porcine left descending coronary artery and coronary anterior interventricular vein in response to CO exposure. Rings of these blood vessels were prepared without endothelium for tension measurements during superfusion with a physiological salt solution; the vessels were precontracted by addition of $PGF_{2\alpha}$. Repeated exposure to 300 ng CO resulted in a sharp decrease in the tension of the rings: 41.1% for the artery and 67.0% for the vein. The addition of 10 μM methylene blue, an inhibitor of sGC, resulted in a substantial decrease in the rate and extent of the relaxation induced by CO. This concentration of methylene blue had an effect in the absence of CO as it produced an increase in tension of the arterial and venous rings by 25.1% and 29.9%, respectively.

As suggested by the authors, these observations indicate that CO-evoked relaxation might be due to sGC activation. Their observations with 8-bromoguanosine-3′,5′-cyclic monophosphate (8-Br cGMP) are not as supportive of this concept. Thus, exposure of tissues precontracted with $PGF_{2\alpha}$, to 10 μM 8-Br cGMP resulted in a relaxation of the arterial and venous rings of 12.0 ± 5.9 and 25.2 ± 2.8%, respectively. The presence of 8-Br cGMP had a modest antagonistic effect on the CO-evoked relaxation of the vein, reducing it to 65.8 ± 2.9% of that observed in the absence of 8-Br cGMP; there was no effect on the artery.

Since 8-Br cGMP is used as a more membrane-permeant analog of cGMP, one might have expected full relaxation of the vascular rings to be induced at a concentration of 10 μM if this analog entered the smooth muscle cells efficiently. On the other hand, one might postulate that 8-Br cGMP entered the cells but was only a partial agonist at the target cGMP kinases. If this were so, then 8-Br cGMP would be anticipated to block relaxation of vascular smooth muscle elicited by increased cGMP levels. These observations do not illuminate the physiological role of cGMP in porcine coronary vessels.

In comparison, Furchgott and Jothianandan,[6] who studied the effects of CO on rabbit aortic rings without endothelium precontracted with phenylephrine, are consistent in their support of cGMP mediation of CO-induced vascular relaxation. In the rabbit aorta, the ED_{50} value observed was 20 to 40 μM CO; in dog coronary artery, similar observations were made with an ED_{50} value of approximately 12 μM CO. With respect to the effects of CO on cGMP content in the rabbit aorta, they observed that 100 μM CO elevated cGMP by about 50% after 30 sec from a basal value of approximately 60 pmol/g protein. In comparison, the content of this cyclic nucleotide in the presence of 20 nM NO was more than 15 times greater, namely, 1580 pmol/g protein. These observations led the authors to suggest that CO was like NO in activating sGC by combining with the heme moiety of the enzyme; the smaller magnitude of the CO effect was attributed to the likelihood "that its affinity and/or efficacy are much less than those of NO."

Heterogeneity in CO-induced vascular responses was observed by Brian, Heistad, and Faraci[7] in their experiments on rabbit and dog cerebral arteries and rabbit aorta. NO, ACh, and nitroprusside all induced relaxation with EC_{50} values in the range 0.1 to 1 μM in the rabbit basilar artery. In contrast, CO was unable to evoke relaxation at concentrations exceeding 100 μM. Similar observations were made in the rabbit and dog cerebral arteries.

In contrast to this absence of CO responsiveness of blood vessels in the brain, these researchers found that the rabbit aorta was relaxed by exposure to CO, which is in agreement with our previous observations.[8] These authors considered the possibility that the heterogeneity of sGC in these different arteries might account for this heterogeneity in responsiveness to CO, but observed that all these blood vessels responded to NO and to sodium nitroprusside, an NO prodrug. As an alternative, it was suggested that the effects of CO might be mediated by a cGMP-independent mechanism in responsive blood vessels.

Jing et al.[9] reported on the effects of CO on rat aortic rings without endothelium in the context of their studies on the effects of halothane and enflurane. Thoracic aortic rings were prepared as conventional isolated preparations with isometric recording. In norepinephrine-precontracted rings, dose–response curves for CO-induced relaxations were obtained in the presence of two concentrations each of halothane and enflurane. Both anesthetics decreased the sensitivity and maximum response elicited by CO. The highest concentration of CO used (176 μM) relaxed the aortic rings by 85% of the norepinephrine-induced contraction.

This concentration of CO elevated tissue cGMP content from 4.2 to 7.9 pmol/mg protein. IBMX (1 mM) was added to Krebs' solution and the tissues were not under tension for the cGMP experiments. No phosphodiesterase inhibitor was added to the Krebs' solution for the vascular relaxation experiments. The authors discussed their results primarily in the context of the ability of halothane and enflurane to interfere with CO-induced vascular relaxation, using the CO/GC model of vascular relaxation. They interpreted their results in terms of the potential direct inhibition of sGC by these anesthetic agents and the possibility that the agents might generate an active metabolite which would then interfere with cGMP generation via sGC. They concluded that the weight of their observations came down on the side of a direct interaction of halothane and enflurane with sGC. On the other hand, it should be noted that not all of their data are consistent with the CO/GC relaxation model; the combination of the highest concentrations of halothane and CO resulted in a decrease in tissue cGMP, and apparently a small amount of tissue relaxation. On the basis of the cGMP content, one might have anticipated either no relaxation or a modest contraction. Unfortunately, the authors did not report a statistical analysis of the questions.

Studies conducted in the authors' laboratory exploited an sGC inhibitor 1H-[1,2,4]oxadiazolo[4,3-a]quinoxalin-1-one (ODQ) in an attempt to determine the role of the cGMP axis in CO-, NO-, and GTN-induced vascular relaxation.[10] Rabbit aortic rings without endothelium were mounted in organ baths for monitoring of isometric tension. CO, NO, and GTN all produced dose-related relaxations of the phenylephrine-precontracted rings. In the case of NO, the presence of ODQ at a concentration of 10 μM resulted in substantial blunting of the relaxation response as evidenced by the shift in the dose–response curve. This concentration of ODQ completely eliminated the relaxation response to a dose of CO that induced a 50%

relaxation in the absence of the sGC inhibitor. This greater effectiveness of ODQ against CO-induced relaxation compared with that induced by NO suggests that the CO effect in rabbit aorta is mediated by the sGC/cGMP axis, whereas the NO effect is only partially due to cGMP.

Coceani et al.[11] suggested that in the ductus arteriosus obtained from near-term fetal lambs, the inhibitory effect of CO is due to its interaction with a cytochrome P450. Accordingly, CO completely relaxed isolated ductus vessels and ductus smooth muscle. This relaxation was reversed by illumination with monochromatic light, with the maximally effective wavelength for photoactivated contraction occurring at 450 nm. This laboratory has conducted a more focused study on the potential role of cGMP in ductus relaxation.[12] They confirmed the almost total relaxation of lamb ductus arteriosus strips upon exposure to CO and an increase in tissue cGMP content. In the presence of the sGC inhibitors, methylene blue and LY-83583, they observed a smaller relaxation effect which was not correlated significantly with the tissue cGMP content. They concluded that the "primary action of CO in the ductus arteriosus is not exerted on the guanylyl cyclase heme and that cyclic GMP may only have an accessory role."

B. CULTURED VASCULAR CELLS

A number of laboratories investigated the effects of CO on vascular cells in culture. Ramos, Lin, and McGrath[13] investigated the effects of CO in primary cultures of smooth muscle cells prepared from the aortas of male Sprague–Dawley rats. These cells were grown in medium 199 supplemented with glutamine and fetal calf serum. Confluent cell cultures were exposed to 5% CO for 30 or 60 min in the presence of 50 mM IBMX; the cells were harvested and cGMP content was determined by radioimmunoassay. Under these conditions, the cGMP content of the cells increased by approximately 50% in 30 min and almost doubled in 60 min. These observations were viewed as consistent with the postulate that an increase in cGMP mediates CO-induced relaxation of vascular smooth muscle.

In a further example, Morita and Kourembanas[14] used a co-culture system to investigate the effects of CO derived from vascular smooth muscle cells on endothelial cells. The experimental procedure allowed these investigators to determine the influence of substances released by the smooth muscle cells on the metabolism of the endothelial cells. The durations of exposure to CO were much longer than in the intact tissue experiments described earlier. Human umbilical vein endothelial cells (HUVECs) were exposed to CO produced by rat aortic smooth muscle cells (under a hypoxic stimulus) for durations of 6, 12, 24, or 48 h. IBMX (1 mM) was added to the medium 20 min before the cells were harvested, and cGMP content was determined by radioimmunoassay for each time point. At the longer time points, cGMP levels tripled, compared with basal control conditions of approximately 1 pmol/mg protein. This elevation in cGMP was obtunded by inhibition of CO generation when a heme oxygenase inhibitor, tin protoporphyrin IX (SnPP), was added or when CO was sequestered by the addition of hemoglobin.

A remarkable feature of these studies was the observation of cGMP elevations maintained over long periods of time in contrast to other studies in which cGMP elevations were maintained for only short periods even in the continued presence of a relaxing agent; see, for example, Keith et al.[15]

In a related study by this laboratory, Morita et al.[16] demonstrated similar but larger elevation of cGMP content in cultured rat aortic smooth muscle cells. The peak elevation of cGMP was obtained after 12 h of hypoxic stimulation; this was maintained through 24 h and waned to near-basal values by 48 h. These observations were discussed in the context of the ability of CO to alter the expression of a number of genes, including those for endothelin-1, vascular endothelial growth factor, and heme oxygenase-1, which would, of course, alter the functioning of blood vessels with a duration of action measured in days.

Concurrently, in their studies on rat cell cultures, Christodoulides et al.[17] examined the effects of elevating heme oxygenase activity on the levels of cGMP in vascular smooth muscle cells and platelets. Conditions of CO production resulted in a modest elevation in cGMP content of vascular smooth muscle cells in the presence of hemin (an HO inducer), and a greater than three-fold increase in the presence of arsenite (also an HO inducer). Platelets were studied in co-culture and showed an elevation of cGMP of 23.6% with hemin and 111% with sodium arsenite. IBMX (100 μM) was added to the cells 45 min before harvesting. These investigators suggested the possibility that heme oxygenase/CO might function in the circulatory system by acting on platelets as well as on vascular smooth muscle.

Suematsu et al.[18] investigated the possibility that HO-derived CO may regulate vascular resistance in the rat isolated perfused liver. They found that liver vascular resistance more than doubled upon the addition of 1 μM zinc protoporphyrin (ZnPP) to the perfusion medium. This increase in resistance was blunted in the presence of either CO or 8Br cGMP. These observations were interpreted to support the idea that cGMP mediates the relaxant effect of CO on hepatic resistance vessels.

On the other hand, these authors point out that the concentration of CO required to induce an increase in the cGMP content of cultured Ito cells was 20 μM or at least 100-fold higher than that measured in the hepatic effluent. In addition, cGMP was determined in the presence of 0.5 mM IBMX. They thus suggested that the mechanism of CO-induced relaxation in the liver might be cGMP independent, and raised the possibility of CO action on K^+ channels. In a subsequent study, this laboratory[19] studied the mechanism of CO control of the bile canaliculi of cultured rat hepatocytes. Bile canaliculi contraction was observed using time lapse videography. At concentrations of CO (2 or 20 μM) that decreased bile canaliculi contractility, there was no change in the cGMP content of the hepatocytes. Thus, the control cGMP content was 0.36 ± 0.07 pmol/10^7 cells, and in the presence of 2 μM CO, it was 0.39 ± 0.07 pmol/10^7 cells; these experiments were conducted in the presence of IBMX. The positive control, 100 μM S-nitroso-N-acetylpenicillamine, produced a cGMP content of 3.04 ± 0.60 pmol/10^7 cells. Thus, these investigators considered that bile canalicular regulation by CO is "through a cGMP-independent mechanism."

In consideration of these observations, it seems likely that cGMP plays a significant role in mediating the CO-induced relaxation of at least some blood vessels. As the larger vessels appear to show the best correlations between relaxation and cGMP content, it may be that they represent one end of a spectrum of dependence on cGMP with other (smaller) blood vessels showing independence from cGMP representing the other end of the spectrum. It is unfortunate that some studies involved the use of phosphodiesterase inhibitors such as IBMX and others did not. Since vascular smooth muscle relaxation induced by CO does not require the presence of phosphodiesterase inhibitors, their use in cGMP determinations seems an unnecessary complicating variable.

III. POTENCY OF CO AND CO ENHANCERS

The concept that CO might have a physiological function has been criticized because of the much lower potency of CO as an inhibitor of vascular smooth muscle tone compared with NO. Thus, considerable interest was piqued by reports of a novel agent that enhanced the potency of CO so that it compared favorably with NO, at least in some systems. Much of the work on 3-(5′-hydroxymethyl-2′-furyl)-1-benzylindazole (YC-1) that caught the attention of the HO/CO community was performed in the Koesling laboratory. YC-1 is an activator of sGC that operates through a novel mechanism and enhances the effectiveness of CO as an sGC activator.[20]

In experiments conducted in our laboratory,[21] rat aortic spiral strips mounted for conventional isolated vascular smooth muscle tension monitoring demonstrated the ability of YC-1 to potentiate CO. After contraction with phenylephrine (PE), the inhibition of tone by various doses of CO was elicited in the absence and presence of a concentration of YC-1 that did not alone produce relaxation. YC-1 increased the potency of CO by approximately 10-fold, and increased the maximum relaxation obtained by the highest concentration of CO by 50%. In the same study, we determined the concentration of CO in the artificial bathing medium using gas chromatography on a molecular sieve column with detection by reduction of HgO (see Chapter 1). The measured concentrations of CO were less than half of the theoretical concentrations, indicating that most laboratories would have underestimated the potency of CO by a factor of two or more. These observations and the fact that some small blood vessels are much more sensitive to CO than the aorta raises an interesting question: whether an endogenous molecule sensitizes cells to CO and whether this molecule is distributed heterogeneously among blood vessels.

The history of pharmacologically active substances leads to the prediction that an endogenous enhancer of CO-induced relaxation will be discovered. This is based on analogies with examples such as morphine and the enkephalins. Morphine was used for centuries and much was learned about its receptors prior to the discovery of its endogenous ligands. Unfortunately, this hypothesis does not lend itself to clean experimental testing because any negative result can be countered with the argument that the appropriate endogenous substance has yet to be tested.

IV. EFFECT OF CO ON CGMP KINASE IN ISOLATED BLOOD VESSELS

Wang, Wang, and Wu[22] addressed the role of the cGMP axis in vascular smooth muscle relaxation of rat tail artery in comparison to effects mediated by actions at K$^+$ channels. These investigators observed CO-induced relaxations of helical strips of these arteries contracted with either PE or the prostaglandin analog, U-46619. They then used a series of pharmacological tools to determine the relative importance of cGMP signal transduction in comparison with K^+ channels. Charybdotoxin and apamin were used as K^+ channel blockers while R-8-bromoguanosine-3',5'-cyclic monophosphorothiolate (Rp-8-Br-cyclic GMPS) was used as a membrane permeable inhibitor of cGMP-dependent protein kinase. Rp-8-Br-cyclic GMPS at a concentration of 30 μM decreased the CO-induced relaxation by only one third. Even when Rp-8-Br-cyclic GMPS was used in the presence of the sGC inhibitor, methylene blue, the CO-induced relaxation was not further compromised. Apamin was found to have little effect while charybdotoxin was almost perfectly complementary with Rp-8-Br-cyclic GMPS in antagonizing CO-induced relaxation. These results indicate that big conductance K^+ channels that are inhibitable by charybdotoxin in rat tail artery mediate the majority of the CO effect, with cGMP accounting for the balance of its effect.

In studies on rat aorta, van der Zypp and Majewski[23] found that the concentration of Rp-8-Br-cyclic GMPS required to completely block glyceryl trinitrate-induced relaxation was 500 μM, with corresponding smaller antagonisms at 50 and 100 μM concentrations. This suggests that Wang, Wang, and Wu[22] might have observed complete inhibition of the CO-induced relaxation of the rat tail artery if they used high concentrations of the protein kinase inhibitor. This does not appear to be the case as they tested higher concentrations of Rp-8-Br-cyclic GMPS and found that the 100 μM concentration was not more effective in blocking CO-induced relaxation than the 30 μM concentration. Thus, it is unlikely that higher concentrations of Rp-8-Br-cyclic GMPS would support a greater role for cGMP in CO-induced relaxations of the rat tail artery.

V. ROLE OF CROSSTALK WITH OTHER CELL SIGNALING MECHANISMS

Durante et al.[24] raised the issue of crosstalk between cAMP and cGMP systems using their cultures of rat aortic smooth muscle cells described earlier. They addressed the possibility of crosstalk at the level of heme oxygenase induction. When these cells were treated with dibutyryl cAMP, forskolin, or isoproterenol, Durante et al. observed a significant increase in both HO-1 mRNA and HO-1 protein. As dibutyryl cAMP is used as a membrane permeant analog of cAMP, and forskolin and isoproterenol both activate adenylyl cyclase, these results indicate that cAMP mediates induction of HO-1.

Sammut et al.[25] investigated the possibility of crosstalk between NO and the HO/CO system in rat isolated aortic ring preparations with intact endothelium. It was found that a 1-hour exposure to the NO prodrug, S-nitroso-N-acetylpenicillamine (SNAP) at a concentration of 500 μM followed by 4 h of incubation in Krebs' solution resulted in an increase in the synthesis of both HO-1 mRNA and protein. This treatment almost obliterated the ability of phenylephrine to contract the aortic rings. When the SNAP stimulus was conducted in the presence of NOS inhibition with N^G-monomethyl-L-arginine (L-NMMA) or HO inhibition with SnPP (10 μM), only the latter allowed the return of the PE contraction. Thus, an NO agonist (SNAP) was able to induce an activation of the HO/CO system showing crosstalk between NO and CO in the rat thoracic aorta. These investigators observed that SNAP-treated aorta had a cGMP content 10-fold higher than baseline in the absence of such treatment; the effect on cGMP was blocked by SnPP (10 μM) but not by L-NMMA (100 μM). At the same time, a single 30-sec exposure to 1% CO gas resulted in a similar 10-fold increase in cGMP above the basal value of 1 fmol/mg tissue. The use of a phosphodiesterase inhibitor was not mentioned. The present results are consistent with a functional interaction between NO and CO, and with the mediation of these responses through elevations in tissue cGMP content.

VI. ROLE OF CA^{++} IN CO ACTIONS ON THE VASCULATURE

Smith and McGrath[26] had previously shown that CO relaxed vascular smooth muscle of the rat heart. In their 1988 study,[27] Lin and McGrath explored the effect of CO on vascular Ca^{++} content. Thoracic aortic rings obtained from Sprague–Dawley rats were immersed in calcium-free, Krebs'–Henseleit solution for 60 min. The aortic segments were then loaded with ^{45}Ca^{++} in the presence of 2.95 mM CaCl$_2$ and 39.2 mM KCl. Aeration was conducted in the presence or absence of 10% CO. After 1 h, Ca^{++} accumulation in the presence of CO (369 ± 18 nmol/g tissue) was 29% lower than in the controls (488 ± 35 nmol/g tissue). These results were interpreted as indicative of CO altering the disposition of Ca^{++}, and consequently inducing relaxation of vascular smooth muscles by decreasing their content of Ca^{++}.

VII. MECHANISM OF CO ACTIVATION OF SGC

One of the criteria described above for hypothesizing the involvement of sGC/cGMP in vascular relaxation was that the enzyme should be activated in broken cell preparations in the presence of CO. In the case of NO, there is a substantial history of documentation of this criterion and the involvement of heme therein, dating back to the early work of Craven and DeRubertis[28] and Ignarro et al.[29] Parallel logic dictates that sGC might also be acted upon by CO. Evidence for this may be found in the report of Brune, Schmidt, and Ullrich,[30] who observed CO activation of crude preparations of human platelet sGC.

Stone and Marletta[31] confirmed the ability of CO to interact with and activate sGC purified from bovine lung; sGC was purified using a multi-step chromatographic strategy which resulted in a greater than 2800-fold purification. The UV-visible spectrum of the enzyme in 5 mM dithiothreitol under air revealed a sharp Soret peak at 431 nm. In the presence of NO, the Soret peak shifted to 398 nm, and in the presence of CO, the Soret peak was observed at 423 nm. Such observations are indicative of interactions of both NO and CO with the heme moiety of sGC. Nevertheless, they noted differences in the ways in which NO and CO interacted with the heme. Their observations led them to conclude that NO breaks the axial bond between heme and imidazole, resulting in a five-coordinate ferrous-nitrosyl-heme complex. CO, on the other hand, participated in a six-coordinate complex in which CO and imidazole comprised the axial ligands. In addition, the extent of enzyme activation differed substantially in response to NO and CO. CO induced about a four-fold increase in activity from 221 to 966 nmol cGMP/min/mg protein, while NO induced a 127-fold increase in activity.

Similar observations were reported by Burstyn et al.,[32] who conducted studies on partially purified bovine lung sGC. They observed a Soret peak at 426 nm for the ferrous enzyme, which shifted to 420 nm upon exposure to CO. While NO markedly activated sGC, CO elicited only a modest increase in activity of no more than two-fold. In a subsequent report,[33] this laboratory compared the turnover values of CO–sGC obtained by their own and three other laboratories. The turnover levels were considered too low to result in a physiologically relevant increase in enzyme activity.

In further studies on bovine sGC, Kharitonov et al.[34] found that the dissociation rate constant of the sGC–CO complex was much higher than predicted for a six-coordinate structure. For sGC–CO, they calculated a rate constant of 28/sec which stands out in comparison with the rate constants reported for CO–myoglobin of 0.02/sec and for CO–horseradish peroxidase of 0.00007/sec. They suggest that a four-fold activation of sGC by CO could be accomplished if 1.5 to 3.0% of the CO–sGC was present as the five-coordinate complex in equilibrium with the six-coordinate species.

Recently, Sharma and Magde[35] reviewed the evolution of the model describing the interaction of NO and CO with sGC and its subsequent activation. Importantly, they raise caveats regarding the model in terms of the limitations of the spectroscopic and kinetic data as well as the sGC preparations. Many more studies must be undertaken before we truly comprehend the mechanism of action of CO as it applies to sGC activation *in vivo*.

A. ACTIVATION OF sGC BY YC-1

As discussed in Chapter 1, a major limitation to the acceptance of a physiological regulatory role for CO has been its lower potency to activate sGC in comparison with NO. The arrival of YC-1 as a pharmacological tool in the study of sGC has given considerable impetus to the consideration of CO as an important regulatory molecule in the vasculature. Since the early studies that identified YC-1 as an inhibitor of platelet aggregation capable of elevating cGMP content, several laboratories embarked on investigations of the interaction of YC-1 with sGC in the presence of CO.

Friebe, Schultz, and Koesling[20] demonstrated that YC-1 alone could activate bovine lung sGC with maximal activation of about 12-fold at 200 μM and at an EC_{50} of 20 μM. The observation that piqued our interest was the synergism between YC-1 and CO in the activation of sGC. The activity increased from a basal value of 64 nmol/min/mg in the absence of activators to 6840 nmol/min/mg in the presence of both CO and YC-1. This was the first demonstration of activation of sGC by CO that was equivalent to that of NO. Friebe et al. also suggested that the existence of an endogenous YC-1-like substance would provide the "molecular basis for a physiological role for CO in the regulation of sGC."

Wegener et al.[36] investigated the actions of YC-1 on rat aortic rings with endo-thelium present. YC-1 relaxed phenylephrine-induced contractions fully at concentrations in excess of 10 μM; this relaxation was antagonized by the addition of Rp-8-Br-cGMPS and enhanced in the presence of zaprinast, a phosphodiesterase inhibitor. In addition, 30 μM YC-1 tripled the cGMP content in these aortic rings, and this increase was blocked in the presence of 30 μM ODQ. The cGMP experiments were conducted in the presence of 100 μM IBMX. These observations are consistent with the idea that YC-1 alone induced relaxation of the aorta by activation of sGC. Freibe et al.[37] determined that the binding of YC-1 to sGC was independent of the heme moiety as YC-1 was able to activate sGC even after it had been stripped of heme by treatment with Tween 20®.

The mechanism by which YC-1 could enhance the ability of CO to activate sGC may involve alterations to the interaction of CO with the heme of sGC. Stone and Marletta[38] have shown that this was not the case, as YC-1 did not change the binding of CO to sGC; their spectroscopic studies did not reveal any differences in K_{on}, K_{off}, or K_d, where K_{on} and K_{off} are the on-rate and off-rate constants of CO for binding to sGC. In their studies on sGC expressed in a baculovirus/Sf9 system, Hoenicka et al.[39] also showed that CO and YC-1 together effected a large increase in enzyme activity; on the basis of spectroscopic studies, they concluded that YC-1 was an allosteric regulator of sGC.

In contrast, Friebe and Koesling[40] suggested that YC-1 dramatically decreases the rate of dissociation of CO from sGC. This was based on their observation that the addition of oxyHb during an sGC assay immediately blocked further formation of cGMP in the absence of YC-1; this would be consistent with oxyHb binding, and therefore inactivating, CO that dissociated quickly from sGC. Addition of oxyHb during the sGC assay in the presence of YC-1 only partially blocked further cGMP accumulation; this can be interpreted as indicative that YC-1 slows the dissociation of CO from sGC.

This apparent discrepancy in the conclusions reached by these two laboratories may be resolvable on consideration of the methods used to address this question. Thus, it may be possible that CO dissociates unimpaired and quickly from the inactive six-coordinate sGC, which would result in the spectroscopic observation. The effect of YC-1 on the less abundant, but active, pentacoordinate form of sGC might be observable only in functional enzyme assays. Further reports from the Koesling laboratory[34] indicate that YC-1 caused a major increase in the affinity of CO for sGC based on spectroscopic data; these investigators based their determination on the intensity of light absorption at the Soret band for sGC–CO (424 nm) and the change therein in the presence of YC-1 (420 nm). We look forward to further research reports that will reveal the details of the mechanism of YC-1 action.

As this chapter goes to press, we are not aware of any reports on the existence of an endogenous YC-1-like factor. Schmidt et al.[41] may have discovered an explanation for the discrepancy between the large increase in cGMP content of intact cells upon stimulation with NO plus YC-1 and the more moderate activation of sGC. They observed that the addition of endothelial homogenate to purified sGC activated with a combination of NO (contributed by diethylamine NO, DEA/NO) and YC-1 resulted in further increases in cGMP production. The putative sGC activator was destroyed by boiling, which was interpreted as indicative of a YC-1-like cooperative sGC binding protein or a metabolite of YC-1 generated by a heat-labile component of the homogenate.

VIII. LIMITATIONS OF DRUGS USED FOR INVESTIGATIONS OF CO ACTION

The bane of pharmacologists is the insufficient specificity of the tools of the trade — in this case, the drugs used in studies on sGC and CO. Unfortunately, YC-1 is not an exception. For example, Galle et al.[42] reported the inhibition of phosphodiesterase (PDE) activity by YC-1. PDE1 (Ca^{++}/calmodulin-dependent), PDE2 (cGMP-stimulated), PDE4 (cAMP-specific), PDE3 (cGMP-inhibited), and PDE5 (cGMP-specific) were derived from bovine brain, rat heart, human polymorphonuclear neutrophils (PMNs), and human platelets (both PDE3 and PDE5), respectively. All five isozymes were fully inhibited in the presence of 100 μM YC-1. PDE4 and PDE5 appeared somewhat more sensitive to YC-1 inhibition with ID_{50} values less than 10 μM.

Two papers recently documented an effect of YC-1 on K^+ channels that appears to be independent of cGMP. Wu et al.[43] reported that in rat pituitary lactotrophs, YC-1 inhibited the Ca^{++}-activated K^+ current as well as the voltage-dependent K^+ current. In the case of the former, YC-1 appeared to increase the probability of K^+-channel opening at a concentration of 10 μM. For the latter, the IC_{50} was 1 μM. Seitz et al.[44] found that the relaxant effect of YC-1 on rat aorta was attenuated by high conductance K_{Ca} channel blocking agents, tetraethylammonium, charybdotoxin, and iberiotoxin, but not by the K_{ATP} channel blocking agent, glibenclamide. These studies did not address the combined effect of YC-1 and CO on K^+ channels; these experiments should be undertaken. In summary, YC-1 has provided the stimulus for much excellent and relevant research, but there is a great need to find successor molecules that possess the key property of greater selectivity.

IX. SUMMARY

To conclude this chapter, it is instructive to return to the criteria articulated several pages earlier: (1) CO has been demonstrated to stimulate the activity of sGC in broken cell preparations of blood vessels that are relaxed by CO; (2) in many blood vessels, CO-induced relaxation is accompanied by increases in cGMP content; and (3) drugs that alter sGC also alter CO-induced relaxation of certain blood vessels. The weight of currently available evidence is consistent with a functional role for CO acting through the sGC/cGMP axis in at least some blood vessels, especially larger vessels. While this concept is subject to criticism on the basis of the relatively low potency of CO compared with NO in many vascular preparations, the advent of YC-1 has resulted in broader consideration of CO-induced regulation of vascular tone through mediation with cGMP.

On the other hand, serious consideration of a regulatory role for CO does not rest on the existence of an endogenous YC-1-like molecule because Nasjletti[45] and Leffler et al.[46] reported the vasodilatory effects of CO on small blood vessels at very low concentrations (see Chapter 1). There has been great interest in the mechanisms by which YC-1 alters the mechanical activity of vascular tissue, which resulted in identification of inhibitory activities of this drug on phosphodiesterases and K^+ channels. Historical precedent suggests that the present information will stimulate the development of more selective drugs as well as drugs that act on new target sites relevant to the hypothesis articulated at the beginning of this chapter: "CO-induced relaxation of blood vessels is mediated by enhanced production of cGMP content."

ACKNOWLEDGMENT

This work was supported by the Heart and Stroke Foundation of Ontario, Canada (Grant No. NA-4438).

REFERENCES

1. Marks, G.S. et al., Does carbon monoxide have a physiological function? *Trends Pharmacol. Sci.*, 12, 185, 1991.
2. Sutherland, E.W., Robison, G.A., and Butcher, R.W., Some aspects of the biological role of adenosine 3′,5′-monophosphate (cyclic AMP), *Circulation*, 37, 279, 1968.
3. Nakatsu, K. and Diamond, J., Role of cGMP in relaxation of vascular and other smooth muscle, *Can. J. Physiol. Pharmacol.*, 67, 251, 1989.
4. Brune, B. and Ullrich, V., Inhibition of platelet aggregation by carbon monoxide is mediated by activation of guanylate cyclase, *Mol. Pharmacol.*, 32, 497, 1987.
5. Graser, T., Vedernikov, Y.P., and Li, D.S., Study on the mechanism of carbon monoxide induced endothelium-independent relaxation in porcine coronary artery and vein, *Biomed. Biochim. Acta*, 49, 293, 1990.
6. Furchgott, R.F. and Jothianandan, D., Endothelium-dependent and -independent vasodilation involving cyclic GMP: relaxation induced by nitric oxide, carbon monoxide and light, *Blood Vessels*, 28, 52, 1991.
7. Brian, J.E., Jr., Heistad, D.D., and Faraci, F.M., Effect of carbon monoxide on rabbit cerebral arteries, *Stroke*, 25, 639, 1994.
8. Liu, Z. et al., Carbon monoxide does not inhibit glyceryl trinitrate biotransformation by or relaxation of aorta, *Eur. J. Pharmacol.*, 211, 129, 1992.
9. Jing, M. et al., Effects of halothane and isoflurane on carbon monoxide-induced relaxations in the rat aorta, *Anesthesiology*, 85, 347, 1996.
10. Hussain, A.S. et al., The soluble guanylyl cyclase inhibitor 1*H*-[1,2,4]oxadiazolo[4,3-*a*]quinoxalin-1-one (ODQ) inhibits relaxation of rabbit aortic rings induced by carbon monoxide, nitric oxide, and glyceryl trinitrate, *Can. J. Physiol. Pharmacol.*, 75, 1034, 1997.
11. Coceani, F. et al., Further evidence implicating a cytochrome P-450-mediated reaction in the contractile tension of the lamb ductus arteriosus, *Circ. Res.*, 62, 471, 1988.
12. Coceani, F., Kelsey, L., and Seidlitz, E., Carbon monoxide-induced relaxation of the ductus arteriosus in the lamb: evidence against the prime role of guanylyl cyclase, *Br. J. Pharmacol.*, 118, 1689, 1996.
13. Ramos, K.S., Lin, H., and McGrath, J.J., Modulation of cyclic guanosine monophosphate levels in cultured aortic smooth muscle cells by carbon monoxide, *Biochem. Pharmacol.*, 38, 1368, 1989.

14. Morita, T. and Kourembanas, S., Endothelial cell expression of vasoconstrictors and growth factors is regulated by smooth muscle cell-derived carbon monoxide, *J. Clin. Invest.*, 96, 2676, 1995.

15. Keith, R.A. et al., Vascular tolerance to nitroglycerin and cyclic GMP generation in rat aortic smooth muscle, *J. Pharmacol. Exp. Ther.*, 221, 525, 1982.

16. Morita, T. et al., Smooth muscle cell-derived carbon monoxide is a regulator of vascular cGMP, *Proc. Natl. Acad. Sci. U.S.A.*, 92, 1475, 1995.

17. Christodoulides, N. et al., Vascular smooth muscle cell heme oxygenases generate guanylyl cyclase-stimulatory carbon monoxide, *Circulation*, 91, 2306, 1995.

18. Suematsu, M. et al., Carbon monoxide: an endogenous modulator of sinusoidal tone in the perfused rat liver, *J. Clin. Invest.*, 96, 2431, 1995.

19. Shinoda, Y. et al., Carbon monoxide as a regulator of bile canalicular contractility in cultured rat hepatocytes, *Hepatology*, 28, 286, 1998.

20. Friebe, A., Schultz, G., and Koesling, D., Sensitizing soluble guanylyl cyclase to become a highly CO-sensitive enzyme, *EMBO J.*, 15, 6863, 1996.

21. McLaughlin, B.E. et al., Potentiation of carbon monoxide-induced relaxation of rat aorta by YC-1 [3-(5′-hydroxymethyl-2′-furyl)-1-benzylindazole], *Can. J. Physiol. Pharmacol.*, 78, 343, 2000.

22. Wang, R., Wang, A., and Wu, L., Carbon monoxide-induced vasorelaxation and the underlying mechanisms, *Br. J. Pharmacol.*, 121, 927, 1997.

23. van der Zypp, A., and Majewski, H., Effect of cGMP inhibitors on the actions of nitrodilators in rat aorta, *Clin. Exp. Pharmacol. Physiol.*, 25, 38, 1998.

24. Durante, W. et al., cAMP induces heme oxygenase-1 gene expression and carbon monoxide production in vascular smooth muscle, *Am. J. Physiol.*, 273, H317, 1997.

25. Sammut, I.A. et al., Carbon monoxide is a major contributor to the regulation of vascular tone in aortas expressing high levels of haeme oxygenase-1, *Br. J. Pharmacol.*, 125, 1437, 1998.

26. McGrath, J.J. and Smith, D.L., Response of rat coronary circulation to carbon monoxide and nitrogen hypoxia, *Exp. Biol. Med.*, 177, 132, 1984.

27. Lin, H. and McGrath, J.J., Carbon monoxide effects on calcium levels in vascular smooth muscle, *Life Sci.*, 43, 1813, 1988.

28. Craven, P.A. and DeRubertis, F.R., Requirement for heme in the activation of purified guanylate cyclase by nitric oxide, *Biochim. Biophys. Acta*, 745, 310, 1983.

29. Ignarro, L.J. et al., Activation of purified guanylate cyclase by nitric oxide requires heme. Comparison of heme-deficient, heme reconstituted and heme-containing forms of soluble enzyme from bovine lung, *Biochim. Biophys. Acta*, 718, 49, 1982.

30. Brune, B., Schmidt, K.U., and Ullrich, V., Activation of soluble guanylate cyclase by carbon monoxide and inhibition by superoxide anion, *Eur. J. Biochem.*, 192, 683, 1990.

31. Stone, J.R. and Marletta, M.A., Soluble guanylate cyclase from bovine lung: activation with nitric oxide and carbon monoxide and spectral characterization of the ferrous and ferric states, *Biochemistry*, 33, 5636, 1994.

32. Burstyn, J.N. et al., Studies of the heme coordination and ligand binding properties of soluble guanylyl cyclase (sGC): characterization of Fe(II)sGC and Fe(II)sGC(CO) by electronic absorption and magnetic circular dichroism spectroscopies and failure of CO to activate the enzyme, *Biochemistry*, 34, 5896, 1995.

33. Vogel, K.M. et al., Variable forms of soluble guanylyl cyclase: protein–ligand interactions and the issue of activation by carbon monoxide, *J. Biol. Inorg. Chem.*, 4, 804, 1999.

34. Kharitonov, V.G. et al., Basis of guanylate cyclase activation by carbon monoxide, *Proc. Natl. Acad. Sci. U.S.A.,* 92, 2568, 1995.

35. Sharma, V.S. and Magde, D., Activation of soluble guanylate cyclase by carbon monoxide and nitric oxide: a mechanistic model, *Methods,* 19, 494, 1999.

36. Wegener, J.W. et al., Activation of soluble guanylyl cyclase by YC-1 in aortic smooth muscle but not in ventricular myocardium from rat, *Br. J. Pharmacol.,* 122, 1523, 1997.

37. Friebe, A. et al., YC-1 potentiates nitric oxide- and carbon monoxide-induced cyclic GMP effects in human platelets, *Mol. Pharmacol.,* 54, 962, 1998.

38. Stone, J.R. and Marletta, M.A., Synergistic activation of soluble guanylate cyclase by YC-1 and carbon monoxide: implications for the role of cleavage of the iron–histidine bond during activation by nitric oxide, *Chem. Biol.,* 5, 255, 1998.

39. Hoenicka, M. et al., Purified soluble guanylyl cyclase expressed in a baculovirus/Sf9 system: stimulation by YC-1, nitric oxide, and carbon monoxide, *J. Mol. Med.,* 77, 14, 1999.

40. Friebe, A. and Koesling, D., Mechanism of YC-1-induced activation of soluble guanylyl cyclase, *Mol. Pharmacol.,* 53, 123, 1998.

41. Schmidt, K. et al., Molecular mechanisms involved in the synergistic activation of soluble guanylyl cyclase by YC-1 and nitric oxide in endothelial cells, *Mol. Pharmacol.,* 59, 220, 2001.

42. Galle, J. et al., Effects of the soluble guanylyl cyclase activator, YC-1, on vascular tone, cyclic GMP levels and phosphodiesterase activity, *Br. J. Pharmacol.,* 127, 195, 1999.

43. Wu, S.N. et al., The mechanism of actions of 3-(5'-hydroxymethyl-2'-furyl)-1-benzyl indazole (YC-1) on Ca^{2+}-activated K^+ currents in GH_3 lactotrophs, *Neuropharmacology,* 39, 1788, 2000.

44. Seitz, S. et al., Involvement of K^+ channels in the relaxant effects of YC-1 in vascular smooth muscle, *Eur. J. Pharmacol.,* 382, 11, 1999.

45. Nasjletti, A., Carbon monoxide of vascular origin is an inhibitory regulator of vasoconstrictor responsiveness to myogenic and hormonal stimuli, *Acta Haematol.,* 103, 68, 2000.

46. Leffler, C.W. et al., Carbon monoxide and cerebral microvascular tone in newborn pigs, *Am. J. Physiol.,* 276, H1641, 1999.

5 Carbon Monoxide, Vascular Contractility, and K⁺ Channels

Kun Cao and Rui Wang

CONTENTS

I. INTRODUCTION

Vascular contractility is closely related to the structural and functional integrity of K⁺ channels in vascular smooth muscle cells (SMCs). SMCs have a high input resistance. K⁺ efflux resulting from the activation of even a small number of K⁺ channels will hyperpolarize cell membrane, which in turn inhibits the agonist-induced increase in inositol triphosphate (IP_3), reduces Ca^{2+} sensitivity and resting

0-8493-1041-5/02/$0.00+$1.50

Ca^{2+} levels, inactivates voltage-dependent Ca^{2+} channels, and relaxes vascular SMCs.[1] Conversely, the closing of K^+ channels causes vasoconstriction by the depolarization of cell membrane.

K^+ channels are far more complex and versatile than any other types of ionic channels expressed in vascular SMCs, including Ca^{2+} channels, Na^+ channels, and Cl^- channels. At least four sub-families of K^+ channels have been identified in vascular SMCs: (1) K_V, voltage-dependent; (2) K_{ATP}, ATP-sensitive; (3) K_{Ca}, Ca^{2+}-activated; and (4) Kir, inward rectifier. A wide spectrum of K^+ channel distribution is found in different tissue preparations. The molecular compositions of K^+ channels also vary in a tissue-specific fashion. Now that the molecular bases of K^+ channels in many tissues, including brain and heart, have been extensively studied, we still do not know much about their sequence features, subunit expression patterns, multimeric assembly formats, and their structure–function relationships in vascular SMCs.

Interestingly, many recent studies have designated different types of K^+ channels as the molecular targets of carbon monoxide (CO). The direct or indirect modulation of K^+ channels in vascular SMCs constitutes an important mechanism for the vascular effect of CO. In this chapter, we briefly review the state-of-art knowledge about the molecular bases of various sub-families of K^+ channels, especially K_V, K_{Ca}, and K_{ATP} channels, in vascular SMCs. From this background, the modulation of K^+ channels by CO is described in detail.

II. ROLES OF VARIOUS K⁺ CHANNELS IN REGULATION OF THE FUNCTIONS OF VASCULAR SMCs

A. The Coupling of Membrane Potential Change to SMC Contraction — The Role of K_V Channels

K_V channels in vascular SMCs play a significant role in control of arterial diameter and vascular resistance[2] by setting the resting membrane potential and dampening cellular excitation. When the membrane potential of vascular SMCs is depolarized by increased sheer stress of blood vessel wall or by the surge of vasoconstrictors, K_V channels are activated to allow efflux of K^+ ions, which in turn hyperpolarizes membrane and maintains the resting membrane potential at –40 to –60 mV under physiological situations. The vascular tone is closely coupled to the membrane potential changes. A small change in membrane potential would induce a great alteration in the opening probability (Po) of K_V channels and therefore the contractile status of SMCs. K_V channels are also vital in the regulation of the hypoxia-induced depolarization of SMC membrane. The hypoxic pulmonary vasoconstriction involves the inhibition of K_V channels in the pulmonary vascular SMCs.[3] Incidental reports showed the involvement of K_V channels in action potential repolarization in electrically excitable smooth muscle tissues, such as portal veins.[4] SMCs in most resistance arteries, however, do not fire action potential and have stable resting membrane potentials under physiological conditions.

K_V channel currents have two major components, I_K and I_A. I_K is a slowly inactivating outward delayed rectifier that is activated at membrane potential more positive than −40 mV, present in almost all types of vascular SMCs. Within the physiological range of membrane potential and normal intracellular Ca^{2+} level, I_K represents the dominant repolarizing conductance.[5,6] The sensitivity of I_K to tetra-ethylammonium (TEA) varies according to different reports. I_K in vascular SMCs is sensitive to 4-aminopyridine (4-AP); but 4-AP-insensitive I_K current has been observed.[2,7] Interestingly, I_K in ventricular myocytes is only sensitive to TEA, not to 4-AP.[8-10] I_A, another major K_V current, activates and inactivates very rapidly and can be reversibly blocked by 4-AP, but is not sensitive to TEA. I_A co-exists with I_K in some types of vascular SMCs, including those from renal microvascular beds,[11] rat pulmonary artery and mesenteric artery,[12] rabbit pulmonary artery,[13] human mesenteric artery,[14] rabbit coronary artery,[15] portal vein,[4] and rabbit aorta.[16] The resting membrane potential in vascular SMCs is around −50 mV, at which more than half the I_A is inactivated. Moreover, the inactivation of I_A is too fast to exert significant stable influence on membrane potentials of vascular SMCs that do not normally generate action potentials. Therefore, the major function of I_A in vascular SMCs may be to act as a "brake" to counteract quickly any depolarizing influence[16] that may induce spontaneous action potential activity or oscillatory vasoconstriction under physiological or pathophysiological situations. I_A has not been detected in freshly isolated rat kidney resistance artery[17] or rat mesenteric artery.[18] Studies from our laboratory and others showed that the predominant K_V current in rat mesenteric artery SMCs[18,19] or tail artery SMCs is I_K.[20]

B. THE COUPLING OF INTRACELLULAR CALCIUM CHANGE TO SMC CONTRACTION — THE ROLE OF K_{CA} CHANNELS

Calcium-activated potassium (K_{Ca}) channels are expressed in many excitable and non-excitable cells and are functionally heterogeneous. Calcium influx resulting from the opening of voltage-dependant Ca^{2+} channels will increase intracellular calcium concentration. The increase will cause K_{Ca} channels to open. This process counteracts the membrane depolarization-induced vasoconstriction, leading to vasorelaxation.[21] K_{Ca} channels are divided into three groups according to their single-channel conductance with symmetrical $[K^+]$ across cell membranes: big-conductance (BK_{Ca}) (~250 pS), intermediate-conductance (IK_{Ca}) (20 to 80 pS) and small-conductance (SK_{Ca}) (10 to 15 pS) channels.[22] BK_{Ca} channels in vascular SMCs are blocked by micromolar ranges of external TEA and more specifically by nanomolar ranges of charybdotoxin (ChTX) and iberiotoxin (IbTX).[21] SK_{Ca} channels can generate long-lasting hyperpolarization or slow after-hyperpolarization (sAHP) after an action potential in most brain neurons.

Apamin is a selective SK_{Ca} channel blocker having an IC_{50} value of 0.3 nM. However, apamin-insensitive SK_{Ca} channels were also reported in hippocampal pyramidal neurons[23] and in neocortical neurons.[24] Apamin-sensitive SK_{Ca} channels are found in the brain and also in some porcine vascular beds, indicating their possible contributions to the maintenance of intrinsic vascular tone.[25,26] Human IK_{Ca}

channels were recently detected at high levels in lung, placenta, trachea and salivary gland, liver, bone marrow, and colon.[27] IK_{Ca} channels were also cloned from non-excitable human B and T lymphocytes, indicating the possible association of IK_{Ca} channels with immune reactions.[28,29] Nevertheless, IK_{Ca} channels are undetectable in excitable tissues, such as brain, heart muscle, and aortic smooth muscles.[27] IK_{Ca} channels can be blocked by ChTX ($IC_{50} = 28$ nM) and clotrimazole ($IC_{50} = 153$ nM), but not by apamin.[27]

BK_{Ca} channels sense the changes of both intracellular calcium concentrations and membrane potentials, whereas IK_{Ca} and SK_{Ca} channels are voltage-independent and gated only by cytoplasmic calcium. The expression of the α-subunit of BK_{Ca} channel alone yields Ca^{2+} independent current when the intracellular calcium concentration is lower than 100 nM, turning the channels into pure voltage-dependent pores.[30] The functional coupling of the BK_{Ca} β-subunit with the α-subunit greatly increases sensitivity to the cytoplasmic calcium and confers the inactivation properties of BK_{Ca} channels.[30-32]

Many endogenous vasoactive substances regulate K_{Ca} channel activities. Vaso-constrictors such as angiotensin II and a thromboxane A2 agonist (U46619) inhibit the channel opening.[33,34] The phosphorylation of the channel protein mediated by a cAMP-dependent protein kinase (PKA),[35] G protein coupled pathway,[36] or cGMP-dependent protein kinase (PKG)[37] also activates K_{Ca} channels in vascular smooth muscles.

Endothelium-derived hyperpolarizing factor (EDHF) is defined as a non-NO, non-prostaglandin substance released by acetylcholine (ACh) that induces smooth muscle hyperpolarization.[38,39] Although the candidacy of K^+ ion,[40] epoxyeicosa-trienoic acid (EET), or endocannabinoids[41] has been proposed, the real nature of EDHF has not yet been identified. EDHF-mediated vasorelaxation in many vascular beds is believed to occur through activating K^+ channels, especially K_{Ca} channels, as the EDHF effect can be abolished by ChTX[42] and by apamin[43] in rat mesenteric arteries. Recent studies have shown that a combination of ChTX and apamin (but not either one alone) can abolish the EDHF-induced vasorelaxation in guinea pig coronary, carotid, and basilar arteries.[40,44,45] However, whether this combination of ChTX and apamin targets a novel K_{Ca} channel subtype or multi-K_{Ca} channels in vascular SMCs needs to be further elucidated. The regulation mechanisms for K_{Ca} channels are summarized in Figure 5.1.

C. The Coupling of Cellular Metabolic Change to SMC Contraction — The Role of K_{ATP} Channels

K_{ATP} channels play an important role in cells like pancreatic β-cell,[46] cardiomyocytes,[47] skeletal muscle cells,[48] and vascular SMCs.[49,50] Single-channel conductance of K_{ATP} channels in vascular SMCs is about 20 to 50 pS with symmetric $[K^+]$ across cell membranes.[51] Large conductance K_{ATP} channels, however, were also reported.[50,52] The controversy over single-channel conductance may be caused by multiplicity of the isoforms of K_{ATP} channels and by varying experimental configurations.

Functionally, K_{ATP} channels coordinate the metabolism and electrical excitability of cells. Accumulating evidence has showed that K_{ATP} channels contribute to the

K_{Ca} Channels

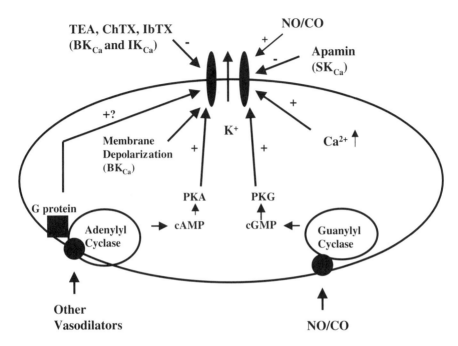

FIGURE 5.1 Modulation of the gating of K_{Ca} channels in vascular SMCs. Some vasodilators (such as adenosine) activate K_{Ca} channels through the G-protein-coupled adenylyl cyclase pathway, while nitric oxide and carbon monoxide activate K_{Ca} channels through the cGMP pathway or by directly acting on the channel protein.

maintenance of basal vascular tone in some vascular beds, including mesenteric arteries[53] and coronary arteries.[54] The vasodilation mediated by the opening of K_{ATP} channels can be abolished by glibenclamide (a K_{ATP} channel blocker), leading to vasoconstriction. K_{ATP} channels are regulated by intracellular ATP, ADP, or the ATP/ADP ratio, and by some vasoactive substances such as CGRP, adenosine,[55] or NO[56] (Figure 5.2). When binding to the pore-forming Kir6.x subunit, intracellular ATP inhibits the channel opening (ligand action). In contrast, when ATP is associated with SUR subunit of the K_{ATP} channel complex, it stimulates the channel.[57,58]

ADP and many other nucleoside diphosphates (NDPs), in the absence of Mg^{2+}, also inhibited the activity of K_{ATP} channels. In the presence of Mg^{2+}, the inhibitory effect of ADP reversed to a stimulatory effect on K_{ATP} channels.[59,60] The importance of K_{ATP} channels to the regulation of cellular functions can be exemplified in the case of hypoxia. Hypoxia or ischemia suppresses the cellular production of ATP, which may activate K_{ATP} channels. The consequent membrane hyperpolarization would relax blood vessels to increase the blood supply to the hypoxic cells. Thus, the balance of oxygen supply and demand may be restored.

K_{ATP} channels are inhibited by sulphonylurea drugs, such as glibenclamide and tolbutamide, with different sensitivities. The widely used K^+ channel openers

K$_{ATP}$ channels

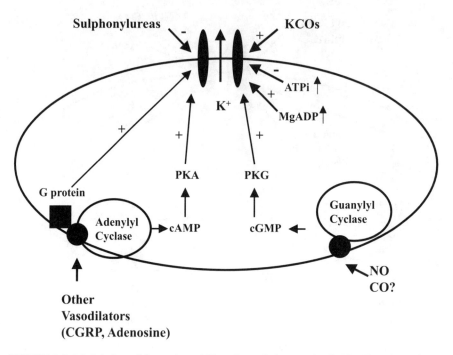

FIGURE 5.2 Modulation of the gating of K$_{ATP}$ channels in vascular SMCs. The channels are selectively inhibited by sulphonylureas such as glibenclamide and tolbutamide and opened by KCOs such as pinacidil, dizoxide, cromakalim, and nicorandil.

(KCOs), such as pinacidil, cromakalim, and nicorandil act to stimulate K$_{ATP}$ channels.[60,61] The pharmacological sensitivities of K$_{ATP}$ channels to different agents are largely determined by the molecular composition of the K$_{ATP}$ channel complex. K$_{ATP}$ channels reconstituted with Kir6.x and SUR1 subunits are far more sensitive to glibenclamide-related inhibition than the reconstituted Kir6.x/SUR2A channels. Biochemical data show that the SUR1 subunit binds glibenclamide with a dissociation constant (K_d) about 1 nM, whereas the SUR2A subunit has a K_d near 1.2 μM.[62]

On the other hand, Isomoto et al.[63] indicated that SUR2B is also a low-affinity SUR. Therefore, the differential responses to sulphonylureas can be utilized to classify K$_{ATP}$ channel subtypes in different tissues. The target site of KCOs in the K$_{ATP}$ channel complex is also assumed to be the SUR subunit, considering that the response of reconstituted K$_{ATP}$ channels to either diazoxide or pinacidil is correlated with the presence of SUR subtypes. The C-terminal end of the SUR appears to be a critical determinant for KCO pharmacology. SUR1 and SUR2B C-termini, for example, are similar, and channels formed from these subunits appear to share similar responsiveness to diazoxide. The Kir6.2/SUR2A channel showed essentially no response to diazoxide because of the different C-terminus in SUR2A. The molecular basis for K$_{ATP}$ channel subtype-specific properties will be discussed further below.

III. MOLECULAR BASIS OF K⁺ CHANNELS

A. K_V CHANNELS

K_V channels represent the most sophisticated ion channel superfamily found in mammals. At least ten subfamilies of K_V channels have been characterized in a variety of tissues, including the K_V 1 to K_V 4 (KCNA to KCND) subfamilies (corresponding to *shaker, shab, shaw,* and *shal* gene subfamilies in *Drosophila Melanogaster*), K_V 5 [K_V 5.1 (KCNF1)], K_V 6 [K_V 6.1 (KCNG1) and K_V 6.2 (KCNF2)], K_V 8, K_V 9, K_V LQT1 (KCNQ1), and Erg (ether a go-go gene) (KCNH1) subfamilies. For unknown reasons, the K_V7 family does not appear in literature.

In terms of electrophysiological properties, K_V α-subunits can be further divided into two subtypes. K_V 1.1, 1.2, 1.3, 1.5, 1.6, 2.1, 3.1, and 3.2 may underlie the functional I_K (outward delayed rectifier) current. K_V 1.4, 1.7,[64] K_V 3.3, 4.1, 4.2, and 4.3 may generate I_A (rapid inactivation transient rectifier) current.[65] This superfamily also includes some accessory K_V subunits, i.e., K_V β-subunits, I_{SK} (KCNE1), and minK related peptide 2 (MiRP2 or KCNE3).[66,67] Structurally, K_V channels are composed of four pore-forming α-subunits (homogeneous or heterogeneous tetramers) with or without the associated cytoplasmic β-subunit tetramer to form an $\alpha_4\beta_4$ octameric structure or an α4 tetrameric structure.

Each monomer of the α-subunit has six putative transmembrane domains (S1 through S6) with its hydrophilic amino and carboxyl termini located inside the cell. The S5 and S6 domains form a structural core surrounding a pore loop containing a "signature" sequence. The crystal structure of KcsA [a bacteria K⁺ channel protein having two (M1 and M2) transmembrane domains] has revealed that S6 (corresponding to KcsA M2) has a Pro–Val–Pro motif resulting in flexibility for the pore-lining helix as a molecular hinge.[68,69] The charged residues in the S4 domain are essential for the channel to sense voltage changes across the cell membrane.[70] The resulting conformational changes and cooperative interactions in the secondary and tertiary structures of these transmembrane segments are vital in affecting the voltage dependence of channel gating (Figure 5.3).

Altering amino acid residues (introduction of mutations or deletions) in these segments has proven to be very useful in studying K_V channel gating mechanisms.[71-73] The cytoplasmic T1 domain of the K_V channel α-subunits, which is about 100-residues long and located on the amino terminal side of the S1 transmembrane helix, has drawn great attention recently for its key roles in regulating the gating of channels. Miller and colleagues suggested a "hanging gondola" structure for the T1 domain; the tetrameric T1 forms four 20-Å^2 window-like holes through which selective K⁺ ions can access the inner entrance of the pole. Mutagenesis of some residues in the T1 domain may result in changes of the tetrameric conformation and thus open the channels.[74]

To date, three subfamilies of K_V β-subunits (K_V β1, K_V β2, and K_V β3) have been reported in mammalian tissue preparations including rat and bovine brain and human heart.[75-77] The cytoplasmic β-subunits associate with and alter the kinetics of K_V channel α-subunits. For instance, the rat β 1-subunit induces a rapid inactivation (N-type inactivation) of the delayed rectifier K_V 1.1 channel. However, the rat β 2.1-subunit

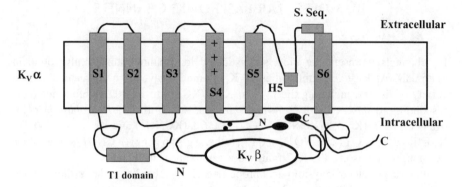

FIGURE 5.3 Schematic topology of K_V channels. The monomer of the α-subunit contains six putative transmembrane domains (S1 through S6) with intracellular N- and C-termini. S5 and S6 domains form a structural core (H5) and a "signature" sequence (S.Seq). Positively charged residues in the S4 domain are essential for channel sensitivity to cell membrane voltage changes. The cytoplasmic 100-residue T1 domain has key roles in regulating the gating of channels. The accessory β-subunit is important in modulating gating of the channels. The K_V β-subunit may plug its "ball-like" segment onto the N- or C-terminus to the cytoplasmic entrance of the K_V α-subunit pore-forming domain. It may also bind to the amino terminal side of the T1 domain. Additionally, its N-terminal amino acid residues may interact with the residues at the loops between the S4 and S5 domains of α-subunits.

isoform does not change K_V current phenotypes (delayed rectifiers K_V 1.1 and 1.4) in the heterologous expression system.[77]

Another report indicates that rat β 3.1-subunit can confer partial inactivation of the *shaker* related K_V 1 family.[76] At least three alternatively spliced mRNA variants (K_V β 1.1, β 1.2 and β 1.3) were identified in the K_V β1 subfamily. They have distinctive sequences at the N-terminus (66 to 91 aa) (inactivation domain) while sharing identical sequences near the C terminus (328 aa).[75]

Several mechanisms for the K_V β-subunit related modulation of K_V channels have been proposed. K_V β-subunit may plug its "ball-like" segment on the N or C terminus to the cytoplasmic entrance of the K_V α-subunit pore-forming domain.[78] It may also bind to the amino terminal side of the T1 domain.[74,79,80] Additionally, Lombardi and co-workers[81] proposed that a protein–protein interaction between K_V β1 amino terminal residues (Arg20 and Leu21) and the S4–S5 loop of K_V 1.1 (Arg324 and Leu328) might be responsible for β-subunit-mediated K_V channel inactivation. Nevertheless, Yang et al.[82] reported that K_V β2 might increase the expression level of a *shal*-related subfamily (K_V 4.3) when co-expressed in HEK-293 cells rather than affect K_V channel gating and current patterns through their molecular interactions at the C-terminus. K_V β-subunit diversity is thought at least partially to underlie K_V channel functional diversity and its tissue specificity under physiological conditions.

K_V 1.1, 1.2, 1.4, 1.5, 2.1, and 4.2 have been identified in rat aorta at mRNA level.[83] K_V 2.1 and 1.5 proteins were immunolocalized in rat cerebral, coronary, and renal arteries,[84] and in human aorta (K_V 1.5).[85] The first systematic characterization of K_V gene expression in vascular SMCs was carried out in our laboratory. We screened the expression of 18 K_V channel genes using RT-PCR based techniques.

Six I_K-encoding genes (K_V 1.2, K_V 1.3, K_V 1.5, K_V 2.1, K_V 2.2, and K_V 3.2) were expressed in rat mesenteric artery, but K_V 1.1, K_V 1.6, and K_V 3.1 were not detected. Although no transient outward K_V currents (I_A) were recorded in the studied SMCs, transcripts of multiple I_A-encoding genes including K_V 1.4, K_V 3.3, K_V 3.4, K_V 4.1, K_V 4.2, and K_V 4.3 as well as I_A-facilitating K_V β-subunits (K_V β 1.1, K_V β 2.1, and K_V β 3.1) were detected in the same tissue preparation. Western blot analysis demonstrated that four I_K-related K_V channel proteins (K_V 1.2, K_V 1.3, K_V 1.5, and K_V 2.1), but not the protein for K_V 3.2, were detected in rat mesenteric artery tissues. The presence of K_V 1.2, K_V 1.3, K_V 1.5, and K_V 2.1 channel proteins in primary cultured SMCs was further confirmed by immunocytochemistry.[86] The same expression pattern of K_V channel genes was also recognized in SMCs from rat tail arteries.[87]

Mutations appearing in certain K_V channel α-subunit, β-subunit, or other auxiliary subunit genes are related to certain pathophysiological situations. Zuberi et al.[88] reported that a novel mutation at nucleotide position 677 in the human K_V 1.1 gene on chromosome 12p13 was associated with inherited episodic ataxia type 1. The down-regulation of K_V 1.5 and 2.1 at mRNA level in pulmonary arterial SMCs may contribute to primary pulmonary hypertension.[89] Abbott and co-workers[90] reported that a mutant MiRP2 (KCNE3) that complexes with K_V 4.3 in skeletal muscle was associated with inherited periodic paralysis because the K_V channel exhibited reduced current density and diminished capacity to set resting membrane potential.

B. K_{Ca} Channels

Like many other ionic channels, voltage-dependent or -independent, K_{Ca} channels are composed of tetrameric $\alpha_4\beta_4$ in membrane stoichiometry. Among BK_{Ca}, IK_{Ca}, and SK_{Ca} channels, BK_{Ca} channels are best described and characterized in various tissues including vascular SMCs. BK_{Ca} channels are believed to be encoded from a single gene rather than many homogeneous genes. The single gene origin with a family of alternatively spliced variants can explain the wide difference in unitary conductance, calcium sensitivity, and gating of BK_{Ca} channels in different tissues and even within the same tissue.[91,92]

BK_{Ca} α-subunits were first cloned from *Drosophila* (dSlo)[93] and later from mammalian animals: human (hSlo),[94] rat (rSlo) [GenBank Accession No.U55995], mouse (mSlo),[95] and canine (cSlo) [GenBank Accession No.U41001]. Human BK_{Ca} α-subunit (hSlo) is mapped to chromosome 10q23.1.[94] The transmembrane segments (S0 through S6) near the N-terminus of the BK_{Ca} channel α-subunit have similar amino acid sequences to those of the voltage sensors and the pore domains of K_V channels. The charged residues (Arg) in the S4 transmembrane domain move outward when the cell membrane depolarizes and interact with negative residues in the S2 and S3 domains. Gene expression of the hSlo α-subunit with the pore region between S5 and S6 (H5 domain) replaced by dSlo (known as an IbTX insensitive channel) showed that the chimera can abolish the IbTX-blocking sensitivity of hSlo, indicating the structural importance for the binding of IbTX to the pore domain of BK_{Ca} channels.[96]

In addition to the seven transmembrane domains (S0 through S6), BK_{Ca} channels have four extra hydrophobic domains (S7 through S10) at the C terminus, which are conservative among species.[93,95,97] The S9 and S10 regions are associated with intracellular calcium sensitivity and calcium binding.[96,98,99] A more recent topology model for the BK_{Ca} channel α-subunit suggested that an additional S0 transmembrane segment leads to the extracellular location of the N terminus. The exoplasmic N terminal end and S0 transmembrane domain of the channel are associated with the β-subunit regulation in mammalian BK_{Ca} gene.[100] The amino acid sequence of the human BK_{Ca} gene (1113 aa) shares very high identity rate with that of the rat (1178 aa) and the mouse (1180 aa) (96 to 97%), but relates only distantly to *Drosophila* (1175 aa) (49%).

At least four types of β-subunits that couple with BK_{Ca} channel α-subunits have been cloned in human tissues ($\beta1$ to $\beta4$). The β-subunit family of BK_{Ca} channels regulates several critical aspects of channel phenotype such as inactivation and apparent Ca^{2+} sensitivity. Structurally, BK_{Ca} channel β-subunits are about 192 to 310 amino acid residues in length, having two transmembrane domains (TM1 and TM2) with a long extracellular loop between the domains and two N-linked glycosylation sites (Figure 5.4). TM1 and TM2 are similar in amino acid sequence, suggesting a common structure. The $\beta1$-subunit increases the apparent calcium sensitivity at micromolar range of the BK_{Ca} channel α-subunit and it is mainly expressed in smooth muscle tissues.[30] Co-expression of $\beta2$-subunit (a neuronal β-subunit) with the BK_{Ca} α-subunit may cause the non-inactivating hyperpolarizing K^+ current to become a rapidly inactivating K^+ current.[31]

Similarly, Xia et al.[32] reported that the $\beta3$-subunit confers very fast but incomplete inactivating K^+ current compared with that of the $\beta2$-subunit. The intracellular amino acid residues at the N termini of β-subunits are thought to have the "ball-like" structure that is vital for BK_{Ca} channel phenotypes.[32] Overexpression of the human $\beta3$-subunit (3q26.3–q27 segment duplication) is reported to cause a syndrome characterized by multiple congenital neurological anomalies.[101] On the other hand, the $\beta4$-subunit is abundant in adult brain tissues and appears to be essential for the formation of a ChTX-insensitive channel with a BK_{Ca} α-subunit. This feature is associated with its long extracellular loop that may affect the binding of the BK_{Ca} blocker to the pore region of the α-subunit.[102]

In contrast to BK_{Ca} channels, intermediate and small conductance K_{Ca} channels (IK_{Ca} and SK_{Ca}) are activated solely by surges in intracellular calcium. Several genes encoding SK_{Ca} channels have been cloned recently from human brain ($hSK_{Ca}1$), rat brain ($rSK_{Ca}2$ and $rSK_{Ca}3$),[25] human pancreas ($hSK_{Ca}4$),[103] and porcine vascular SMCs.[26] The amino acid sequence homology among rat SK_{Ca} channel isoforms is about 46%. Similar percentages were also found between human $SK_{Ca}1$ and $SK_{Ca}4$, indicating tissue-specific channel properties. IK_{Ca} channels share very high amino acid identity with some SK_{Ca} channels from the same animal species: $rIK_{Ca}1$ to $rSK_{Ca}4$, 98.6%, (GenBank Accession Nos. AF156554 and AJ133438); $hIK_{Ca}1/hIK_{Ca}4$ to $hSK_{Ca}4$, 100% (GenBank Accession Nos. AF022150, AF033021, and AF000972). The structures of IK_{Ca} and SK_{Ca} channels have not been fully elucidated, but a consensus claims that they also have six membrane-spanning domains (Figure 5.4).

IK_{Ca} and SK_{Ca} channels have calmodulin, rather than classical BK_{Ca} β-subunits, to be constitutively associated with the C-terminus of the IK_{Ca}/SK_{Ca} α-subunit as a high-affinity Ca^{2+} sensor. Calmodulin has four EF-hand (a calcium binding motif

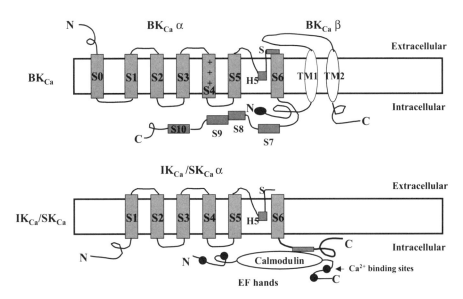

FIGURE 5.4 Schematic topology of K_{Ca} channels. The monomer of the BK_{Ca} channel α-subunit has seven putative transmembrane domains (S0 through S6) in which the charged residues in S4 are crucial for the responsiveness to voltage changes across the membrane. BK_{Ca} channel α-subunits also have four putative cytoplasmic hydrophobic domains (S7 through S10) which are responsible for intracellular Ca^{2+} sensing. The BK_{Ca} channel β-subunit has two putative transmembrane domains with a long extracellular loop that may interact with the pore regions of the α-subunits. The N-terminal end of the β-subunit has a "ball-like" structure that can regulate the gating properties of the channels by plugging or unplugging the cytoplasmic entrances of the channels. The interaction of the N terminal end, S0, and β-subunit is not shown in this figure. The IK_{Ca}/SK_{Ca} channels interact with cytoplasmic calmodulin instead of specific β-subunits.

containing a 12-aa loop and a 12-aa helix at either end providing octahedral coordination for calcium ion) motifs for calcium binding (two each at the N- and C-termini). Calcium that binds to the N terminal end of calmodulin leads to the conformational changes in calmodulin and C termini of the IK_{Ca}/SK_{Ca} channels, thus resulting in channel opening.[104,105]

Although understanding of the molecular structures of K_{Ca} channels has greatly improved recently, many details of the relationships between K_{Ca} channel α- and β-subunits and their molecular structures and functions remain to be elucidated.

C. K_{ATP} CHANNELS

K_{ATP} channels are hetero-octamer complexes of four pore-forming subunits and four regulatory sulphonylurea binding subunits. The former (Kir6.1 and Kir6.2) belong to a class of inwardly rectifying K^+ channel subunits and the latter (SURs) to the ATP-binding cassette (ABC) superfamily.[62,63] The channels are assembled with a 1:1 tetrameric stoichiometry of Kir6.x and SUR subunits (Kir6.x/SUR)$_4$. Although Kir6.x and SUR subunits are structurally distinct, they have to physically interact

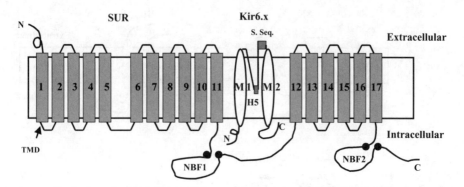

FIGURE 5.5 Schematic topology of K_{ATP} channels. K_{ATP} channels are hetero-octamer complexes of four pore-forming subunits (Kir6.x) and four regulatory sulphonylurea binding subunits (SURs). Kir6.x subunits have two putative transmembrane domains (M1 and M2) with N- and C-termini positioning inside the cell. Accessory SUR subunits have 17 putative transmembrane domains (TMDs). The nucleotide binding folds (NBF1 and NBF2) are located in the intracellular loop between TMD11 and 12 and near the C-terminus.

with each other to constitute functional K_{ATP} channels.[106] Kir6.1 was first cloned from a rat pancreatic islet cDNA library using Kir3.1 cDNA as a probe, whereas Kir6.2 (BIR) was cloned from a human genomic library and MIN6 cDNA library using Kir6.1 cDNA as a probe.[48,62] Kir6.1 and Kir6.2, encoding 424 aa and 390 aa proteins, respectively, have membrane topologies of two putative transmembrane segments (M1 and M2) surrounding a pore-forming domain (H5).

Kir6.1 shares about 70% amino acid sequence homology with Kir6.2. Phylogenetic analysis showed that Kir6.1 and Kir6.2 were clustered into a group located next to the G protein-activated Kir3.x subfamily.[107] A conservative Gly–Tyr–Gly (G–Y–G) motif in the pore-forming H5 domains among various K^+ channels is replaced by a Gly–Phe–Gly (G–F–G) motif in both Kir6.1 and Kir6.2 genes. The motif is thought to be critical for K^+ selectivity for the channel.[108,109] Both the C and N termini of Kir6.1 and Kir6.2 are located inside the cell and are thought important for intracellular ATP binding and interactions with SUR subunits. SUR subunits are large proteins with 17 putative transmembrane domains (TMD1 through 17) having an extracellular N terminus and an intracellular C terminal end[110] (Figure 5.5).

Five SUR subunits have been identified in various mammalian tissues. SUR1 which encodes a protein of 177 kDa was first cloned from insulinoma cells.[111] More recently, SUR1B was cloned from a rat insulinoma cell line (GenBank Accession No. AF039595). SUR1B has a 38-amino acid deletion (Glu[1253] to Met[1291]) within the third group of TMDs (TMD12 through 17), compared to the original SUR1 and SUR1 cloned from rat mesenteric artery smooth muscle in our laboratory (GenBank Accession No. AB052294).

A SUR2A subunit has been isolated from rat brain tissue by Inagaki et al.[112] A novel alternative spliced variant of this SUR2 from a mouse heart cDNA library was later named SUR2B. Both SUR2A and SUR2B proteins contain 1545 amino acids (174 kDa), yet they differ at the C-terminus for 42 amino acid residues. The

C-terminal 42-aa sequence of SUR2B exhibits about 75% identity with that of SUR1. This segment is responsible for diazoxide activation and may be the key element in distinguishing SUR2A from SUR2B in their distinct sensitivity to diazoxide.[63]

One more splicing variant of SUR2 was recently cloned and named SUR2C. It has a 35-amino acid deletion between the second and third groups of TMDs (TMD11 and 12), but its functional implication is not known.[113] The binding pockets for KCOs and sulphonylureas are located between TMD12 and 17 of the SUR proteins. The affinity of KCOs or sulphonylurea to the binding pockets in the SUR subunits determines the pharmacological sensitivity of the native K_{ATP} channels.[114] SUR proteins also have protein kinase A- and C-dependent phosphorylation sites and two N (Asn)-linked glycosylation sites (Asn[10] and Asn[1050]).[49]

Human K_{ATP} channel genomic mappings revealed that SUR and Kir6.x genes may come in pairs. SUR1 and Kir6.2 are on the short arm of chromosome 11 at 11p15.1. The distance between them is about 4.5 kb. On the other hand, SUR2 gene is paired with Kir6.1 in the short arm of chromosome 12 at 12p11.12 and Kir6.1 is at 12p11.23. The distance in between is too great to be amplified by conventional PCR.[62,115]

Studies on the tissue distribution of K_{ATP} channel subunits by RT-PCR and Northern blot analysis have showed that Kir6.2 and SUR1 are mainly expressed in pancreatic β-cells and Kir6.2 and SUR2A in cardiomyocytes[112]; Kir6.1 and SUR2B are functionally paired in vascular SMCs.[63] We have found that Kir6.2 and SUR1 were also expressed at mRNA level in rat mesenteric artery smooth muscles (unpublished data). These data imply that heterogeneous Kir6.x tetramer may be co-assembled in native vascular tissues. Cui and co-workers[116] showed a chimeric Kir6.1–Kir6.2 co-expressed with SUR2 in HEK-293 cells to form functional K_{ATP} channels.

The expression of pore-forming Kir6.1 or Kir6.2 alone did not elicit functional K_{ATP} channel currents in *Xenopus* oocytes.[117] A truncated Kir6.2 gene, Kir6.2ΔN44, inhibits functional expression of K_{ATP} channels, indicating possible involvement of this region in co-assembly with SUR subunits.[57] On the other hand, truncation of Kir6.2ΔC26 formed ATP-inhibited potassium channels in the absence of SUR subunits, implying that the C terminus of Kir6.2 subunit may function as a "molecular plug" to close the channel. Furthermore, a segment near the Kir6.2 C terminus (Glu[179] through Leu[355]) forming a low-affinity nucleotide-binding pocket may be associated with K_{ATP} channel gating.[118]

Taken together, the reconstitution and mutagenesis studies on SUR/Kir6.x channels show that the potassium selectivity, inward rectification, and unitary conductance of the K_{ATP} channels are determined by the Kir6.x subunit, whereas their nucleotide and pharmacological sensitivity depend on the SUR subunits. The functional diversity of K_{ATP} channels may be implied by the multiplicity of Kir6.x/SUR channel constitutions in native vascular SMCs.

IV. THE EFFECTS OF CO ON K⁺ CHANNELS IN VASCULAR SMCs

Many studies have reported the modulation of ion channels by CO in different cell preparations and proposed different working hypotheses. In most cases, CO acts on

K_{Ca} channels. Therefore, our discussion will focus on the interaction of CO and K_{Ca} channels in vascular SMCs.

A. The Effects of CO on K_{CA} Channels in Vascular SMCs and Other Types of Cells

We have previously shown that CO induced a concentration-dependent relaxation of isolated rat tail artery tissues precontracted with phenylephrine or U46619. The CO-induced vasorelaxation was partially inhibited by blocking either the cGMP pathway or BK_{Ca} channels. When both the cGMP pathway and K_{Ca} channels were blocked, the CO-induced vasorelaxation was completely abolished.[119] These results suggest that CO may activate both a cGMP signaling pathway and K_{Ca} channels in the same vascular tissues. We further showed the direct effect of CO on K_{Ca} channels in isolated rat tail artery SMCs.[120] CO enhanced the whole-cell K^+ channel currents at more depolarized membrane potentials in a reversible manner. At +10 mV, the amplitude of whole-cell K^+ channel currents was increased by $130 \pm 45\%$ by 10 μM CO. Interestingly, CO had no effect on whole-cell K^+ channel currents in N1E-115 cells. In these neuroblastoma cells, only medium-conductance (98 pS) and small-conductance (5.4 pS), but not the big-conductance K_{Ca} channels have been identified,[121] which might explain the lack of effect of CO on whole-cell K^+ channel currents in this cell preparation.

The nature of the CO-sensitive whole-cell K^+ channel current was further examined using single channel recording technique.[120] In rat tail artery SMCs, a K_{Ca} channel was identified, of which the single channel conductance is around 239 ± 8 pS with symmetric 145 mM KCl on both sides of the patch membrane. The addition of EGTA to or the increase in calcium concentration of the intracellular solution decreased or increased, respectively, the opening probability (NPo) of the channel. The NPo activity of K_{Ca} channels was also inhibited by 92% by external applied ChTX (100 nM), but not by apamin (100 nM). Extracelluarly or intracellularly applied CO increased the NPo of single big-conductance K_{Ca} channels in a concentration-dependent fashion without affecting the single channel conductance. The effect of CO on the NPo was also antagonized by ChTX (100 nM).

Two mechanisms can explain the CO-increased activity of K_{Ca} channels. An increased intracellular calcium concentration in the presence of CO was first examined. We found that CO had no effect on the resting intracellular free calcium concentrations in acutely isolated rat tail artery SMCs. Alternatively, the calcium sensitivity of K_{Ca} channels might have been enhanced by CO so that, even with the same intracellular calcium concentration, K_{Ca} channels may increase their activity. This hypothesis was tested by comparing the relationship of NPo and intracellular free calcium concentrations, $[Ca^{2+}]_i$, using the equation NPo = $[Ca^{2+}]_i^h/(K+[Ca^{2+}]_i^h)$, where K is the overall dissociation constant and h is the Hill coefficient. With different concentrations of CO, the Hill coefficient increased from a control value of 0.88 to 1.70 and 3.07, respectively. With $[Ca^{2+}]_i$ at 3 μM, the K_{Ca} channels spent about 40% of the time in their open state in the absence of CO, whereas in the presence of CO (10 μM), the NPo increased significantly so that the channels were open about 90% of the time. Thus, calcium sensitivity of K_{Ca} channels in the cell-free patches increased in the presence of a CO, which can be correlated to CO-induced increase in the NPo levels of K_{Ca} channels.

Our results show that CO directly affects K_{Ca} channels in vascular SMCs, an effect not mediated by cGMP or other intracellular second messengers. This conclusion was reached not only because the CO effect was observed in either inside–out or outside–out cell-free patch clamp recordings, but also because the absence of GTP and cGMP-dependent protein kinase in the patch-clamp recording solutions excludes the indirect effect of CO on K_{Ca} channel via the activation of cGMP-dependent protein kinases.

If the effects of CO on single K_{Ca} channels in cell-free membrane patches were mediated by membrane-bound G proteins, application of GTP-γ-S alone to cell-free membrane patches should stimulate G proteins possibly attached to the isolated membrane patches, thus modulating the activity of K_{Ca} channels. This hypothesis was not proven in our experiments since GTP-γ-S (400 μM) did not affect K_{Ca} channel currents or the excitatory effects of CO on K_{Ca} channels. In outside–out membrane patches, pertussis toxin (200 ng/ml), which catalyzes ADP ribosylation and prevents the activation of Gi or Go, had no effect on the basal activities of K_{Ca} channels.

We also tested the effect of cholera toxin, which irreversibly activates Gs, and this toxin (200 ng/ml) did not alter the basal activities of K_{Ca} channels. The stimulatory effect of CO on K_{Ca} channels was not changed after pretreatment of excised patches with either pertussis toxin or cholera toxin. These observations indicate that even if the co-existence of different types of G proteins, especially Gi/Go or Gs, with K_{Ca} channel proteins were possible, those G proteins may not affect the basal activities of K_{Ca} channels; neither was the effect of CO on K_{Ca} channels mediated by Gi/Go or Gs proteins in excised membrane patches from vascular SMCs.

Leffler et al.[122] showed that topically applied CO dose-dependently dilated piglet pial arterioles *in vivo*. This effect of CO was completely abolished by treatment with the K_{Ca} channel inhibitors TEA and IbTX. The HO substrate heme-L-lysinate also produced a dose-dependent dilation that is sensitive to TEA inhibition. It was concluded that CO dilated pial arterioles exclusively via activation of K_{Ca} channels.

The direct modulation of big-conductance K_{Ca} channels in vascular SMCs by CO may constitute a novel mechanism for the vascular effect of CO. The opening of K_{Ca} channels can lead to vasorelaxation if cell membrane is hyperpolarized and voltage-gated Ca^{2+} channels inactivated. In agreement with this reasoning, CO (10 μM) effectively hyperpolarized primarily cultured SMCs from –62 mV to –84 mV.[120]

In addition to the study of vascular SMCs, the effects of CO on K_{Ca} channels in other types of cells have also been reported. For example, in cultured urinary bladder SMCs, CO inhibited a whole-cell K_{Ca} channel current.[123] Werkstrom et al.[124] reported that CO relaxed the inner smooth muscle of the oesophagogastric junction (OGJ) isolated from pigs. Although apamin or ChTX alone did not alter the CO effect, a combination of both reduced CO-induced relaxation. This result suggests that a specific type of K_{Ca} channels located in smooth muscles partially mediated the relaxant effect of CO on the OGJ. It has been reported that the relaxation of rat hepatic artery induced by an endothelium-derived hyperpolarizing factor (EDHF) is also inhibited by the combined application of apamin and ChTX.[125] Therefore, the relationship of CO and EDHF should be further investigated.

B. THE CHEMICAL MODIFICATION OF SINGLE K_{Ca} CHANNELS BY CO

As a gaseous molecule, CO can freely penetrate plasma membrane and interact with the membrane-spanning K_{Ca} channel proteins. Different amino acid residues that are constitutive components of the channel protein determine the electrical properties of K_{Ca} channels. A direct reaction between CO and certain amino acid residues may significantly affect the function of K_{Ca} channels. In this regard, the interaction of CO and heme-containing proteins may be revealing. CO forms a complex with heme via forming hydrogen bonds with the distal histidine residue (His^{64}) in myoglobin[126] or histidine[25] in heme oxygenase.[127] To extrapolate the interaction of CO and heme-containing proteins, we decided to test whether CO can chemically interact with certain amino acid residues of K_{Ca} channel proteins, thus modulating the activities of these channels. Similarly, the modification of sulfhydryl groups in cysteine has been shown to inhibit the conduction of an anion-selective channel in oocytes.[61]

Modification of histidine residues: We used diethyl pyrocarbonate (DEPC) to modify histidine residues located on the external or cytoplasmic surfaces of K_{Ca} channel proteins. DEPC is not membrane permeable. Application of DEPC to different sides of plasma membranes can provide information on the topological differences of certain membrane proteins across membranes. Exposure of the cytoplasmic surfaces of cell membranes to DEPC (0.5 mM) did not affect the characteristics of K_{Ca} channels nor modify the stimulatory effect of CO on K_{Ca} channels in cell-free membrane patches from rat tail artery SMCs. In contrast, when DEPC was applied to the external surfaces of cell membranes, the opening probability of K_{Ca} channels was reduced. This inhibitory effect of DEPC, if specific for histidine residues, should be a function of pH, since DEPC reacts only with the unprotonated imidazole ring. At pH 6.3, a 46% inhibition of the NPo of K_{Ca} channels by DEPC was observed. At pH 5.2, the NPo of K_{Ca} channels only slightly decreased by DEPC treatment (6%). The pH dependence of the effect of DEPC indicated the specific modification of histidine residues.

A kinetic analysis of the effect of DEPC on K_{Ca} channels revealed that the NPo of K_{Ca} channels began to decrease 1 min after the DEPC application and decreased by 50% 4 min after the DEPC treatment. The decrease in the NPo of K_{Ca} channels by DEPC was also concentration-dependent, following a pseudo-first-order kinetics. The reaction order obtained from the slope of the double logarithmic plot was 1.0, indicating that one histidine residue per channel protein might be involved in the modifying effect of DEPC.[128]

After characterizing the chemical modification of K_{Ca} channel proteins by DEPC, we continued to investigate the interaction of CO and DEPC on K_{Ca} channels. DEPC treatment abolished the CO-induced increase in the NPo of single K_{Ca} channels in outside–out membrane patches, but not in inside–out patches. The inactivated DEPC did not affect the stimulatory effect of CO on K_{Ca} channels, indicating the specific involvement of histidine in this interaction. We also applied hydroxylamine to remove DEPC from imidazoles after treatment of the membrane patch with DEPC.

In one case, we found that the inhibitory effect of DEPC on the CO-induced modification of single K_{Ca} channel currents was removed. An interaction between CO and DEPC on histidine residue was also demonstrated by the CO-induced protection of K_{Ca} channels from inhibition by DEPC.

To further confirm the involvement of histidine residues in the modifying effect of CO on K_{Ca} channels, the cells were exposed to illuminated Rose Bengal, a treatment specifically modifying histidine residues. Photooxidation of the histidine residue located on the external membrane surface abolished the CO-induced activation of K_{Ca} channels. However, CO still significantly increased the NPo of K_{Ca} channels in outside–out patches isolated from cells which were preincubated with Rose Bengal in the absence of light or exposed to illumination in the absence of the dye for 15 min. These results ruled out possible non-specific damage of K_{Ca} channels induced by non-illuminated dye or by photoinactivation of the K_{Ca} channels.

All these results demonstrate that the CO-induced increase in the opening probability of K_{Ca} channels may be specifically altered by the chemical modification of histidine residues. Yet, the chemical modification of the externally located histidine residue may not fully account for the interaction of CO with K_{Ca} channels. For instance, whether the modification of external histidine residue is responsible for the CO-induced increase in the calcium-sensitivity of K_{Ca} channels in vascular SMCs is unknown. Although the structural information about Ca^{2+}-binding sites of K_{Ca} channels is lacking, the Ca^{2+}-binding sites should be located on the cytoplasmic surfaces of K_{Ca} channel proteins. It is possible that the externally located histidine residue is the modulator site, the activation of which will induce necessary conformational changes in the channel-forming protein, either changing the apparent calcium affinity of the existing binding sites or unmasking new binding sites.

Alternatively, CO may modify the externally located histidine residue to change the gating mechanism and modify other cytoplasmic located amino acid residues to change the calcium-sensitivity of K_{Ca} channels. Increasing the concentration of CO would simply increase the probability that the modulator sites or Ca^{2+}-binding sites would be modified. Also worth noting are the obvious differences between the effects of CO and DEPC on K_{Ca} channels. DEPC decreased the NPo of K_{Ca} channels in a relatively irreversible manner because this reagent is involved in the covalent modification of histidine. On the other hand, CO increased the NPo in a reversible fashion, probably due to a relatively weak reaction between CO and the imidazole group of histidine via hydrogen bonds.

Modification of sulfhydryl groups: The permeation and gating mechanisms of K_{Ca} channels are not only determined by histidine residues. The interaction of CO and amino acid residues other than histidines with K_{Ca} channels has not been examined. For instance, sulfhydryl groups of cysteinyl residues of peptides and proteins are generally the most reactive of all amino acid side chains under normal physiological conditions. Among the irreversible modifying agents for sulfhydryl groups, N-ethylmaleimide (NEM) has been the most commonly used.[129] Pretreatment of membrane patches with NEM has been shown to prevent the NO-induced activation of K_{Ca} channels.[130] It is suggested for future studies to use NEM to modify sulfhydryl groups located on the cytoplasmic or external surfaces of the membrane patches. Subsequently, the direct effects of NEM and the effects of CO after NEM treatment on single-channel activity and calcium-sensitivity of K_{Ca} channels in vascular SMCs can be studied.

Modification of carboxyl groups: It has been suggested that the calcium-sensing and -binding sites of K_{Ca} channels are probably on carboxyl groups located on cytoplasmic domain of the channel protein.[131] Since CO mainly changes the calcium sensitivity of K_{Ca} channels, it is reasonable to hypothesize that the cytoplasmic-located carboxyl groups may also be affected by CO. These important issues should be further examined.

Trimethyloxonium (TMO) is a highly reactive agent that specifically esterifies carboxyl groups, such as those contained in aspartic or glutamic acid residues.[132] This reaction converts a normally negatively charged hydrophilic group to a neutral and more hydrophobic residue. It has been reported that TMO modification reduced the single-channel conductance of Na^+ channels[133,134] and K_{Ca} channels.[135] Thus, TMO can be used to probe the interaction of CO and the possible Ca^{2+}-binding sites of K_{Ca} channels in vascular SMCs.

In addition to the chemical modification of K_{Ca} channels, different mutants of K_{Ca} channel genes can be generated with specifically deleted or replaced target amino acid residues. The altered effect of CO on these mutated K_{Ca} channels will more specifically reveal the targets of CO on K_{Ca} channel proteins.

C. THE EFFECTS OF CO ON K_{ATP} OR K_V CHANNEL CURRENTS

Whether CO affects K_{ATP} channel activity in vascular SMCs has been unclear. Werkstrom et al.[124] reported that the CO-evoked relaxations of urethra and the OGJ inner smooth muscle of pig were not significantly reduced by treatment with glibenclamide, a blocker of K_{ATP} channels. Therefore, K_{ATP} channels were not considered to play an important role in the effect of CO on these tissues. However, the role of K_{ATP} channels in the regulation of contractility in these tissues was nominal since the addition of glibenclamide had no effect on spontaneous tension development at resting conditions.

An interaction of CO and K_{ATP} channels in SMCs cannot be excluded based on this report due to the putative absence of K_{ATP} channels in this tissue preparation. Future studies should be carried out at the tissue level to examine the relaxant effects of CO in the presence of K_{ATP} channel blockers or openers on the vascular tissues. At the cellular level, electrophysiological recording of transmembrane K^+ currents and their modulation by CO should be carried out with micromolar concentrations of ATP in the pipette solution and with K_{Ca} channel activity eliminated. Until these experiments are accomplished, the role played by K_{ATP} channels in the effect of CO cannot be ascertained. Another scenario that should also be considered is that CO may interfere with cellular metabolism to induce ATP level fluctuation, and may indirectly modulate K_{ATP} channels in vascular SMCs.

Also in the study by Werkstrom et al.,[124] urethra and the OGJ inner smooth muscle of pig developed spontaneous contractile tension in the presence of 4-aminopyridine, a K_V channel blocker. This signifies the presence of K_V channels in these tissues. However, the CO-induced relaxation was not affected by 4-aminopyridine.

An interaction between CO and K_V channels, therefore, is unlikely in this setting. To date, the mediation of the vascular effects of CO by K_V channels in vascular SMCs has not been reported.

V. CONCLUSIONS AND FUTURE DIRECTIONS

Different types of K^+ channels influence the contractility of vascular SMCs differentially. The voltage sensors of K_V channels, buried inside the plasma membranes, react to the membrane potential change, altering the conformation and the gating of K_V channel proteins. The calcium sensors of K_{Ca} channels detect the changes in free calcium concentration of the microzone on the intracellular side of the membrane. Consequently, K_{Ca} channels will open or close. The K_{ATP} channel complex also has its ATP sensor located on the intracellular side. Cellular metabolism leads to the fluctuation of ATP level, which in turn controls the gating of K_{ATP} channels. The trigger for the opening of different K^+ channels varies, but opening of K^+ channels leads to the same outcome, i.e., relaxation of vascular SMCs. The presence of multiple subfamilies of K^+ channels in vascular SMCs provides fine-tuned mechanisms for the modulation of vascular tone in the face of different stimuli and under different situations. The interaction among different types of K^+ channels in vascular SMCs is schematically presented in Figure 5.6. Different types of K^+ channels are interrelated, not only in their similar core molecular structures, but also in their functional connections.

The stimulatory effect of CO on K_{Ca} channels has been demonstrated. The most plausible mechanism for this effect resides in the chemical modifications of K_{Ca} channel proteins by CO. On the other hand, the cGMP-mediated effect of CO on K_{Ca} channels has also been reported. Accumulating evidence also substantiates the tissue specific distribution of different types of K_{Ca} channels. The vascular effect of CO as well as its stimulatory effect on K_{Ca} channels exhibits reasonably tissue specific features. The effect of CO on K_{ATP} channels, however, remains unsettled.

Elucidation of the interaction of CO and K^+ channels can generate two lines of important information. It will help to understand the vasoactive mechanisms of CO and shed light on the altered vascular effect of CO in different pathophysiological situations. It will also give clues pertinent to the interaction of CO and membrane protein, thus showing a "probing" role for CO. As reported previously, NO also acts on K_{Ca} channels in vascular SMCs. Unlike the CO-targeted parts of K_{Ca} channel proteins (histidine residues), NO acts on the sulfydryl groups of K_{Ca} channel proteins. Are the targets of CO and NO located on the same subunits (α or β) of K_{Ca} channel proteins or the same sides of cell membranes (external vs. internal sides)? What is the relationship of the CO-targeted residues to the calcium-binding and sensing residues of K_{Ca} channels? Will the effect of CO on K^+ channels be affected by the presence of NO or vice versa? What is the effect of CO on K^+ channels located on vascular endothelial cells? Answers to these and other related questions will no doubt be greatly welcomed by CO physiologists and ion channel electrophysiologists.

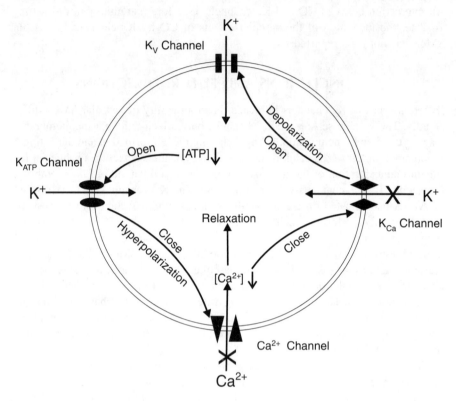

FIGURE 5.6 Interactions of different types of K^+ channels in vascular SMCs. A decrease in intracellular ATP level opens K_{ATP} channels, which hyperpolarizes the membrane and closes the voltage-gated Ca^{2+} channels. The resulting decrease in intracellular free calcium levels shuts down the K_{Ca} channels and depolarizes the membrane. Subsequently, the K_V channel opens and the membrane tends to be depolarized.

ACKNOWLEDGMENTS

This work is supported by research grants from the Smokeless Tobacco Research Council, and the Canadian Institute of Health Research (CIHR). K. Cao is supported by a post-doctoral fellowship award from Health Services Utilization and Research Commission of Saskatchewan. R. Wang is supported by a scientist award from CIHR.

REFERENCES

1. Quast, U. et al., Binding of the K^+ channel opener [^{3}H] P1075 in rat isolated aorta: relationship to functional effects of openers and blockers, *Mol. Pharmacol.*, 43, 474, 1993.
2. Cole, W.C., Clement–Chomienne, O., and Aiello E.A., Regulation of 4-aminopyridine-sensitive, delayed rectifier K^+ channels in vascular smooth muscle by phosphorylation, *Biochem. Cell Biol.*, 74, 439, 1996.

3. Post, J. et al., Direct role for potassium channel inhibition in hypoxic pulmonary vasoconstriction, *Am. J. Physiol.*, 262, C882, 1992.

4. Beech, D.J. and Bolton, T.B., A voltage-dependent outward current with fast kinetics in single smooth muscle cells isolated from rabbit portal vein, *J. Physiol. (Lond.)*, 412, 397, 1989.

5. Fleischmann, B.K., Washabau, R.J., and Kotlikoff, M.I., Control of resting membrane potential by delayed rectifier potassium currents in ferret airway smooth muscle cells, *J. Physiol. (Lond.)*, 469, 625, 1993.

6. Gelband, C.H. and Hume, J.R., $[Ca^{2+}]i$ inhibition of K^+ channels in canine renal artery. Novel mechanism for agonist-induced membrane depolarization, *Circ. Res.*, 77, 121, 1995.

7. Volk, K.A., Matsuda, J.J., and Shibata, E.F., A voltage-dependent potassium current in rabbit coronary artery smooth muscle cells, *J. Physiol. (Lond.)*, 439, 751, 1991.

8. Apkon, M. and Nerbonne, J.M., Characterization of two distinct depolarization-activated K^+ currents in isolated adult rat ventricular myocytes, *J. Gen. Physiol.*, 97, 973, 1991.

9. Jourdon, P. and Feuvray, D., Calcium and potassium currents in ventricular myocytes isolated from diabetic rats, *J. Physiol. (Lond.)*, 470, 411, 1993.

10. Magyar, J. et al., Action potentials and potassium currents in rat ventricular muscle during experimental diabetes, *J. Mol. Cell. Cardiol.*, 24, 841, 1992.

11. Gordienko, D.V., Clausen, C. and Goligorsky, S., Ionic currents and endothelin signaling in smooth muscle cells from rat renal resistance arteries, *Am. J. Physiol.*, 266, F325, 1994.

12. Yuan, X.J. et al., Inhibition of cytochrome P-450 reduces voltage-gated K^+ currents in pulmonary arterial myocytes, *Am. J. Physiol.*, 268, C259, 1995.

13. Smirnov, S.V. and Aaronson, P.I., Inhibition of vascular smooth muscle cell K^+ currents by tyrosine kinase inhibitors genistein and ST 638, *Circ. Res.*, 76, 310, 1995.

14. Smirnov, S.V. and Aaronson, P.I., Ca^{2+}-activated and voltage-gated K^+ currents in smooth muscle cells isolated from human mesenteric arteries, *J. Physiol. (Lond.)*, 457, 431, 1992.

15. Vogalis, F. and Lang, R.J., Identification of single transiently opening ("A-type") K channels in rabbit coronary artery smooth muscle cells, *Pflügers Arch.*, 429, 160, 1994.

16. Halliday, F.C. et al., The pharmacological properties of K^+ currents from rabbit isolated aortic smooth muscle cells, *Br. J. Pharmacol.*, 116, 3139, 1995.

17. Martens, J.R. and Gelband, C.H., Ion channels in vascular smooth muscle: alterations in essential hypertension, *Proc. Soc. Exp. Biol. Med.*, 218, 192, 1998.

18. Criddle, D.N., Greenwood, I.A., and Weston, A.H., Levcromakalim-induced modulation of membrane potassium currents, intracellular calcium and mechanical activity in rat mesenteric artery, *Naunyn-Schmiedeberg's Arch. Pharmacol.*, 349, 422, 1994.

19. Lu, Y. et al., Voltage-dependent K^+ channel current in vascular smooth muscle cells from rat mesenteric arteries, *J. Memb. Biol.*, 180, 163, 2001.

20. Tang, G. and Wang, R., Differential expression of K_V and K_{Ca} channels in vascular smooth muscle cells during one-day culture, *Pflügers Arch.*, 442, 124, 2001.

21. Brayden, J.E. and Nelson, M.T., Regulation of arterial tone by activation of calcium-dependent potassium channels, *Science*, 256, 532, 1992.

22. Benham, C.D. et al., Calcium-activated potassium channels in single smooth muscle cells of rabbit jejunum and guinea pig mesenteric artery, *J. Physiol.(Lond.)*, 371, 45, 1986.

23. Nicoll, R.A., The coupling of neurotransmitter receptors to ion channels in the brain, *Science*, 241, 545, 1988.

24. Lorenzon, N.M. and Foehring, R.C., Relationship between repetitive firing and afterhyperpolarizations in human neocortical neurons, *J. Neurophysiol.*, 67, 350, 1992.

25. Köhler, M. et al., Small-conductance, calcium-activated potassium channels from mammalian brain, *Science*, 273, 1709, 1996.

26. Sokol, P.T., Cloning of an apamin binding protein of vascular smooth muscle, *J. Prot. Chem.*, 13, 117, 1994.

27. Jensen, B.S. et al., Characterization of the cloned human intermediate-conductance Ca^{2+}-activated K^+ channel, *Am. J. Physiol.*, 275, C848, 1998.

28. Grissmer, S., Nguyen, A.N., and Cahalan, M.D., Calcium-activated potassium channels in resting and activated human T lymphocytes, *J. Gen. Physiol.*, 102, 601, 1993.

29. Partiseti, M. et al., Differential regulation of voltage- and calcium-activated potassium channels in human B lymphocytes, *J. Immunol.*, 148, 3361, 1992.

30. Meera, P. et al., A calcium switch for the functional coupling between α (*hslo*) and β subunits (K_V, Ca β) of maxi K channels, *FEBS Lett.*, 382, 84, 1996.

31. Wallner, M., Meera, P., and Toro, L., Molecular basis of fast inactivation in voltage and Ca^{2+}-activated K^+ channels: a transmembrance β-subunit homolog, *Proc. Natl. Acad. Sci. U.S.A.*, 96, 4137, 1999.

32. Xia, X.M., Ding, J.P., and Lingle, C.J., Molecular basis for the inactivation of Ca^{2+}- and voltage-dependent BK channels in adrenal chromaffin cells and rat insulinoma tumor cells, *J. Neurosci.*, 19, 5255, 1999.

33. Scornik, F. S and Toro, L., U46619, a thromboxane A_2 agonist, inhibits K_{Ca} channel activity from pig coronary artery, *Am. J. Physiol.*, 262, C708, 1992.

34. Toro, L., Amador, M., and Stefani, E., ANG II inhibits calcium-activated potassium channels from coronary smooth muscle in lipid bilayers, *Am. J. Physiol.*, 258, H912, 1990.

35. Sadoshima, J.I. et al., Cyclic AMP modulates Ca-activated K channel in cultured smooth muscle cells of rat aortas, *Am. J. Physiol.*, 255, H754, 1988.

36. Kume, H., Graziano, M.P., and Kotlikoff, M.I., Stimulatory and inhibitory regulation of calcium-activated potassium channels by guanine nucleotide-binding proteins, *Proc. Natl. Acad. Sci. U.S.A.*, 89, 11051, 1989.

37. Taniguchi, J., Furukawa, K.I., and Shigekawa, M., Maxi K^+ channels are stimulated by cyclic guanosine monophosphate-dependent protein kinase in canine coronary artery smooth muscle cells, *Pflügers Arch.*, 463, 167, 1993.

38. Furchgott, R.F. and Zawadzki, J.V., The obligatory role of endothelial cells in the relaxation of arterial smooth muscle by acetylcholine, *Nature*, 288, 373, 1980.

39. Garland, C.J. et al., Endothelium-dependent hyperpolarization: a role in the control of vascular tone, *Trends Pharmacol. Sci.*, 16, 23, 1995.

40. Edwards, G. et al., K^+ is an endothelium-derived hyperpolarizing factor in rat arteries, *Nature*, 396, 269, 1998.

41. Mombouli, J.V. and Vanhoutte, P.M., Endothelium-derived hyperpolarizing factor(s): updating the unknown, *Trends Pharmacol. Sci.*, 18, 252, 1997.

42. Hwa, J.J. et al., Comparison of acetylcholine-dependent relaxation in large and small arteries of rat mesenteric vascular bed, *Am. J. Physiol.*, 266, H952, 1994.

43. Chen, G. and Cheung, D.W., Effect of K^+-channel blockers on ACh-induced hyperpolarization and relaxation in mesenteric arteries, *Am. J. Physiol.*, 272, H2306, 1997.

44. Corriu, C. et al., Endothelium-derived factors and hyperpolarization of the carotid artery of the guinea pig, *Br. J. Pharmacol.*, 119, 959, 1996.

45. Yamanaka, A., Ishikawa, T., and Goto, K., Characterization of endothelium-dependent relaxation independent of NO and prostaglandins in guinea pig coronary artery, *J. Pharmacol. Exp. Ther.*, 285, 480, 1998.

46. Cook, D.L. and Hales, C.N., Intracellular ATP directly blocks K^+ channels in pancreatic β-cells, *Nature*, 311, 271, 1984.

47. Noma, A., ATP-regulated K^+ channels in cardiac muscle, *Nature*, 305, 147, 1983.

48. Inagaki, N. et al., Cloning and functional characterization of a novel ATP-sensitive potassium channel ubiquitously expressed in rat tissues, including pancreatic islets, pituitary, skeletal muscle, and heart, *J. Biol. Chem.*, 270, 5691, 1995.

49. Seino, S., ATP-sensitive potassium channels: a model of heteromultimeric potassium channel/receptor assemblies, *Annu. Rev. Physiol.*, 61, 337, 1999.

50. Standen, N.B. et al., Hyperpolarizing vasodilators activate ATP-sensitive K^+ channels in arterial smooth muscle, *Science*, 245, 177, 1989.

51. Zhang, H. and Bolton, T.B., Activation by intracellular GDP, metabolic inhibition and pinacidil of a glibenclamide-sensitive K-channel in smooth muscle cells of rat mesenteric artery, *Br. J. Pharmacol.*, 114, 662, 1995.

52. Furspan, P.B. and Webb, R.C., Decreased ATP-sensitivity of a K^+ channel and enhanced vascular smooth muscle relaxation in genetically hypertensive rats, *J. Hypertens.*, 11, 1067, 1993.

53. Quayle, J.M. et al., Pharmacology of ATP-sensitive K^+ currents in smooth muscle cells from rabbit mesenteric artery, *Am. J. Physiol.*, 269, C1112, 1995.

54. Samaha, F.F. et al., ATP-sensitive potassium channel is essential to maintain basal coronary vascular tone *in vivo*, *Am. J. Physiol.*, 262, C1220, 1992.

55. Brayden, J.E., Potassium channels in vascular smooth muscle, *Clin. Exp. Pharmacol. Physiol.*, 23, 1069, 1996.

56. Quayle, J.M., Nelson, M.T., and Standen, N.B., ATP-sensitive and inwardly rectifying potassium channels in smooth muscle, *Physiol. Rev.*, 77, 1165, 1997.

57. Babenko, A.P., Gonzalez, G., and Bryan, J., Pharmaco-topology of sulfonylurea receptors: separate domains of the regulatory subunits of K_{ATP} channel isoforms are required for selective interaction with K^+ channel openers, *J. Biol. Chem.*, 275, 717, 2000.

58. Yokoshiki, H. et al., ATP-sensitive K^+ channels in pancreatic, cardiac, and vascular smooth muscle cells, *Am. J. Physiol.*, 274, C25, 1998.

59. Dunne, M.J. and Petersen, O.H., Intracellular ADP activates K^+ channels that are inhibited by ATP in an insulin-secreting cell line, *FEBS Lett.*, 208, 59, 1986.

60. Terzic, A. et al., Dualistic behavior of ATP-sensitive K^+ channels toward intracellular nucleoside diphosphates, *Neuron*, 12, 1049, 1994.

61. Xu, M. and Akabas, M.H., Amino acids lining the channel of the γ-aminobutyric acid type A receptor identified by cysteine substitution, *J. Biol. Chem.*, 268, 21505, 1993.

62. Inagaki, N. et al., Reconstitution of I_{KATP}: an inward rectifier subunit plus the sulfonylurea receptor, *Science*, 270, 1166, 1995.

63. Isomoto, S. et al., A novel sulfonylurea receptor forms with BIR (Kir6.2) a smooth muscle type ATP-sensitive K^+ channel, *J. Biol. Chem.*, 271, 24321, 1996.

64. Kalman, K. et al., Genomic organization, chromosomal localization, tissue distribution, and biophysical characterization of a novel mammalian shaker-related voltage-gated potassium channel, K_V 1.7, *J. Biol. Chem.*, 273, 5851, 1998.

65. Deal, K.K., England, S.K., and Tamkun, M.M., Molecular physiology of cardiac potassium channels, *Physiol. Rev.*, 76, 49, 1996.

66. Chandy, K.G. and Gutman, G.A., Voltage-gated K^+ channels, in *Handbook of Receptors and Channels: Ligand- and Voltage-Gated Ion Channels*, North, R.A., Ed., CRC Press, Boca Raton, FL, 1995, 1.

67. Stocker, M., Hellwig, M., and Kerschensteiner, D., Subunit assembly and domain analysis of electrically silent K^+ channel alpha-subunits of the rat K_V 9 subfamily, *J. Neurochem.*, 72, 1725, 1999.

68. Moczydlowski, E., Chemical basis for alkali cation selectivity in potassium-channel proteins, *Chem. Biol.*, 5, R291, 1998.
69. Shrivastava, I.H. et al., Structure and dynamics of K channel pore-lining helices: a comparative simulation study, *Biophys. J.*, 78, 174, 2000.
70. Starace, D.M., Stefani, E., and Bezanilla, F., Voltage-dependent proton transport by the voltage sensor of the *shaker* K$^+$ channel, *Neuron*, 19, 1319, 1997.
71. Cha, A. et al., Atomic scale movement of the voltage-sensing region in a potassium channel measured via spectroscopy, *Nature*, 402, 809, 1999.
72. Ledwell, J.L. and Aldrich, R.W., Mutations in the S4 region isolate the final voltage-dependent cooperative step in potassium channel activation, *J. Gen. Physiol.*, 113, 389, 1999.
73. Mathur, R. et al., Ile-177 and Ser-180 in the S1 segment are critically important in Kv1.1 channel function, *J. Biol. Chem.*, 274, 11487, 1999.
74. Kobertz, W.R., Williams, C., and Miller, C., Hanging gondola structure of the T1 domain in a voltage-gated K$^+$ channel, *Biochemistry*, 39, 10347, 2000.
75. England, S.K. et al., A novel K$^+$ channel β-subunit (hK$_V$β1.3) is produced via alternative mRNA splicing, *J. Biol. Chem.*, 270, 28531, 1995.
76. Heinemann, S. et al., Molecular and functional characterization of a rat brain K$_V$ beta 3 potassium channel subunit, *FEBS Lett.*, 377, 383, 1995.
77. Rettig, J. et al., Inactivation properties of voltage-gated K$^+$ channels altered by presence of β-subunit, *Nature*, 369, 289, 1994.
78. Morales, M.J. et al., The N-terminal domain of a K$^+$ channel β subunit increases the rate of C-type inactivation from the cytoplasmic side of the channel, *Proc. Natl. Acad. Sci. U.S.A.*, 93, 15119, 1996.
79. Gulbis, J.M. et al., Structure of the cytoplasmic beta subunit-T1 assembly of voltage-dependent K$^+$ channels, *Science*, 289, 123, 2000.
80. Minor, D.L. et al., The polar T1 interface is linked to conformational changes that open the voltage-gated potassium channel, *Cell*, 102, 657, 2000.
81. Lombardi, S.J. et al., Structure-activity relationships of the K$_V$β1 inactivation domain and its putative receptor probed using peptide analogs of voltage-gated potassium channel α- and β-subunits, *J. Biol. Chem.*, 273, 30092, 1998.
82. Yang, E.K. et al., K$_V$β subunits increase expression of K$_V$4.3 channels by interacting with their C termini, *J. Biol. Chem.*, 276, 4839, 2001.
83. Roberds, S.L. and Tamkun, M.M., Cloning and tissue-specific expression of five voltage-gated potassium channel cDNAs expressed in rat heart, *Proc. Natl. Acad. Sci. U.S.A.*, 88, 1798, 1991.
84. Archer, S.L. et al., Differential distribution of electrophysiologically distinct myocytes in conduit and resistance arteries determines their response to nitric oxide and hypoxia, *Circ. Res.*, 78, 431, 1996.
85. Mays, D.J. et al., Localization of the K$_V$1.5 K$^+$ channel protein in explanted cardiac tissue, *J. Clin. Invest.*, 96, 282, 1995.
86. Xu, C. et al., Expression of voltage-dependent K$^+$ channel genes in mesenteric artery smooth muscle cells, *Am. J. Physiol.*, 277, G1055, 1999.
87. Xu, C. et al., Molecular basis of voltage-dependent delayed rectifier K$^+$ channels in smooth muscle cells from rat tail artery, *Life Sci.*, 66, 2023, 2000.
88. Zuberi, S.M. et al., A novel mutation in the human voltage-gated potassium channel gene (K$_V$1.1) associates with episodic ataxia type 1 and sometimes with partial epilepsy, *Brain*, 122, 817, 1999.
89. Archer, S. and Rich, S., Primary pulmonary hypertension: a vascular biology and translational research "work in progress," *Circulation*, 102, 2781, 2000.

90. Abbott, G.W. et al., MiRP2 forms potassium channels in skeletal muscle with K_V 3.4 and is associated with periodic paralysis, *Cell*, 104, 217, 2001.

91. Ha, T.S. et al., Functional characteristics of two BK_{Ca} channel variants differentially expressed in rat brain tissues, *Eur. J. Biochem.*, 267, 910, 2000.

92. Lagrutta, A. et al., Functional differences among alternatively spliced variants of Slowpoke, a *Drosophila* calcium-activated potassium channel, *J. Biol. Chem.*, 269, 20347, 1994.

93. Atkinson, N.S., Robertson, G.A., and Ganetzky, B., A component of calcium-activated potassium channels encoded by the *Drosophila* Slo locus, *Science*, 253, 551, 1991.

94. McCobb, D.P. et al., A human calcium-activated potassium channel gene expressed in vascular smooth muscle, *Am. J. Physiol.*, 269, H767, 1995.

95. Butler, A. et al., mSlo, a complex mouse gene encoding "maxi" calcium-activated potassium channels, *Science*, 261, 221, 1993.

96. Meera, P. et al., Large conductance voltage- and calcium-dependent K^+ channel, a distinct member of voltage-dependent ion channels with seven N-terminal transmembrane segments (S0–S6), an extracellular N terminus, and an intracellular (S9–S10) C terminus, *Proc. Natl. Acad. Sci. U.S.A.*, 94, 14066, 1997.

97. Adelman, J.P. et al., Calcium-activated potassium channels expressed from cloned complementary DNAs, *Neuron*, 9, 209, 1992.

98. Knaus, H.G. et al., Characterization of tissue-expressed alpha subunits of the high conductance Ca^{2+}-activated K^+ channel, *J. Biol. Chem.*, 270, 22434, 1995.

99. Wei, A. et al., Calcium sensitivity of BK-type K_{Ca} channels determined by a separable domain, *Neuron*, 13, 671, 1994.

100. Wallner, M., Meera, P., and Toro, L., Determinant for β-subunit regulation in high-conductance voltage-activated and Ca^{2+}-sensitive K^+ channels: an additional transmembrane region at the N terminus, *Proc. Natl. Acad. Sci. U.S.A.*, 93, 14922, 1996.

101. Riazi, M.A. et al., Identification of a putative regulatory subunit of a calcium-activated potassium channel in the dup (3q) syndrome region and a related sequence on 22q11.2, *Genomics*, 62, 90, 1999.

102. Meera, P., Wallner, M., and Toro, L., A neuronal β subunit (KCNMB4) makes the large conductance, voltage- and Ca^{2+}-activated K^+ channel resistant to charybdotoxin and iberiotoxin, *Proc. Natl. Acad. Sci. U.S.A.*, 97, 5562, 2000.

103. Joiner, W.J. et al., hSK4, a member of a novel subfamily of calcium-activated potassium channels, *Proc. Natl. Acad. Sci. U.S.A.*, 94, 11013, 1997.

104. Keen, J.E. et al., Domains responsible for constitutive and Ca^{2+}-dependent interactions between calmodulin and small conductance Ca^{2+}-activated potassium channels, *J. Neurosci.*, 19, 8830, 1999.

105. Xia, X.M. et al., Mechanism of calcium gating in small-conductance calcium-activated potassium channels, *Nature*, 395, 503, 1998.

106. Lorenz, E. et al., Evidence for direct physical association between a K^+ channel (Kir6.2) and an ATP-binding cassette protein (SUR1) which affects cellular distribution and kinetic behavior of an ATP-sensitive K^+ channel, *Mol. Cell Biol.*, 18, 1652, 1998.

107. Fujita, A. and Kurachi, Y., Molecular aspects of ATP-sensitive K^+ channels in the cardiovascular system and K^+ channel openers, *Pharmacol. Ther.*, 85, 39, 2000.

108. Jan, L.Y. and Jan, Y., Potassium channels and their evolving gates, *Nature*, 371, 119, 1994.

109. Kerr, I.D. and Sansom, M.S.P., Cation selectivity in ion channels, *Nature*, 373, 112, 1995.

110. Raab–Graham, K.F. et al., Membrane topology of the amino-terminal region of the sulfonylurea receptor, *J. Biol. Chem.*, 274, 29122, 1999.

111. Aguilar–Bryan, L. et al., Cloning of the β cell high-affinity sulphonylurea receptor: a regulator of insulin secretion, *Science*, 268, 423, 1995.

112. Inagaki, N. et al., A family of sulphonylurea receptors determines the pharmacological properties of ATP-sensitive K^+ channels, *Neuron*, 16, 1011, 1996.

113. Ashcroft, F.M. and Gribble, F.M., Correlating structure and function in ATP-sensitive K^+ channels, *Trends Neurosci.*, 21, 288, 1998.

114. Uhde, I. et al., Identification of the potassium channel opener site on sulfonylurea receptors, *J. Biol. Chem.*, 274, 28079, 1999.

115. Inagaki, N., Inazawa, J., and Seino, S., cDNA sequence, gene structure, and chromosomal localization of the human ATP-sensitive potassium channel, uKATP-1, gene (KCNJ8), *Genomics*, 30, 102, 1995.

116. Cui, Y. et al., A mechanism for ATP-sensitive potassium channel diversity: functional co-assembly of two pore-forming subunits, *Proc. Natl. Acad. Sci. U.S.A.*, 98, 729, 2001.

117. Gribble, F.M. et al., Properties of cloned ATP-sensitive K^+ currents expressed in *Xenopus* oocytes, *J. Physiol. (Lond.)*, 498, 87, 1997.

118. Tucker, S.J. et al., Truncation of Kir6.2 produces ATP-sensitive K^+ channels in the absence of the sulphonylurea receptor, *Nature*, 387, 179, 1997.

119. Wang, R., Wang, Z.Z., and Wu, L., Carbon monoxide-induced vasorelaxation and the underlying mechanisms, *Br. J. Pharmacol.*, 121, 927, 1997.

120. Wang, R., Wu, L., and Wang, Z.Z., The direct effect of carbon monoxide on K_{Ca} channels in vascular smooth muscle cells, *Pflügers Arch.*, 434, 285, 1997.

121. Leinders, T., Van Kleef, R.G.D.M., and Vijverberg, H.P.M., Divalent cations activate small- (SK) and large-conductance (BK) channels in mouse neuroblastoma cells: selective activation of SK channels by cadmium, *Pflügers Arch.*, 422, 217, 1992.

122. Leffler, C.W. et al., Carbon monoxide and cerebral microvascular tone in newborn pigs, *Am. J. Physiol.*, 276, H1641, 1999.

123. Trischmann, U. et al., Carbon monoxide inhibits depolarization-induced Ca rise and increases cyclic GMP in visceral smooth muscle cells, *Biochem. Pharmacol.*, 41, 237, 1991.

124. Werkstrom, V. et al., Carbon monoxide-induced relaxation and distribution of haem oxygenase isoenzymes in the pig urethra and lower oesophagogastric junction, *Br. J. Pharmacol.*, 120, 312, 1997.

125. Zygmunt, P.M. and Hogestatt, E.D., Role of potassium channels in endothelium-dependent relaxation resistant to nitroarginine in the rat hepatic artery, *Br. J. Pharmacol.*, 117, 1600, 1996.

126. Yang, F. and Phillips, G.N., Jr., Crystal structures of CO-, deoxy- and met-myoglobins at various pH values, *J. Mol. Biol.*, 8, 762, 1996.

127. Sun, J. et al., Resonance Raman and EPR spectroscopic studies on heme–heme oxygenase complexes, *Biochemistry*, 33, 13734, 1994.

128. Wang, R. and Wu, L., The chemical modification of K_{Ca} channels by carbon monoxide in vascular smooth muscle cells, *J. Biol. Chem.*, 272, 8222, 1997.

129. Kenyon, G.L. and Bruice, T.W., Novel sulfhydryl reagents, in *Methods in Enzymology*, Colowick, S.P. and Kaplan N.O., Eds., Academic Press, New York, 1977, 407.

130. Bolotina, V. et al., Nitric oxide directly activates calcium-dependent potassium channels in vascular smooth muscle, *Nature*, 368, 850, 1994.

131. Oberhauser, A., Alvarez, O., and Latorre, R., Activation by divalent cations of a Ca^{2+}-activated K^+ channel from skeletal muscle membrane, *J. Gen. Physiol.*, 92, 67, 1988.

132. Pappone, P.A. and Barchfeld, G.L., Modifications of single acetylcholine-activated channels in BC3H-1 cells, *J. Gen. Physiol.*, 96,1, 1990.

133. Sigworth, F.J. and Spalding, B.C., Chemical modification reduces the conductance of sodium channels in nerve, *Nature*, 283, 293, 1980.
134. Worley, J.F., French, R.J., and Krueger, B.K., Trimethyloxonium modification of single batrachotoxin-activated sodium channels in planar bilayers, *J. Gen. Physiol.*, 87, 327, 1986.
135. MacKinnon, R. and Miller, C., Functional modification of a Ca^{2+}-activated K^+ channel by trimethyloxonium, *Biochemistry*, 28, 8087, 1989.

6 Nitric Oxide and the Heme Oxygenase/Carbon Monoxide System: Cooperation in the Control of Vascular Function

Roberta Foresti, Colin J. Green, and Roberto Motterlini

CONTENTS

I. INTRODUCTION

Although we have known since the 1950s that carbon monoxide (CO) is generated by the human body,[1] only in the last ten years have scientists considered the possibility that this gaseous molecule might have biologically active properties. In fact, many articles now published discuss the role of CO as a modulator of vessel tone,[2-5] platelet aggregation,[6] as an anti-apoptotic agent,[7] and as a neurotransmitter.[8,9] The main endogenous source of CO is heme oxygenase, the enzyme responsible for degradation of heme in tissue.[10] The heme oxygenase (HO) family includes three different isoforms: HO-1 or inducible enzyme, HO-2 or constitutive enzyme, and HO-3, a recently identified constitutive form that is a poor heme catalyst.[11,12] During heme breakdown, HO-2 and HO-1 also release iron (Fe^{2+}) and biliverdin, which is then reduced to bilirubin by biliverdin reductase.[11,13]

Nitric oxide (NO) is another signaling gas produced intracellularly by NO synthase using L-arginine as a substrate.[14,15] The great importance of this molecule has already been established in the control of smooth muscle tone, apoptosis, neurotransmission, host response to infection, and many other physiological processes.[16] It is interesting that both CO and NO possess similar functions and can be simultaneously generated by the same tissue (e.g., cardiovascular system, brain, testis).[11] Even more intriguing is the fact that NO affects the expression and activity of heme oxygenase and that heme oxygenase, by virtue of controlling the availability of intracellular heme, may regulate NO synthase activity and NO function.[17] These observations raise important questions about the relationship between the two systems and suggest a strong interdependence of CO and NO in their physiological actions. This chapter will discuss how the heme oxygenase and the NO synthase pathways are closely interrelated and will highlight the consequences of this relationship in the context of the cardiovascular system.

II. EXPRESSION OF HEME OXYGENASES AND NO SYNTHASES IN THE CARDIOVASCULAR SYSTEM

The protein expression and localization of HO in vascular tissue have been investigated mainly in animal studies. It appears that HO-2 is a subtype of heme oxygenase predominantly expressed in both endothelial and smooth muscle layers of blood vessels under normal conditions.[3,11] Therefore, it seems that the vascular tissue has an intrinsic capacity to produce basal levels of CO, especially if one considers that hemoglobin may also be a readily available source of heme as a substrate for HO activity. HO-2 is not present in cardiac muscle.[18] Apart from glucocorticoids,[19] no other known stimuli up-regulate HO-2 and more investigations are required to explore whether disease states targeting the cardiovascular system also affect the expression or the activity of HO-2 protein. Although further studies are needed to characterize HO-3, Northern hybridization reveals that the message of the enzyme is present in all tissues examined, including the heart.[12] It is not yet possible to make a distinction about the subtype of cells expressing the protein.

Concerning the inducible isoform (HO-1), many reports have shown induction of this enzyme in endothelium, smooth muscle, and even myocytes.[20-27] Thus, HO-1 is hardly detectable in vascular tissue under physiological situations, but many stressful stimuli can strongly up-regulate the protein to very high levels. Conditions that influence HO-1 expression include endotoxins,[28,29] hemorrhagic shock,[30] ischemia–reperfusion,[27] and hypoxia.[31-33] The induction of HO-1 appears to be a fundamental defensive system to counteract cellular and tissue damage and the importance of this protein in the maintenance of vascular function is best exemplified by the first case of human HO-1 deficiency described in the literature.[34] The patient suffered severe growth retardation, hemolytic anemia, and iron deposition in hepatic and renal tissue, but the finding of interest was the presence of persistent endothelial damage and detachment of the endothelium from renal glomeruli membranes.[34] This indicates that expression of HO-1 and the ability to induce HO-1 following stress insults have fundamental consequences for the integrity of the endothelium and may have relevant repercussions for proper vascular activities. In fact, this first internal layer of blood vessels constitutes a barrier for selective absorption of substances from blood and actively contributes to the regulation of many physiological processes such as production of vasoactive factors and expression of adhesion molecules. The HO-1-deficient patient also exhibited hyperlipidemia, with high cholesterol and triglyceride levels, suggesting that lack of HO-1 may predispose an individual to the development of cardiovascular disease. Although few published studies discussed the localization of heme oxygenases in humans, the picture that emerges is that the expression of HO-1 is mainly associated with pathophysiological conditions such as Alzheimer's and Parkinson's diseases,[35-37] atherosclerosis,[38] malignant melanomas,[39] and portal hypertension.[40] HO-1 and HO-2 have also been detected in the myometria of pregnant women[41] and human term placentae.[42]

NO synthase and HO-2 are co-localized in vascular endothelial cells and in some enteric neurons,[3] and NO and CO appear to act as co-neurotransmitters in the enteric nervous system.[43] Smooth muscle cells were depolarized in HO-2 and neuronal NO synthase null mice; the double null mice (HO-2 and neuronal NO synthase) manifested additional depolarization, reflecting additive effects of the two enzymes. Electrical field stimulation of jejunal smooth muscle strips from HO-2 null mice hardly produced any response despite expression of NO synthase. However, application of exogenous CO restored normal relaxation, indicating that the NO system does not function in the absence of CO generation. The authors suggested that CO may sensitize intestinal smooth muscle to the effects of NO. It is possible that NO and HO-2-derived CO act similarly to control vascular tone under normal conditions.

In stress situations characterized by high expression of HO-1, CO may become predominant in the modulation of endogenous processes. Indeed, we have shown that increased vascular CO production following HO-1 up-regulation suppresses acute hypertensive responses *in vivo*[5] and vasoconstriction in a model of isolated aortic rings.[4] Interestingly, the use of NO synthase inhibitors did not restore vessel contractility, emphasizing the concept that some NO functions can be temporarily annulled by the presence of high CO levels. Why and how this happens is uncertain, but it may indicate that an overall balance between the generation of the two signaling molecules must be maintained in order not to exceed a critical threshold — important for preventing tissue damage. In other words, too much of both CO and NO or over-stimulation of the transduction mechanisms by the two gases would probably result in an insult too aggressive to be tolerated by cells or organs.

In some circumstances, however, HO-1 and the inducible isoform of NO synthase (iNOS) are up-regulated in the same tissue by the same stimuli. In fact, HO-1 and iNOS genes are responsive to bacterial endotoxins, cytokines, and reactive oxygen species.[11] Transcriptional activation of iNOS and HO-1 genes was observed upon stimulation of murine macrophages with interferon-γ and lipopolysaccharide[44] and in rat liver subjected to ischemia–reperfusion.[45] We recently reported that hypoxia induces the expression of iNOS and HO-1 in bovine aortic endothelial cells[33]; by analyzing the temporal pattern that characterizes this phenomenon, we found that the increase in iNOS protein precedes HO-1 induction. This peculiarity appears to be extendible also to rat organs, in which endotoxic shock causes iNOS induction before HO-1 expression.[46] Our laboratory found similar preliminary results in rat aorta following endotoxin administration.[29]

These findings point to a direct relationship between the CO- and NO- generating systems and their mutual influence in controlling physiological and non-physiological processes. However, more investigations are necessary to fully elucidate the role of the two pathways in cardiovascular tissue and, ultimately, to determine the significance of CO production in the human body.

III. COMMON TARGETS FOR CO AND NO

One reason to support the hypothesis of cooperation between CO and NO is that the two molecules exert their effects through a common signal transduction mechanism. Soluble guanylate cyclase, which produces cGMP from guanosine triphosphate, is a heme-containing protein that can be activated by CO and NO.[47-49] The interaction of NO with the heme moiety of guanylate cyclase to increase cGMP is an established and powerful mode of action for NO in modulating vasorelaxation, neurotransmission, and platelet aggregation.[49] Admittedly, CO is a relatively weak stimulator of guanylate cyclase in *in vitro* studies when compared to NO[47]; on the other hand, many reports indicate that HO-1 induction and increased CO generation result in augmented cGMP levels in several *ex vivo* and *in vivo* models.[4,5,50] In addition, the co-localization of HO-2 and guanylate cyclase in certain neuron populations strongly suggests a direct role for CO in enhancing cGMP production.[11,51]

Studies have also shown that YC-1, a benzylindazole derivative, can sensitize guanylate cyclase to CO and potentiate CO-mediated stimulation of cGMP production to the same extent as NO.[52] Whether a naturally synthesized substance similar to YC-1 exists intracellularly remains to be ascertained. The fact that NO and CO can up-regulate cGMP levels greatly enhances the magnitude of effects exerted by the two gaseous molecules, since cGMP is a second messenger that regulates the concentration of cAMP by activating or inhibiting cAMP-specific phosphodiesterases, opens cyclic-nucleotide-gated cation channels, and activates a whole series of cGMP-dependent protein kinases.[53]

NO and CO may also act as signaling molecules by utilizing common targets different from guanylate cyclase. For example, calcium-dependent potassium channels in smooth muscle cells can be activated by both gases[54]; chemical modification of sulfhydryl groups present on the channels mediate the action of NO whereas CO seems to specifically affect histidine residues of the channel extracellular domain.[55] The consequence of this interaction is NO- or CO-induced vascular relaxation independent from cGMP.[54,56,57] Experiments performed to evaluate the responses of calcium-dependent potassium channels exposed simultaneously to NO and CO should clarify the contribution of each gas to the vasodilatory effect.

Another protein known to combine with NO and CO is hemoglobin. NO can associate with either the reduced (ferrous) or oxidized (ferric or met) form of the protein, while CO only binds ferrous hemoglobin.[58] The affinity of hemoglobin for NO is 1500 times that for CO, because the rate of CO dissociation from the protein is much faster than that of NO.[58,59] Furthermore, hemoglobin appears capable of binding NO not only to the heme groups, but also to cysteine 93 of the β-chain forming S-nitrosohemoglobin.[60] This reaction has been suggested to provide a protective route for delivery of bioactive NO in the organism.

Oxyhemoglobin can also interact with NO to produce nitrate, thereby inactivating vascular NO and producing methemoglobin.[61] However, Gow and colleagues challenged this generally accepted chemistry of hemoglobin by proposing that, under physiological conditions, NO binds instead to the minor population of the hemoglobin's vacant hemes (nitrosylates or thiols) in a cooperative manner, or reacts with superoxide present in solution.[62] Interestingly, cardiac myoglobin reacts with NO to form metmyoglobin and nitrate, in a mechanism aimed at reducing the effective cytosolic NO concentration and protecting cardiac performance against transient increases in NO levels.[63] Thus, considering that myoglobin is present in the heart and skeletal muscle in large quantities, the authors hypothesize that the protein may underlie a process for NO turnover of the entire organism alternative and additional to hemoglobin. These exciting and new discoveries are rapidly enlarging and shaping our view on the functions of hemoglobin and myoglobin in respect to NO and oxygen.

Little is known about the chemistry of CO and the common perspective of the cellular action of this gas is still based on early studies with hemoglobin and myoglobin. Therefore, CO at non-physiological levels is used in many experiments involving heme-containing proteins, but detailed investigations of the effects of HO-derived CO are still lacking. An important and useful tool that has helped to accelerate the research on NO has been the development of NO donors; likewise, accessibility to CO-releasing molecules that allow us to precisely mimic physiological or pathophysiological conditions of CO production would greatly benefit the fields of CO and HO research. Our laboratory has been working for some time on the development of such compounds and more details can be found in Chapter 14.

Recent reports highlighted the ability of CO to mediate cellular effects via mitogen-activated protein (MAP) kinase pathways.[7,64] Otterbein and colleagues showed that exogenously applied CO selectively inhibits the expression of the proinflammatory cytokines TNF-α, IL-1β and MIP-1β while increasing the antiinflammatory cytokine IL-10 both *in vitro* and *in vivo*.[64] This effect appeared to be independent of CO-induced cGMP production and involved the specific activation of p38 MAP kinase. Similarly, the same group observed that activation of p38 MAP kinase is the mechanism underlying suppression of endothelial apoptosis by CO.[7] In line with the idea that NO and CO interact with common targets, it has been demonstrated that NO and NO-related species promote phosphorylation and activate p38 MAP kinase to modulate a variety of intracellular processes, including apoptosis[65,66] and inflammatory actions.[67] Interestingly, NO seems to induce HO-1 expression via involvement of the MAP kinase ERK and p38 pathways.[68]

Despite the emerging experimental evidence indicating that NO and CO share many signal transduction pathways, more investigations are needed to identify the chemical reactions characterizing these events; it is reasonable to expect diverse modes of action for NO and CO, since their chemical reactivity and redox properties are extremely different.

IV. EFFECTS OF NO ON HEME OXYGENASES

NO exerts different effects on the various isoforms of heme oxygenases. NO and NO donors are strong inducers of HO-1 expression and the mechanism depends on *de novo* synthesis of RNA and protein. We and others established that in many different tissues, in *in vitro*, *ex vivo* and *in vivo* models, exposure to these agents results in increased HO activity,[4,22,23,25,69-74] suggesting that this may be a generalized response elicited by NO. We have postulated that NO may serve as a signaling molecule to modulate the tissue stress response and that the interaction of NO with the HO pathway represents an endogenous adaptation to restore cellular homeostasis.[17]

Recently published observations also emphasize a role for NO in stabilizing HO-1 mRNA in cell culture; an NO scavenger (CPTIO) completely prevented NO-mediated HO-1 induction,[75] pointing to a direct role for NO in this effect. This is not surprising; we previously demonstrated that, by using hydroxocobalamin as another NO scavenger, NO is the essential element in HO-1 up-regulation by NO donors.[23] We found that increased intra- and extra-cellular thiol groups considerably abolish the elevated HO-1 expression obtained after exposure of endothelial cells to sodium nitroprusside (SNP) and S-nitroso-N-penicillamine (SNAP).[23]

A strong correlation between HO-1 induction and thiols was reported in early investigations by Lautier and colleagues, who showed that depletion of endogenous glutathione enhanced HO-1 levels.[76] It is thought that, by diminishing the most abundant intracellular antioxidant defense (glutathione), cells and tissues need to counteract oxidative challenge by increasing alternative antioxidant systems and one of those could be represented by HO-1. However, we believe that NO also occupies a relevant position in this equilibrium, since thiol groups are highly susceptible to attack by NO. In fact, thiols seem to be involved in NO binding, stabilization, and transport in biological systems[60,77]

A striking example of these functions is described by Pawloski and colleagues.[78] They showed that transfer of the NO group can occur between the cysteine residues of S-nitroso-hemoglobin present in red blood cells and cysteines in the membrane-bound anion exchanger AE1,[78] possibly identifying the first step in the export of NO bioactivity from erythrocytes. We confirmed the importance of the NO–thiol interaction in mediating HO-1 induction in endothelial cells subjected to severe hypoxia. Among the various antioxidants used in our study, N-acetylcysteine was the only compound capable of completely suppressing increased HO activity by low oxygen tension.[33] This effect was accompanied by oxidation of glutathione and formation of S-nitrosothiols, paralleled by up-regulation of iNOS and NO synthase activity. These findings indicate that control of HO-1 gene expression may also rely on NO-induced stress (nitrosative stress) in a manner independent from oxidant mediators; we suggest that the HO-1 pathway may represent a cellular adaptation to the threat imposed by increased NO and NO-related species.

Although it has been proven that NO gas and different NO donors are efficient stimulators of HO-1, the fact that NO can exist in many redox activated forms (i.e., NO^+, NO^- and $NO^{\bullet}$) and can react quickly with superoxide to yield peroxynitrite[79] still leaves an open question as to the exact species involved in this effect. We employed NO donors that have (1) strong NO^+ character (SNP)[22,23,71,72]; (2) the ability to release NO^+, NO^-, or $NO^{\bullet}$, depending on reaction conditions (SNAP and S-nitrosoglutathione)[4,22,23,33]; and (3) the ability to release stoichiometric amounts of NO and superoxide (3-morpholinosydnonimine).[22,23,70] We also used pure peroxynitrite[23,80] and recently we tested Angeli's salt, a compound that liberates NO^- in solution (unpublished observations). The strong correlation we have been able to establish is between the levels of heme oxygenase activity and the stability of the different NO donors.[23] Specifically, the more NO group released by the compound, the higher the observed HO activity. We do not know whether any NO-related species liberated by NO donors is transformed extra- or intracellularly into the same unique NO congener that induces HO-1 or whether multiple mechanisms are implicated in this effect.

From a perspective of NO reactivity, HO-1 greatly differs from HO-2. In fact, HO-1 does not contain cysteine residues, whereas two conserved cysteines are present in the heme binding motif of HO-2.[11] HO-3, which awaits further characterization, also possesses cysteines. It can then be inferred that HO-2 may be a more sensitive target than HO-1 with respect to NO. Ding and colleagues published an interesting article on the interaction of HO-2 with NO donors.[81] Exposure of HO-2 purified from *E. coli* to various NO donors (including SIN-1) resulted in a red shift of the Soret band (from 405 nm to 413 to 419 nm) of the protein. NO appears to cause these changes by combining with heme bound to HO-2 heme motifs and this reaction leads to considerable loss of HO-2 catalytic activity. HO-2 mutants (Cys/Cys to Ala/Ala), in which heme motifs are absent, are virtually unaffected by NO donors and the enzymatic activity of purified HO-1 is also refractory to the treatment. Although the mechanism of HO-2 sensitivity to NO is dependent on the high-affinity binding of heme to heme motifs, this work provides evidence that cysteines are important elements in determining the susceptibility of HO-2 to external NO attack.

In a collaborative study investigating diaphragmatic contractility of rats treated with endotoxins, we observed an interesting biphasic pattern of HO activity.[82] During the first 12 h after endotoxin administration, a transient decrease in activity occurred; the effect was particularly evident at 6 h, with a 33% decrement compared to control. However, at 24 and 48 h, heme oxygenase activity increased above basal levels resulting from induction of HO-1. Interestingly, these changes reflected the course of the pathological state. The initial decreased activity was associated with muscle failure and the late increase contributed to the recovery of muscle function. HO-1 and HO-2 were expressed in the control diaphragms and both isoforms likely contributed to basal HO activity. In view of the findings by Ding and co-workers[81] and considering that an early rise in NO production and peroxynitrite has been reported in the diaphragms of endotoxemic rats,[83,84] we postulate that the transient reduction of activity was the consequence of HO-2 protein inactivation, since these nitrogen species do not influence HO-1 catalytic activity.

The effect of NO on heme catabolism may also be independent of the interaction of NO with HO enzymes. In fact, NO can complex with heme and the formation of nitrosyl-heme appears to inhibit heme degradation by HO. Juckett and colleagues[85] showed that incubation of HO-1-rich microsomes with NO donors causes a concentration-dependent inhibition of HO activity. The authors hypothesized that this might be a transient event and, as the concentration of NO declines, the nitrosyl-hemes will dissociate and free heme would be available as substrate for HO and inducers of HO-1.

We recently performed experiments by exposing endothelial cells to hemin in the presence of NO donors. By measuring the accumulation of bilirubin in the culture medium, we found that this treatment enhanced bilirubin production compared to production observed in cells incubated with hemin alone (unpublished observations). In addition, HO activity and heme up-take increased in cells treated with hemin and NO donors compared to hemin alone. Our findings are in sharp contrast with those presented by Juckett and colleagues[85] and more investigations are required to shed light on this complicated issue.

V. EFFECTS OF CO ON NO SYNTHASES

Exogenous CO has been proven to inhibit macrophage and neuronal NO synthase activity,[86] based on the fact that NO synthase is a P-450 type of hemeprotein and the heme present in the enzyme is involved in the mechanism of conversion of L-arginine to citrulline and NO. Further direct *in vitro* measurements of NO production by endothelial NO synthase with an NO-selective microelectrode confirmed that application of CO produces a concentration-dependent suppression of NO generation.[87] Some evidence indicates that endogenous CO derived from HO-2 may exert similar effects.

In internal anal sphincter smooth muscle strips, 1 μM zinc protoporphyrin IX (an inhibitor of HO activity) increased NO production, suggesting that the HO pathway exerts an important counter-regulation of NO synthase under physiological conditions.[88] Another way for CO to modulate NO levels has been described recently. Exposure of endothelial cells to environmentally relevant CO concentrations augmented the release of NO and resulted in formation of cytotoxic NO-related species, such as peroxynitrite.[89,90] CO did not appear to alter NO synthase activity, and the authors reason that CO may increase the steady state levels of NO by competing for intracellular binding sites. A similar conclusion was reached by Thorup and co-workers, who showed that renal resistance arteries release NO upon perfusion with buffer containing low levels of CO and react to this stimulus by vasodilating; they postulate that the source of NO liberated in response to CO is most likely a pre-existing intracellular heme-bound pool of NO.[87] The progress in this field of research is expected to bring exciting new developments for the understanding of physiological processes controlled by the HO/CO pathway.

VI. HEME OXYGENASES:
MODULATORS OF NO FUNCTIONS

NO is a fast-reacting gas molecule and many of its biological functions are likely related to this chemical property. We can imagine that this characteristic of NO may result in the propagation of detrimental effects, especially when the levels of NO exceed thresholds critical for cell survival. Therefore, intracellularly constitutive and inducible systems able to control NO generation and action must exist. Among the potential systems, the HO pathway possesses the prerequisites to fulfill such a role. As mentioned above, exogenous CO inhibits NO synthase activity and it is reasonable to suggest that even HO-derived CO produces a similar inhibition. This blockade of NO formation might become more relevant in stress conditions in which HO-1 is up-regulated and the generation of CO is considerably enhanced. Since NO synthase is a heme-containing protein, the degradation of heme by HO may represent an additional mechanism controlling its activity.

Supporting this idea are interesting results by Albakri and co-workers, who showed that macrophages stimulated by cytokines to express iNOS contain only a small percentage of dimeric active enzyme 8 h after stimulation, and NO appears to mediate this process by preventing heme insertion and heme availability.[91] Since cytokines and NO also induce HO-1 protein, it should not be surprising that HO-1 may contribute to this effect.

Finally, a scientific basis exists for the hypothesis that bilirubin and biliverdin may act as NO scavengers. These bile pigments contain extended systems of conjugated double bonds and reactive hydrogen atoms that are susceptible to a wide range of redox reactions. From a chemical point of view, the carbon at position 10 of the linear tetrapyrrole appears to be the most reactive.

We have already reported that increased bilirubin levels following HO-1 induction in endothelial cells are associated with a marked reduction in apoptosis caused by peroxynitrite, an NO derivative with strong oxidant and nitrosative characteristics.[80] We also demonstrated that bilirubin reacts with different NO-releasing agents, and observed that all redox-activated forms of NO (i.e., NO^+, $NO^\bullet$, and NO^-) interact with bilirubin, albeit to different extents.[92] The kinetics and mechanisms of this reaction are currently under investigation in our laboratory. More studies are needed to confirm these ideas, but the above findings and considerations make it rational to suggest that HO constitutes a fundamental NO-detoxifying system, with the ultimate aim to regulate the action of NO in signal transduction.

VII. CONCLUSIONS

Since the discovery a few years ago that NO and NO donors are capable of inducing HO-1 expression, a new field of investigation has opened for HO research. Many questions remain to be answered, and the overall significance of this phenomenon in the context of the cardiovascular and other systems must be fully established. We believe that the interaction of the NO synthase and the HO pathway is of great importance in the modulation of physiological processes, and progress in this area will depend on advances in NO research.

Although NO can affect cellular functions through a direct pharmacological action on signal transduction pathways, it will become increasingly evident that many long-lasting effects mediated by NO occur through the participation of HO and their CO and bilirubin products. It was not the aim of this chapter to emphasize a role of bilirubin. However, during heme degradation by HO, three distinct products with different characteristics are generated. We can only envision that explanation of many experimental results will be possible if concerted actions of CO, iron, and biliverdin/bilirubin are taken into consideration when analyzing specific physiological or pathophysiological events.

ACKNOWLEDGMENTS

We would like to thank the funding bodies that supported our research: the National Heart Research Fund (to R.M.), the National Kidney Research Fund (R30/1/99 to R.M.), the British Heart Foundation (PG/99005 to R.M. and PG/2000047 to R.F.), the Dunhill Medical Trust, and the Northwick Park Institute for Medical Research. We also thank all our collaborators at the Northwick Park Institute for Medical Research for their contributions to the studies carried out in the laboratory.

REFERENCES

1. Sjostrand, T., Endogenous formation of carbon monoxide in man under normal and pathological conditions, *Scan. J. Clin. Lab. Invest.*, 1, 201, 1949.
2. Furchgott, R.F. and Jothianandan, D., Endothelium-dependent and -independent vasodilation involving cGMP: relaxation induced by nitric oxide, carbon monoxide and light, *Blood Vessels*, 28, 52, 1991.
3. Zakhary, R. et al., Heme oxygenase 2: endothelial and neuronal localization and role in endothelium-dependent relaxation, *Proc. Natl. Acad. Sci. U.S.A.*, 93, 795, 1996.
4. Sammut, I.A. et al., Carbon monoxide is a major contributor to the regulation of vascular tone in aortas expressing high levels of haeme oxygenase-1, *Br. J. Pharmacol.*, 125, 1437, 1998.
5. Motterlini, R. et al., Heme oxygenase-1-derived carbon monoxide contributes to the suppression of acute hypertensive responses *in vivo*, *Circ. Res.*, 83, 568, 1998.
6. Wagner, C.T. et al., Hemodynamic forces induce the expression of heme oxygenase in cultured vascular smooth muscle cells, *J. Clin. Invest.*, 100, 589, 1997.
7. Brouard, S. et al., Carbon monoxide generated by heme oxygenase 1 suppresses endothelial cell apoptosis, *J. Exp. Med.*, 192, 1015, 2000.
8. Verma, A. et al., Carbon monoxide: a putative neural messenger, *Science*, 259, 381, 1993.
9. Maines, M.D., Carbon monoxide: an emerging regulator of cGMP in the brain, *Mol. Cell. Neurosci.*, 4, 389, 1993.
10. Tenhunen, R., Marver, H.S., and Schmid, R., Microsomal heme oxygenase. Characterization of the enzyme, *J. Biol. Chem.*, 244, 6388, 1969.
11. Maines, M.D., The heme oxygenase system: a regulator of second messenger gases, *Annu. Rev. Pharmacol. Toxicol.*, 37, 517, 1997.
12. McCoubrey, W.K., Huang, T.J., and Maines, M.D., Isolation and characterization of a cDNA from the rat brain that encodes hemoprotein heme oxygenase-3, *Eur. J. Biochem.*, 247, 725, 1997.

13. Liu, Y. and Ortiz de Montellano, P.R., Reaction intermediates and single turnover rate constants for the oxidation of heme by human heme oxygenase-1, *J. Biol. Chem.*, 275, 5297, 2000.
14. Ignarro, L.J., Buga, G.M., and Wood, K.S., Endothelium-derived relaxing factor produced and released from artery and vein is nitric oxide, *Proc. Natl. Acad. Sci. U.S.A.*, 84, 9265, 1987.
15. Palmer, R.M.J., Ferrige, A.G., and Moncada, S., Nitric oxide release accounts for the biological activity of endothelium-derived relaxing factor, *Nature*, 327, 524, 1987.
16. Darley–Usmar, V.M. et al., Nitric oxide, free radicals and cell signaling in cardiovascular disease, *Biochem. Soc. Trans.*, 25, 925, 1997.
17. Foresti, R. and Motterlini, R., The heme oxygenase pathway and its interaction with nitric oxide in the control of cellular homeostasis, *Free Rad. Res.*, 31, 459, 1999.
18. Grozdanovic, Z. and Gossrau, R., Expression of heme oxygenase-2 (HO-2)-like immunoreactivity in rat- tissues, *Acta Histochemica*, 98, 203, 1996.
19. Maines, M.D., Eke, B.C., and Zhao, X.D., Corticosterone promotes increased heme oxygenase-2 protein and transcript expression in the newborn rat brain, *Brain Res.*, 722, 83, 1996.
20. Balla, J. et al., Endothelial-cell heme uptake from heme proteins: induction of sensitization and desensitization to oxidant damage, *Proc. Natl. Acad. Sci. U.S.A.*, 90, 9285, 1993.
21. Motterlini, R. et al., Oxidative-stress response in vascular endothelial cells exposed to acellular hemoglobin solutions, *Am. J. Physiol.*, 269, H648, 1995.
22. Motterlini, R. et al., NO-mediated activation of heme oxygenase: endogenous cytoprotection against oxidative stress to endothelium, *Am. J. Physiol.*, 270, H107, 1996.
23. Foresti, R. et al., Thiol compounds interact with nitric oxide in regulating heme oxygenase-1 induction in endothelial cells. Involvement of superoxide and peroxynitrite anions, *J. Biol. Chem.*, 272, 18411, 1997.
24. Durante, W. et al., Nitric oxide induces heme oxygenase-1 expression in vascular smooth cells, *FASEB J.*, 10, 1744, 1996.
25. Hartsfield, C.L. et al., Regulation of heme oxygenase-1 gene expression in vascular smooth muscle cells by nitric oxide, *Am. J. Physiol.*, 273, L980, 1997.
26. Ewing, J.F., Raju, V.S., and Maines, M.D., Induction of heart heme oxygenase-1 (HSP32) by hyperthermia: possible role in stress-mediated elevation of cyclic 3':5'-guanosine monophosphate, *J. Pharmacol. Exp. Ther.*, 271, 408, 1994.
27. Raju, V.S. and Maines, M.D., Renal ischemia/reperfusion up-regulates heme oxygenase-1 (HSP32) expression and increases cGMP in rat heart, *J. Pharmacol. Exp. Ther.*, 277, 1814, 1996.
28. Yet, S.F. et al., Induction of heme oxygenase-1 expression in vascular smooth muscle cells. A link to endotoxic shock, *J. Biol. Chem.*, 272, 4295, 1997.
29. Foresti, R. et al., Heme oxygenase-1 is partially responsible for decreased vascular contractility mediated by endotoxin, in *The Biology of Nitric Oxide, Part 7*, Moncada, S. et al., Eds., Portland Press, London, 2000, 58.
30. Pannen, B.H.J. et al., Protective role of endogenous carbon monoxide in hepatic microcirculatory dysfunction after hemorrhagic shock in rats, *J. Clin. Invest.*, 102, 1220, 1998.
31. Morita, T. et al., Smooth muscle cell-derived carbon monoxide is a regulator of vascular cGMP, *Proc. Natl. Acad. Sci. U.S.A.*, 92, 1475, 1995.
32. Lee, P.J. et al., Hypoxia-inducible factor-1 mediates transcriptional activation of the heme oxygenase-1 gene in response to hypoxia, *J. Biol. Chem.*, 272, 5375, 1997.

33. Motterlini, R. et al., Endothelial heme oxygenase-1 induction by hypoxia: modulation by inducible nitric oxide synthase (iNOS) and S-nitrosothiols, *J. Biol. Chem.*, 275, 13613, 2000.
34. Yachie, A. et al., Oxidative stress causes enhanced endothelial cell injury in human heme oxygenase-1 deficiency, *J. Clin. Invest.*, 103, 129, 1999.
35. Premkumar, D.R. et al., Induction of heme oxygenase-1 mRNA and protein in neo-cortex and cerebral vessels in Alzheimer's disease, *J. Neurochem.*, 65, 1399, 1995.
36. Schipper, H.M., Liberman, A., and Stopa, E.G., Neural heme oxygenase-1 expression in idiopathic Parkinson's disease, *Exper. Neurol.*, 150, 60, 1998.
37. Ham, D. and Schipper, H.M., Heme oxygenase-1 induction and mitochondrial iron sequestration in astroglia exposed to amyloid peptides, *Cell Mol. Biol.*, 46, 587, 2000.
38. Wang, L.J. et al., Expression of heme oxygenase-1 in atherosclerotic lesions, *Am. J. Pathol.*, 152, 711, 1998.
39. Torisu–Itakura, H. et al., Co-expression of thymidine phosphorylase and heme oxygenase-1 in macrophages in human malignant vertical growth melanomas, *Jpn. J. Cancer Res.*, 91, 906, 2000.
40. Makino, N. et al., Altered expression of heme oxygenase-1 in the livers of patients with portal hypertensive diseases, *Hepatology*, 33, 32, 2001.
41. Acevedo, C.H. and Ahmed, A., Hemeoxygenase-1 inhibits human myometrial contractility via carbon monoxide and is up-regulated by progesterone during pregnancy, *J. Clin. Invest.*, 101, 949, 1998.
42. McLean, M. et al., Expression of the heme oxygenase-carbon monoxide signaling system in human placenta, *J. Clin. Endocrinol. Metab.*, 85, 2345, 2000.
43. Xue, L. et al., Carbon monoxide and nitric oxide as coneurotransmitters in the enteric nervous system: evidence from genomic deletion of biosynthetic enzymes, *Proc. Natl. Acad. Sci. U.S.A.*, 97, 1851, 2000.
44. Kurata, S., Matsumoto, M., and Yamashita, U., Concomitant transcriptional activation of nitric oxide synthase and heme oxygenase genes during nitric oxide-mediated macrophage cytostasis, *J. Biochem.*, 120, 49, 1996.
45. Sonin, N.V. et al., Patterns of vasoregulatory gene expression in the liver response to ischemia/reperfusion and endotoxemia, *Shock*, 11, 175, 1999.
46. Tomlinson, A. et al., Temporal and spatial expression of the inducible isoforms of cyclooxygenase, nitric oxide synthase and heme oxygenase in tissues from rats infused with LPS in the conscious state, *Br. J. Pharmacol.*, 123, P178, 1998.
47. Kharitonov, V.G. et al., Basis of guanylate cyclase activation by carbon monoxide, *Proc. Natl. Acad. Sci. U.S.A.*, 92, 2568, 1995.
48. Ignarro, L.J., Heme-dependent activation of soluble guanylate cyclase by nitric oxide: regulation of enzyme activity by porphyrins and metalloporphyrins, *Sem. Hematol.*, 26, 63, 1989.
49. Moncada, S., Palmer, R.M.J., and Higgs, E.A., Nitric oxide: physiology, pathophysiology, and pharmacology, *Pharmacol. Rev.*, 43, 109, 1991.
50. Suematsu, M. et al., Carbon monoxide: an endogenous modulator of sinusoidal tone in the perfused rat liver, *J. Clin. Invest.*, 96, 2431, 1995.
51. Snyder, S.H., Jaffrey, S.R., and Zakhary, R., Nitric oxide and carbon monoxide: parallel roles as neural messengers, *Brain Res. Rev.*, 26, 167, 1998.
52. Friebe, A., Schultz, G., and Koesling, D., Sensitizing soluble guanylyl cyclase to become a highly CO-sensitive enzyme, *EMBO J.*, 15, 6863, 1996.
53. Hofmann, F. et al., Rising behind NO: cGMP-dependent protein kinases, *J. Cell Sci*, 113, 1671, 2000.

54. Bolotina, V.M. et al., Nitric oxide directly activates calcium-dependent potassium channels in vascular smooth muscle, *Nature*, 368, 850, 1994.

55. Wang, R. and Wu, L., The chemical modification of K_{Ca} channels by carbon monoxide in vascular smooth muscle cells, *J. Biol. Chem.*, 272, 8222, 1997.

56. Homer, K.L. and Wanstall, J.C., Cyclic GMP-independent relaxation of rat pulmonary artery by spermine NONOate, a diazeniumdiolate nitric oxide donor, *Br. J. Pharmacol.*, 131, 673, 2000.

57. Wang, R., Wang, Z.Z., and Wu, L.Y., Carbon monoxide-induced vasorelaxation and the underlying mechanisms, *Br. J. Pharmacol.*, 121, 927, 1997.

58. Motterlini, R., Vandegriff, K., and Winslow, R., Hemoglobin-NO interaction and its implications, *Transf. Med. Rev.*, 10, 77, 1996.

59. Gibson, Q.H. and Roughton, F.J.W., The kinetics and equilibria of the reactions of nitric oxide with sheep hemoglobin, *J. Physiol.*, 136, 507, 1957.

60. Jia, L. et al., S-nitrosohaemoglobin: a dynamic activity of blood involved in vascular control, *Nature*, 380, 221, 1996.

61. Pietraforte, D. et al., Role of thiols in the targeting of S-nitroso thiols to red blood cells, *Biochemistry*, 34, 7177, 1995.

62. Gow, A.J. et al., The oxyhemoglobin reaction of nitric oxide, *Proc. Natl. Acad. Sci. U.S.A.*, 96, 9027, 1999.

63. Flogel, U. et al., Myoglobin: a scavenger of bioactive NO, *Proc. Natl. Acad. Sci U.S.A.*, 98, 735, 2001.

64. Otterbein, L.E. et al., Carbon monoxide has antiinflammatory effects involving the mitogen-activated protein kinase pathway, *Nat. Med.*, 6, 422, 2000.

65. Callsen, D. and Brune, B., Role of mitogen-activated protein kinases in S-nitroso-glutathione-induced macrophage apoptosis, *Biochemistry*, 38, 2279, 1999.

66. Jun, C.D. et al., Overexpression of protein kinase C isoforms protects RAW 264.7 macrophages from nitric oxide-induced apoptosis: involvement of c-Jun N-terminal kinase/stress-activated protein kinase, p38 kinase, and CPP-32 protease pathways, *J. Immunol.*, 162, 3395, 1999.

67. Muhl, H. et al., Nitric oxide augments release of chemokines from monocytic U937 cells: modulation by antiinflammatory pathways, *Free Radic. Biol. Med.*, 29, 969, 2000.

68. Chen, K. and Maines, M.D., Nitric oxide induces heme oxygenase-1 via mitogen-activated protein kinases ERK and p38, *Cell Mol. Biol.*, 46, 609, 2000.

69. Durante, W. et al., Nitric oxide induces heme oxygenase-1 gene expression and carbon monoxide production in vascular smooth muscle cells, *Circ. Res.*, 80, 557, 1997.

70. Motterlini, R. et al., A precursor of the nitric oxide donor SIN-1 modulates the stress protein heme oxygenase-1 in rat liver, *Biochem. Biophys. Res. Commun.*, 225, 167, 1996.

71. Clark, J.E., Green, C.J., and Motterlini, R., Involvement of the heme oxygenase–carbon monoxide pathway in keratinocyte proliferation, *Biochem. Biophys. Res. Commun.*, 241, 215, 1997.

72. Vesely, M.J.J. et al., Heme oxygenase-1 induction in skeletal muscle cells: hemin and sodium nitroprusside are regulators *in vitro*, *Am. J. Physiol.*, 275, C1087, 1998.

73. Hara, E. et al., Expression of heme oxygenase and inducible nitric oxide synthase messenger RNA in human brain tumors, *Biochem. Biophys. Res. Commun.*, 224, 153, 1996.

74. Immenschuh, S., Tan, M., and Ramadori, G., Nitric oxide mediates the lipopolysaccharide dependent up-regulation of the heme oxygenase-1 gene expression in cultured rat Kupffer cells, *J. Hepatology*, 30, 61, 1999.

75. Bouton, C. and Demple, B., Nitric oxide-inducible expression of heme oxygenase-1 in human cells. Translation-independent stabilization of the mrna and evidence for direct action of nitric oxide, *J. Biol. Chem.*, 275, 32688, 2000.

76. Lautier, D., Luscher, P., and Tyrrell, R.M., Endogenous glutathione levels modulate both constitutive and UVA radiation/hydrogen peroxide inducible expression of the human heme oxygenase gene, *Carcinogenesis*, 13, 227, 1992.

77. Stamler, J.S. et al., Nitric oxide circulates in mammalian plasma primarily as an S-nitroso adduct of serum albumin, *Proc. Natl. Acad. Sci. U.S.A.*, 89, 7674, 1992.

78. Pawloski, J.R., Hess, D.T., and Stamler, J.S., Export by red blood cells of nitric oxide bioactivity, *Nature*, 409, 622, 2001.

79. Stamler, J.S., Singel, D.J., and Loscalzo, J., Biochemistry of nitric oxide and its redox-activated forms, *Science*, 258, 1898, 1992.

80. Foresti, R. et al., Peroxynitrite induces haem oxygenase-1 in vascular endothelial cells: a link to apoptosis, *Biochem. J.*, 339, 729, 1999.

81. Ding, Y., McCoubrey, W.K., and Maines, M.D., Interaction of heme oxygenase-2 with nitric oxide donors. Is the oxygenase an intracellular "sink" for NO? *Eur. J. Biochem.*, 264, 854, 1999.

82. Taille, C. et al., Protective role of heme oxygenases against endotoxin-induced diaphragmatic dysfunction in rats, *Am. J. Resp. Crit. Care Med.*, 163, 753, 2001.

83. Boczkowski, J. et al., Induction of diaphragmatic nitric oxide synthase after endotoxin administration in rats. Role on diaphragmatic contractile dysfunction, *J. Clin. Invest.*, 98, 1550, 1996.

84. Boczkowski, J. et al., Endogenous peroxynitrite mediates mitochondrial dysfunction in rat diaphragm during endotoxemia, *FASEB J.*, 13, 1637, 1999.

85. Juckett, M. et al., Heme and the endothelium. Effects of nitric oxide on catalytic iron and heme degradation by heme oxygenase, *J. Biol. Chem.*, 273, 23388, 1998.

86. White, K.A. and Marletta, M.A., Nitric oxide synthase is a cytochrome P-450 type protein, *J. Biol. Chem.*, 269, 26390, 1992.

87. Thorup, C. et al., Carbon monoxide induces vasodilation and nitric oxide release but suppresses endothelial NOS, *Am. J. Physiol.*, 277, F882, 1999.

88. Chakder, S. et al., Heme oxygenase inhibitor zinc protoporphyrin-IX causes an activation of nitric oxide synthase in the rabbit internal anal sphincter, *J. Pharmacol. Exp. Ther.*, 277, 1376, 1996.

89. Thom, S.R., Xu, Y.A., and Ischiropoulos, H., Vascular endothelial cells generate peroxynitrite in response to carbon monoxide exposure, *Chem. Res. Toxicol.*, 10, 1023, 1997.

90. Thom, S.R. et al., Adaptive responses and apoptosis in endothelial cells exposed to carbon monoxide, *Proc. Natl. Acad. Sci. U.S.A.*, 97, 1305, 2000.

91. Albakri, Q.A. and Stuehr, D.J., Intracellular assembly of inducible NO synthase is limited by nitric oxide-mediated changes in heme insertion and availability, *J. Biol. Chem.*, 271, 5414, 1996.

92. Kaur, H., Green, C.J., and Motterlini, R., Interaction of bilirubin and biliverdin with reactive nitrogen species, *Free Rad. Biol. Med.*, 27, S78, 1999.

7 Developmental Biology of Heme Oxygenase and Carbon Monoxide in the Cardiopulmonary System

Phyllis A. Dennery

CONTENTS

I. INTRODUCTION

Carbon monoxide (CO), a byproduct of the HO reaction, can have significant prenatal and postnatal effects on the cardiovascular and pulmonary systems. CO produces deleterious effects on fetal growth and teratogenic effects were also reported. In contrast, beneficial vasodilatory effects of CO have been observed when abnormal stimuli for vascular tone such as hypoxia are present. Little is known about the developmental expression of HO in the cardiovascular system, but the lungs demonstrate clear developmental regulation of HO.

In the heart, both heme oxygenase (HO-1 and HO-2) proteins are found under normal and stress conditions.[1] Both isoforms of HO have also been demonstrated in the lung.[2] The many cardiac effects of HO and its CO byproduct in the adult

0-8493-1041-5/02/$0.00+$1.50
© 2002 by CRC Press LLC

TABLE 7.1
Developmental Pattern of HO Regulation

Tissue/Organ	Peak HO Expression	Reference
Liver	Postnatal day 1 (HO-1 mRNA)	Lin, 1989[9]
Brain	Postnatal day 7 (HO-1 protein and mRNA) Adulthood (HO-2 mRNA)	Bergeron, 1998[11] Sun, 1990[51]
Lung	Prenatal day 20 (HO-1 protein) Postnatal day 5 (HO-2 protein) Postnatal days 1 and 5 (HO activity)	Dennery, 2000[10]

animal[3-6] are discussed in detail in other chapters. Another role for CO generated from HO may be activation of baroreceptors in the brain which mediate changes in cardiovascular function.[7] Other byproducts of the HO reaction, such as bilirubin, have been implicated in protection against the risk of coronary heart disease.[8] What is less understood is the role of HO and/or CO in the development of the cardio-pulmonary system and the role of HO/CO in placental function.

II. DEVELOPMENTAL EXPRESSION OF HO

Developmental patterns of HO expression have been shown in liver, lung, and brain (Table 7.1). However, no evidence documents the developmental expression of HO-1 in the heart. It is likely that newborns show higher levels of heart HO protein and activity than adults if the developmental pattern observed in other tissues is also seen in the heart. In the rat liver, HO-1 mRNA levels reach a maximum 24 h after birth and the levels are highest in neonates, compared to adults throughout matura-tion.[9] Similarly, in the lungs, HO activity and protein are increased in neonates as compared to adults, remain elevated during the suckling period, then decrease to adult values.[10] With hyperoxic induction, lung HO-1 is differentially regulated in the newborn as HO-1 increases at the post-transcriptional level in neonates; tran-scriptional regulation is observed in adults.[2]

What mediates these maturational differences in modes of HO-1 regulation is not clearly understood. HO activity and HO-1 protein expression in the brain are highest on postnatal day 7 in most regions of the brain compared to levels in adults.[11] The adult pattern of expression is reached by postnatal day 21, with HO-1 localized exclusively to the dentate region of the hippocampus and some hypothalamic and thalamic nuclei.[11] In certain selected areas of the brain, the pattern of HO-1 expression is reversed such that little HO-1 staining is found at day 7 and HO-1 increases toward adulthood.[11] Overall, these data show that HO-1 expression is differentially regulated in specific cells and that HO is clearly developmentally regulated in most tissues.

TABLE 7.2
Effects of CO on the Fetus or Neonate

Prenatal	Postnatal
Decreased birthweight	Cardiomegaly/myocyte hyperplasia
Decreased brain protein/microcephaly/skull malformations	Behavioral abnormalities
Decreased heart weight (CO exposure prior to day 18 of gestation)	
Increased heart size (CO exposure until birth)	
Medullary changes in cholinergic pathways	
Decreased neuroreceptors (with hypothermia)	
Cleft lip and palate	
Scoliosis	
CHARGE association/heart defects	

III. EFFECTS OF HO/CO ON THE DEVELOPING CARDIOPULMONARY SYSTEM

Table 7.2 summarizes the effects of CO on the fetus or neonate. These prenatal and postnatal actions are further discussed in detail below.

A. PRENATAL EFFECTS OF HO/CO

1. Effects on Growth

Despite a lack of understanding of the developmental expression of HO in the heart, it is clear that CO, a byproduct of the HO reaction, significantly alters the fetal cardiovascular system. An important source of CO is maternal cigarette smoking. In fetal blood, a significant correlation between the numbers of cigarettes smoked and maternal carboxyhemoglobin (HbCO) has been identified.[12] This affects the fetus, fetal hemoglobin, and hematocrit.[12] Experimental models demonstrate that maternal smoke exposure results in alteration of fetal blood vessels at the ultrastructural level.[13,14] Cigarette smoke is complex and contains toxins other than CO. Therefore, it cannot be implied that the effects of smoking on the fetus are strictly related to CO.

Several models used inhaled maternal CO to demonstrate similar effects. As early as the 1970s, prenatal exposure to moderate CO levels was demonstrated to decrease birthweight and increase neonatal mortality.[15] In rats prenatally exposed to low concentrations of CO, reduced birthweight, decreased postnatal weight gain, altered brain protein at birth, and neurobehavioral abnormalities were noted.[16,17] In pregnant rats exposed to 200 ppm of CO for 17 out of 22 days of gestation, fetal birthweight, heart weight, and heart weight to body weight ratio were decreased.[18] In contrast, when the fetuses were kept in high CO environments until the end of gestation, cardiomegaly was present at birth and associated with increased DNA content.[18] This increase in cardiovascular size may relate to increased work of breathing associated with CO.[19]

Prenatal exposure to CO (200 ppm CO for 10 h/day) for the latter half of pregnancy affects cholinergic and catecholaminergic pathways in the medullas of guinea pig fetuses.[20] These important cardiorespiratory centers may be compromised in sudden infant death syndrome (SIDS). In addition, prenatal CO exposure followed by postnatal hypothermic stress results in decreased neuroreceptors in the brain, and this may also have implications for the etiology of SIDS.[21]

Oxygen transport is partially carrier-mediated and oxygen competes with CO for the same carrier in transport across the placenta.[22] In the placental equilibration of CO, fetal hemoglobin initially lags behind maternal hemoglobin; however, during CO uptake, fetal HbCO overtakes maternal levels and approaches an equilibrium value as much as 10% higher than the mother's levels[23] This suggests that inspired maternal CO has a profound effect on fetal oxygenation and fetal HbCO levels.

2. Teratogenic Effects

Epidemiologic evidence suggests an increased incidence of cleft lip with or without cleft palate in infants of mothers who smoke cigarettes, suggesting a teratogenic effect of CO from cigarette smoke.[24] This was further documented in an animal model susceptible for cleft lip and palate. Significant increases in the incidence of cleft lip and palate and fetal reasorbtion were demonstrated upon exposure to both hypoxia and CO.[25] Cleft lip and cleft palate as well as heart defects were observed in a male infant after exposure to CO during the first trimester of pregnancy.[26]

When CO exposure is compounded by protein deficiency in mice, the teratogenic effects are even more pronounced. Mice fed low protein diets and exposed to CO demonstrated increased fetal resorption and gross malformations at all levels of CO tested (65 to 500 ppm). The most common malformations were microcephaly, microstomia, and brachygnathia, as well as increased incidence of skull malformations, scoliosis, and lack of ossification in the limbs.[27] This has implications for malnourished smokers. One publication reports the CHARGE association (coloboma, heart disease, atresia choanae, retarded growth and development, genital hypoplasia and ear anomalies) in a child exposed to CO *in utero*.[28] This may imply that CO also affects the development of the cardiovascular system.

3. Role of CO in Closure of the Ductus Arteriosus

Another important aspect of cardiovascular development is the ability of the ductus arteriosus to close in the transition to birth. The fetus begins breathing continuously at birth and this is accompanied by a decrease in pulmonary vascular resistance, increased pulmonary blood flow, and closure of the ductus arteriosus, thereby allowing for increased circulation of oxygenated blood to organs. The contractile tension of the ductus arteriosus is completely reversed by pharmacologic levels of CO, at both high and low partial pressures of oxygen.[29]

Treatment with inhibitors of HO, such as ZnPP, had no effect on the tone of the ductus under normal conditions, but contracted endotoxin-treated ductuses and hypoxic vessels. ZnPP was also able to diminish the relaxation induced by CO after treatment with indothemacin, a vasoconstrictor, or bradykinin, a potent vasodilator, but did not affect the response obtained with sodium nitroprusside, an exogenous nitric oxide (NO) donor. This suggests that the mechanism by which CO induces relaxation is not through cGMP, but rather from cytochrome p450-based mono-oxygenase reactions.[30]

A recent publication[31] evaluated whether CO exerted an inhibitory effect on endothelin-1 (ET-1), a factor that contributes to high basal pulmonary vascular resistance in the normal fetus. Previously it was shown that inhibition of CO synthesis by zinc protoporphyrin (ZnPP) did not have any effect on ET-1.[32] In the more recent study, treatment with CO at pharmacologic doses (65 μM) curtailed ET-1 release; therefore, the conclusion was that endogenous CO has little or no role in the regulation of ET-1.[31] Similarly, another publication demonstrated that inhaled CO (5 to 2500 ppm) did not cause pulmonary vasodilation in late gestation lambs.[33] No change in the vasodilatory response of NO was observed with CO.[33] Treatment with ZnPP, an inhibitor of HO, had no effect on pulmonary vascular resistance or the gradient across the ductus arteriosus.[33] These observations suggest that although CO is a vasodilator in the ductus arteriosus, it is only effective in the presence of vasoconstricor stimuli such as hypoxia and does not appear to promote vasodilation under normal circumstances.

The ductus venosus is another fetal circulatory channel that closes at birth or shortly thereafter. The role of CO in the contractile tension of the ductus venosus of mature fetal lambs was evaluated. When preparations were precontracted with indomethacin, CO was able to completely relax the ductus venosus.[34] This was seen also when the ductus was denuded of endothelium,[34] suggesting a direct effect of CO on the smooth muscle.

B. Postnatal Effects of HO/CO

In adult rats, high levels of expression of HO-1 prevent the development of hypoxic pulmonary hypertension and inhibit structural remodeling of the pulmonary vessels, suggesting a vasodilatory and antiproliferative role for endogenous CO in adaptive responses toward hypoxia.[35] Young animals exposed to high altitudes show altered lung growth,[36] but young rats exposed to 208 ppm CO for 30 days showed no changes in lung dimensions, arguing against the role of CO in altering lung growth.[37]

The hypertrophic effects of CO on cardiac growth observed prenatally can be sustained with postnatal exposure to CO in some animal models. Compared with control animals, right ventricular weight was increased in rats exposed to 200 ppm CO during the fetal period.[38] Postnatal CO exposure caused a further increase in left ventricular weight. By 12 days of age, the heart weight-to-body weight ratios of animals exposed to CO postnatally only gradually increased to reach those of the group exposed to CO prenatally and postnatally.[38] CO exposure after birth also resulted in left ventricular myocyte hyperplasia.[38] These effects were not observed in guinea pigs.[39]

IV. PLACENTAL HEMODYNAMICS AND HO/CO

Another important organ in the regulation of fetal blood flow is the placenta. Many publications demonstrate that HO is found in the placentae of humans and other mammals.[40-44] HO is localized in the syncytiotrophoblasts and umbilical blood vessels of the placenta.[43] This is also the site where NO synthase is found.[42]

A recent publication demonstrates that the α-2 subunit of guanylate cyclase is also found at this location.[45] This suggests that NO or CO derived from HO may act upon guanylate cyclase to generate cyclic cGMP[45] and thus alter vascular tone.

In the human placenta, HO activity was present in various regions, thus supporting a role for the HO/CO pathway in placenta hemodynamics.[40] HO activity was also detected in human umbilical cord, suggesting that CO can play a role in fetal placental vascular tone.[46] It appears that human placental HO-1 mRNA is constitutively expressed in the first trimester and at term, whereas HO-2 mRNA is found at higher levels at term than in the first trimester.[41] HO-1 is found in the villous trophoblastic cells and HO-2 is found in the endothelial and smooth muscle cells.[41] In the rat, HO-1 protein levels are increased toward the latter third of gestation and decrease at birth.[44] This coincides with the expression of vascular endothelial growth factor[44] and the peak of erythropoiesis.[47] The placenta can hypertrophy in response to CO[48]; this may suggest that CO is a vasodilator in the fetoplacental circulation and also serves as a stimulus for villous growth.

With increased placental vascular resistance such as in preeclampsia, one would anticipate a decrease in CO and other vasodilators. In a model of TNF-β-induced placental damage, hemin, an HO inducer, reduced vascular tension by 61% in U46619 preconstricted placental arteries, and this reduction was inhibited by tin protoporphyrin, an HO inhibitor.[49] In placentas from pregnancies complicated with preeclampsia, HO-1 expression was significantly reduced, suggesting that HO-1 activation may prevent placental cellular injury and endothelial cell activation.[49] In other studies, the end-tidal CO breath levels of pregnant women with preeclampsia were significantly lower than in control groups suggesting that CO may have a contributing role in protection against preeclampsia.[50] Overall, HO and CO contribute to the maintenance of normal fetoplacental circulation. Disruption of CO production results in abnormal placental vascular tone.

ACKNOWLEDGMENT

This work was funded by the National Institutes of Health (Grants HD39248 and HL58752) and by the US–Israeli Binational Foundation.

REFERENCES

1. Ewing, J.F., Raju, V.S., and Maines, M.D., Induction of heart heme oxygenase-1 (HSP32) by hyperthermia: possible role in stress-mediated elevation of cyclic 3′:5′-guanosine monophosphate, *J. Pharmacol. Exp. Ther.*, 271, 408, 1994.
2. Dennery, P.A. et al., Hyperoxic regulation of lung heme oxygenase in neonatal rats, *Pediatr. Res.*, 40, 815, 1996.
3. Hangaishi, M. et al., Induction of heme oxygenase-1 can act protectively against cardiac ischemia/reperfusion *in vivo*, *Biochem. Biophys. Res. Commun.*, 279, 582, 2000.

4. Pataki, T. et al., Regulation of ventricular fibrillation by heme oxygenase in ischemic/reperfused hearts, *Antioxid. Redox Signal.*, 3, 125, 2001.
5. Soares, M.P. et al., Expression of heme oxygenase-1 can determine cardiac xenograft survival, *Nat. Med.*, 4, 1073, 1998.
6. Yet, S.F. et al., Hypoxia induces severe right ventricular dilatation and infarction in heme oxygenase-1 null mice, *J. Clin Invest.*, 103, R23, 1999.
7. Johnson, R.A. et al., Role of endogenous carbon monoxide in central regulation of arterial pressure, *Hypertension*, 30, 962, 1997.
8. Mayer, M., Association of serum bilirubin concentration with risk of coronary artery disease, *Clin. Chem*, 46, 1723, 2000.
9. Lin, J.H. et al., Expression of rat liver heme oxygenase gene during development, *Arch. Biochem. Biophys.*, 270, 623, 1989.
10. Dennery, P.A., Regulation and role of heme oxygenase in oxidative injury, *Curr. Top. Cell. Regul.*, 36, 181, 2000.
11. Bergeron, M., Ferriero, D.M., and Sharp, F.R., Developmental expression of heme oxygenase-1 (HSP32) in rat brain: an immunocytochemical study, *Brain Res. Dev. Brain Res.*, 105, 181, 1998.
12. Bureau, M.A. et al., Maternal cigarette smoking and fetal oxygen transport: a study of P50, 2,3-diphosphoglycerate, total hemoglobin, hematocrit, and type F hemoglobin in fetal blood, *Pediatrics*, 72, 22, 1983.
13. Bnait, K.S. and Seller, M.J., Ultrastructural changes in 9-day old mouse embryos following maternal tobacco smoke inhalation, *Exp. Toxicol. Pathol.*, 47, 453, 1995.
14. Kaufmann, R.C., Amankwah, K.S., and Weberg, A.D., The effect of maternal smoke exposure on the ultrastructure of fetal peripheral blood vessels in the mouse, *J. Perinat. Med.*, 14, 309, 1986.
15. Astrup, P. et al., Moderate hypoxia exposure and fetal development, *Arch. Environ. Health*, 30, 15, 1975.
16. Woody, R.C. and Brewster, M.A., Telencephalic dysgenesis associated with presumptive maternal carbon monoxide intoxication in the first trimester of pregnancy, *J. Toxicol. Clin. Toxicol.*, 28, 467, 1990.
17. Fechter, L.D., Mactutus, C.F., and Storm, J.E., Carbon monoxide and brain development, *Neurotoxicology*, 7, 463, 1986.
18. Penney, D.G. et al., Cardiac response of the fetal rat to carbon monoxide exposure, *Am. J. Physiol.*, 244, H289, 1983.
19. Oparil, S., Bishop, S.P., and Clubb, F.J., Jr., Myocardial cell hypertrophy or hyperplasia, *Hypertension*, 6, III38, 1984.
20. Tolcos, M. et al., Chronic prenatal exposure to carbon monoxide results in a reduction in tyrosine hydroxylase-immunoreactivity and an increase in choline acetyltransferase-immunoreactivity in the fetal medulla: implications for Sudden Infant Death Syndrome, *J. Neuropathol. Exp. Neurol.*, 59, 218, 2000.
21. Tolcos, M. et al., Exposure to prenatal carbon monoxide and postnatal hyperthermia: short and long-term effects on neurochemicals and neuroglia in the developing brain, *Exp. Neurol.*, 162, 235, 2000.
22. Gurtner, G.H., Traystman, R.J., and Burns, B., Interactions between placental O_2 and CO transfer, *J. Appl. Physiol.*, 52, 479, 1982.
23. Hill, E.P. et al., Carbon monoxide exchanges between the human fetus and mother: a mathematical model, *Am. J. Physiol.*, 232, H311, 1977.
24. Ericson, A., Kallen, B., and Westerholm, P., Cigarette smoking as an etiologic factor in cleft lip and palate, *Am. J. Obstet. Gynecol.*, 135, 348, 1979.

25. Bailey, L.J., Johnston, M.C., and Billet, J., Effects of carbon monoxide and hypoxia on cleft lip in A/J mice, *Cleft Palate Craniofac. J.*, 32, 14, 1995.
26. Hennequin, Y. et al., *In utero* carbon monoxide poisoning and multiple fetal abnormalities, *Lancet*, 341, 240, 1993.
27. Singh, J., Aggison, L., Jr., and Moore–Cheatum, L., Teratogenicity and developmental toxicity of carbon monoxide in protein-deficient mice, *Teratology*, 48, 149, 1993.
28. Courtens, W. et al., CHARGE association in a neonate exposed *in utero* to carbon monoxide, *Birth Defects Orig. Artic. Ser.*, 30, 407, 1996.
29. Coceani, F. et al., Cytochrome P 450-linked monooxygenase: involvement in the lamb ductus arteriosus, *Am. J. Physiol.*, 246, H640, 1984.
30. Coceani, F., Kelsey, L., and Seidlitz, E., Carbon monoxide-induced relaxation of the ductus arteriosus in the lamb: evidence against the prime role of guanylyl cyclase, *Br. J. Pharmacol.*, 118, 1689, 1996.
31. Coceani, F. and Kelsey, L., Endothelin-1 release from the lamb ductus arteriosus: are carbon monoxide and nitric oxide regulatory agents? *Life Sci.*, 66, 2613, 2000.
32. Coceani, F. et al., Carbon monoxide formation in the ductus arteriosus in the lamb: implications for the regulation of muscle tone, *Br. J. Pharmacol.*, 120, 599, 1997.
33. Grover, T.R. et al., Inhaled carbon monoxide does not cause pulmonary vasodilation in the late-gestation fetal lamb, *Am. J. Physiol.* 278, L779, 2000.
34. Adeagbo, A.S. et al., Lamb ductus venosus: evidence of a cytochrome P-450 mechanism in its contractile tension, *J. Pharmacol. Exp. Ther.*, 252, 875, 1990.
35. Christou, H. et al., Prevention of hypoxia-induced pulmonary hypertension by enhancement of endogenous heme oxygenase-1 in the rat, *Circ. Res.*, 86, 1224, 2000.
36. Thurlbeck, W.M., Lung growth and alveolar multiplication, *Pathobiol. Annu.*, 5, 1, 1975.
37. Bartlett, D., Jr., Postnatal growth of the mammalian lung: lack of influence by carbon monoxide exposure, *Respir. Physiol.*, 23, 343, 1975.
38. Clubb, F.J., Jr. et al., Cardiomegaly due to myocyte hyperplasia in perinatal rats exposed to 200 ppm carbon monoxide, *J. Mol. Cell. Cardiol.*, 18, 477, 1986.
39. Schirmer, E. and Schwartze, H., Effect of mild chronic hypoxia on the infantile heart: ECGs of guinea pigs pre- and postnatally treated with carbon monoxide, *Biomed. Biochim. Acta*, 48, S118, 1989.
40. McLaughlin, B.E. et al., Heme oxygenase activity in term human placenta, *Placenta*, 21, 870, 2000.
41. Yoshiki, N., Kubota, T., and Aso, T., Expression and localization of heme oxygenase in human placental villi, *Biochem. Biophys. Res. Commun.*, 276, 1136, 2000.
42. Odrcich, M.J. et al., Heme oxygenase and nitric oxide synthase in the placenta of the guinea pig during gestation, *Placenta*, 19, 509, 1998.
43. Lyall, F. et al., Heme oxygenase expression in human placenta and placental bed implies a role in regulation of trophoblast invasion and placental function, *FASEB J.*, 14, 208, 2000.
44. Kreiser, D. et al., Heme oxygenase-1 modulates fetal growth in the rat, *Pediatr. Res.*, 49, 58A, 2001.
45. Bamberger, A.M. et al., Expression and tissue localization of soluble guanylyl cyclase in the human placenta using novel antibodies directed against the alpha(2) subunit, *J. Clin. Endocrinol. Metab.*, 86, 909, 2001.
46. Vreman, H.J. et al., Haem oxygenase activity in human umbilical cord and rat vascular tissues, *Placenta*, 21, 337, 2000.
47. Joshima, H., Decrease of erythropoiesis in the fetal liver of X-ray irradiated pregnant mice, *J. Radiat. Res. (Tokyo)*, 37, 177, 1996.

48. Lynch, A.M. and Bruce, N.W., Placental growth in rats exposed to carbon monoxide at selected stages of pregnancy, *Biol. Neonate*, 56, 151, 1989.

49. Ahmed, A. et al., Induction of placental heme oxygenase-1 is protective against TNFalpha- induced cytotoxicity and promotes vessel relaxation, *Mol. Med.*, 6, 391, 2000.

50. Baum, M. et al., End-tidal carbon monoxide measurements in women with pregnancy-induced hypertension and preeclampsia, *Am. J. Obstet. Gynecol.*, 183, 900, 2000.

51. Sun, Y. and Maines, M.D., Heme oxygenase-2 mRNA: developmental expression in the rat liver and response to cobalt chloride, *Arch. Biochem. Biophys.*, 282, 340, 1990.

8 Carbon Monoxide Signaling in the Heart

Dipak K. Das and Nilanjana Maulik

CONTENTS

I. INTRODUCTION

Carbon monoxide (CO) is a soluble gas that activates guanylate cyclase and thereby promotes smooth muscle relaxation and vasodilation.[1,2] CO is generated during the conversion of heme into biliverdin, and biliverdin is rapidly reduced to bilirubin. The reaction is catalyzed by the heme oxygenase (HO) enzyme. HO functions as the rate-limiting enzyme in heme catabolism, which results in the loss of iron and the elimination of the α-methene carbon bridge of the porphyrin ring as CO.[3] Although CO was initially believed to maintain intracellular cGMP levels, it has now been shown to augment these levels.[4]

CO was shown to function in the brain as a retrograde messenger by stimulating or inhibiting corticotropin-releasing hormone, stimulating gonadotropin-releasing hormone, and modulating neurohypophyseal hormones.[5,6] In vascular tissues, CO exerts vasodilatory actions through the up-regulation of cGMP.[7] Evidence also supports a role for prostaglandins in CO-mediated vasodilation.[8]

A recent study demonstrated a role of the activation of the HO–CO pathway in the pathogenesis of cirrhotic cardiomyopathy.[9] In heart failure and cardiac hypertrophy, the induction of HO-1 expression and activity abrogates the effects of CO, reduces second messenger cGMP production, and improves cardiac contractility. Thus, the functional importance of HO-1 expression and activity in cardiac failure, hypertrophy, and cardiomyopathy merits further investigations.

Inhibition of HO-1 activity by tin protoporphyrin caused graft rejection in 3 to 7 days, and this rejection was associated with platelet sequestration, thrombosis of coronary arterioles, cardiac infarction, and development of apoptosis in endothelial and cardiac cells.[10] However, during inhibition of HO-1 by tin protoporphyrin, the application of exogenous CO suppressed graft rejection, restored long-term graft survival, and prevented platelet aggregation, thrombosis, myocardial infarction, and apoptosis. Thus, it is reasonable to assume that the action of the HO-1 is mediated through the generation of CO. The importance of the HO system was stressed in another study in which the overexpression of HO-1 by cobalt protoporphyrin resulted in the inhibition of several immune effector functions, and thus provided an explanation for stress-induced immunosuppression.[11] HO is also a major player in the skin's defense mechanisms against UVB (280 to 320 nm) immunosuppression.[12]

This review will focus on the signal transduction pathway triggered by CO in the heart. The heart is a unique organ in which CO signaling is likely to play a crucial role because all the necessary substrates and enzymes are present. In pathologic conditions like ischemia, the available NO may be reduced and CO may compensate for the loss of NO.

II. HEME OXYGENASE: A HIGHLY INDUCIBLE ENZYME IN THE HEART

HO represents a predominant source for CO in the heart.[13] HO catalyzes the initial rate-limiting step of heme catabolism. Formation of bilirubin from the oxidative degradation of heme is catalyzed by two microsomal enzymes in sequence: heme oxygenase and biliverdin reductase. HO comprises three isoenzymes: HO-1, HO-2, and HO-3. HO-1 is known to be regulated by various endogenous as well as exogenous factors such as hemoglobin, metals, and oxygen free radicals.[14] HO-1 was found to be synonymous with heat shock protein 32 (HSP 32) based on the fact that HO-1 can be transcriptionally controlled by HSP.[15] Highly coordinated 20- to 40-fold increases in the level of 1.8 kb mRNA within a short time (approximately 1 h) make HSP 32 distinct from other HSPs. Very little is known about HO-3.

The presence of heme oxygenase appears to be ubiquitous and highly conserved. It catalyzes equimolar production of CO and bilirubin for each molecule of heme degraded. HO can be induced by free radicals or the oxidative stress developed from free radical generation in the heart.[16,17] HO-1 is not induced by ischemia, but can be easily induced upon reperfusion following an ischemic insult[17,18] (Figure 8.1).

The induction of HO-1 is a function of the duration of reperfusion, and the induction can be blocked by preperfusing the heart with oxygen free radical scavengers, superoxide dismutase, and catalase. Immunohistochemical localization revealed that HO-1 is primarily accumulated in the perivascular region and in the cardiomyocytes. This suggests that oxygen free radicals produced during the reperfusion serve as the stimulus for the expression of HO-1 in the ischemic reperfused myocardium.

HO-1 is also easily induced in the heart in other pathologic conditions. For example, HO mRNA levels are increased in cardiovascular tissues of stroke-prone

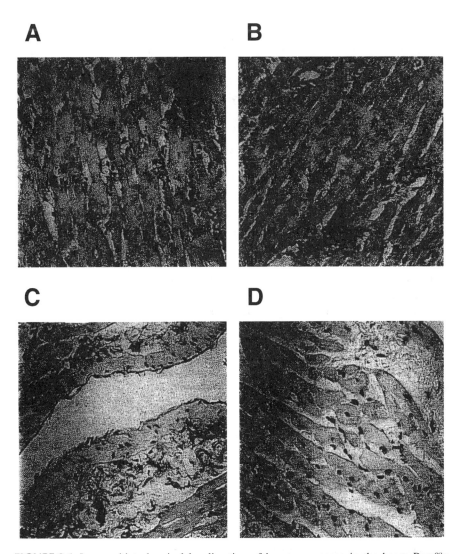

FIGURE 8.1 Immunohistochemical localizartion of heme oxygenase in the heart. Paraffin sections 5 μ*M* thick of rat left ventricular tissue were incubated with the polyclonal antibody against purified rat liver HO-1 followed by visualization after immunoperoxidase color reaction. Panel A shows a representative micrograph of myocardial biopsy obtained at 60 min of reperfusion after 5 min of ischemia and stained with HO-1 antibody. The results demonstrate moderate staining in the cardiomyocytes and intense staining in the interstitial spaces. Panel B shows homogeneous cytoplasmic staining of HO-1 in the perivascular region of a blood vessel and moderate staining in cardiomyocytes of a myocardial biopsy obtained after 60 min of reperfusion following 20 min of ischemia. Panel C demonstrates intense immunoreactivity of HO-1 in the perivascular region of a blood vessel and moderate staining in cardiomyocytes of a myocardial biopsy obtained after 20 min of ischemia and 60 min of reperfusion. Panel D shows a microphotograph of the myocardial tissue obtained from a rat after 20 min of ischemia followed by 60 min of reperfusion; primary antibody (anti-HO-1) was omitted.

spontaneously hypertensive (SHR-SP/Izm) rats.[19] HO was also found to be induced by hemodynamic stress.[20,21] Administration of HO substrate or induction of HO in young spontaneously hypertensive rats (SHRs) resulted in a lowering of blood pressure.[22,23] Interestingly, heme-bearing preparations were found to lower blood pressure via HO-mediated formation of CO in mature SHRs, deoxycorticosterone acetate salt hypertensive rats, and phenylephrine-induced hypertensive rats.[24] Evidence also supports the anti-atherogenic potential of HO-1.[25]

III. VASODILATORY EFFECTS OF CARBON MONOXIDE IN THE HEART

CO is also involved in the modulation of vascular tone.[26] It induces endothelium-independent relaxation of preconstricted arteries and veins *in vitro*.[27,28] Inhaled CO was reported to inhibit hypoxic pulmonary vasoconstriction in an isolated perfused cat lung preparation.[29] This report was subsequently confirmed for perfused pig lung[30] and rat lung[31,32] preparations. In a recent study, however, endogenous CO was found to modulate canine hypoxic pulmonary vasoconstriction only in the absence of NO.[33] The notion that the heme oxygenase–CO system serves a vasodepressor function received additional support from the reports that CO of vascular smooth muscle origin inhibits endothelial cell expression of endothelin-1,[34] and that treatment with heme lowers blood pressure in hypertensive rats via a heme oxygenase-dependent mechanism.[35] This implies that CO formed by heme oxygenase plays a role in the central regulation of arterial pressure.

The coordinated regulation of NO and HO-induced CO production was revealed by a recent study that showed the mechanisms by which NO regulates HO-1 gene expression.[36] The study demonstrated that NO donors are potent inducers of HO-1 mRNA and protein expression in aortic vascular smooth muscle cells. Increased HO-1 gene expression by NO resulted from an increased rate of the HO-1 gene transcription and increased stability of HO-1 mRNA transcript. Conversely, the induction of HO-1 expression by NO was independent of the cGMP

Several recent studies demonstrated that HO-catalyzed CO production by vascular smooth muscle cells is associated with intracellular cGMP production.[37,38] Thus, vascular smooth muscle cells have the capacity to generate two distinct guanylate cyclase-activating molecules (NO and CO). As mentioned earlier, NO can induce the expression of HO-1 and potentiate the formation of CO.[39] NO, either exogenously administered or endogenously generated from cytokine-treated cells, selectively induced HO-1 gene expression and CO release in vascular smooth muscle cells. The induction of HO mRNA expression and activity by NO in vascular smooth muscle cells may have a pathophysiological value. In response to endothelial injury, smooth muscle cells express inducible nitric oxide synthase (iNOS),[40] an isoform of NOS that is capable of producing cytotoxic amounts of NO.[41] The formation of CO following HO activation may limit NO release because CO directly inhibits iNOS mRNA expression and activity by binding to the heme moiety of the enzyme.[42]

Heme is essential for iNOS activity. Thus, an increase in HO activity may reduce intracellular heme levels, leading to the limitation of active iNOS enzyme. Significantly lower cellular heme levels were found in rat hepatocytes after iNOS induction.[43] As a result, NO-induced HO-1 mRNA expression may provide a negative feedback regulation that limits the formation of cytotoxic levels of NO by smooth muscle cells, while preserving blood flow at sites of vascular injury by releasing guanylate cyclase-stimulatory CO production. This implies that NO-induced HO activity may provide cytoprotection from oxidative stress associated with elevated rates of NO synthesis in vascular smooth muscle cells.[44,45] Thus, the HO-catalyzed formation of guanylate cyclase-stimulatory CO may provide vascular smooth muscle cells an additional mechanism by which blood flow and fluidity are maintained at sites of vascular injury.

IV. CARBON MONOXIDE SIGNALING

A growing body of evidence suggests that CO may function as a chemical messenger in neuronal transmission. CO signaling has been demonstrated in the central nervous system where CO may be involved in the potentiation of long-term memory function.[46] The second messenger role of CO is evidenced by its ability to function as an endogenous regulator of cGMP.[47,48] Although, CO is known to stimulate cGMP levels, recent studies revealed differential effects on cGMP. For example, cGMP levels in the cultured neuronal cells remained unchanged when endogenous CO production was blocked with HO inhibitors.[49] The validity of this result was confirmed by the finding that exogenous CO at the physiological level of 7.5 pmol/mg protein only minimally elevated cGMP levels. Interestingly, in the presence of NO, endogenous CO appears to modulate the NO–cGMP signaling system. The same investigators found that exogenous CO at low concentrations of 1.5 to 5 μM inhibited NO-mediated guanylyl cyclase activation, whereas at higher concentrations of 150 to 500 μM, CO actually potentiated this NO-mediated activation.

In another recent study, CO was found to selectively block the expression of proinflammatory cytokines, TNFα, IL-1β and MIP-1β, as well as increase the production of the antiinflammatory cytokine, Il-10.[50] CO at low concentrations *in vivo* and *in vitro* differentially and selectively inhibited or stimulated the expression of lipopolysaccharide-induced proinflammatory and antiinflammatory cytokines. The effects of CO were independent of cGMP and NO, and were mediated through a mitogen-activated protein kinase (MAP kinase) signal transduction pathway.

cGMP-independent effects of CO are further evidenced from the finding that CO can modulate vascular tone independent of cGMP. CO-mediated inhibition of hypoxic pulmonary vasoconstriction is generally attributed to a reduction in function of the cytochromes of the electron transport chain or to an effect of CO on a hemoprotein O_2 sensor.[51,52] In contrast, a low concentration of inhaled CO was recently shown to inhibit hypoxic pulmonary vasoconstriction.[53] Most of the studies in the literature used much higher CO concentrations. At low concentration, CO is unlikely to affect mitochondrial cytochromes or hemoprotein or activate soluble guanylate cyclase. This suggests a different mechanism of CO action in the vascular tissues.

Several recent studies further supported the role of CO as a signaling molecule in the ischemic myocardium. NO appears to function in ischemic myocardium as a

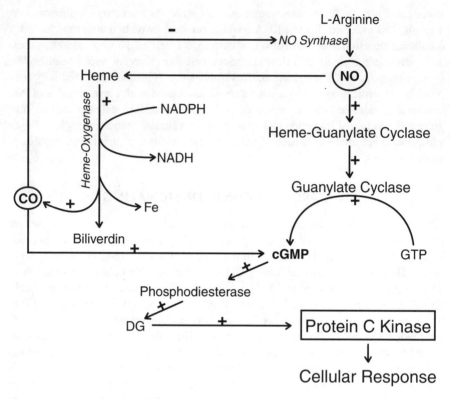

FIGURE 8.2 Proposed mechanism for CO signaling in the ischemic heart.

retrograde messenger for CO signaling.[54] The level of endogenous NO falls significantly during an ischemic insult, and augmentation of NO with its precursor L-
arginine increased the level of cGMP in the heart. The NO-mediated augmentation
of the cGMP was reduced by protoporphyrin, thus suggesting that part of the effect
was mediated by CO generated through the heme oxygenase pathway (Figure 8.2).
As shown in the figure, this study suggested the existence of a feedback loop between
NO–CO signaling.[55] When NO signaling is augmented in the heart, it directly
stimulates soluble guanylate cyclase, activating cGMP and leading to the activation
of protein kinase C. Activation of NO generates CO through the stimulation of HO,
and once generated, the CO can activate cGMP. However, increase in iNOS can
negatively regulate CO signaling of cGMP.

Several lines of evidence indicate that endogenous CO production is associated
with physiologic maintenance of endogenous cGMP concentration. An increased
HO mRNA expression in concert with the modulation of cGMP content was noticed
in the ischemic/reperfused myocardium.[55] Myocardial cGMP content, the second
messenger for NO signaling, was also increased in L-arginine-treated groups, and
was reduced in rats treated with zinc protoporphyrin. These findings also suggest
that NO contributes to myocardial preservation by both cGMP-dependent and
cGMP-independent mechanisms; the former is modulated by CO signaling and the

latter by virtue of its antioxidant mechanism. The same results and conclusions were stressed and obtained by others[56,57] in different models of ischemia/reperfusion. It is therefore reasonable to assume that NO and CO may act on the same mechanism in the regulation of smooth muscle tone as well as myocardial cells, although NO is a free radical and CO is not. It has become increasingly evident that regulation of HO activity leading to CO production and NO formation by nitric oxide synthase are intimately linked. For instance, the interaction of NO with cytochrome heme iron may lead to the inactivation of cytochromes and inability to interact with oxygen; thus, NO has a higher affinity for heme iron than O_2 does. Therefore, observations of the regulation of nitric oxide synthase and HO systems could support the concept that NO production is related to the HO system.[58]

V. INDUCTION OF GENE EXPRESSION BY CARBON MONOXIDE

Hypoxic hypoxia induced by CO was found to induce a number of immediate early gene expressions. For example, after 6-h exposure to CO, c-*Jun*, c-*myc*, and *Egr* mRNA levels in the vital organs of rats including the heart were found to increase by 100%.[59] A more dramatic increase was noticed for c-*fos* mRNA levels in the heart which increased about 20-fold after 6 h of CO exposure.

Exposure of the animals to 0.1% CO did not alter the expression of c-*Jun* mRNA in the vital organs including heart, lung, and kidney within 1 h. After 6 h of exposure to CO, a two-fold increase in the induction of c-Jun mRNA was observed. In contrast, in liver, the induction of c-*Jun* mRNA increased by about seven-fold within 1 h of CO exposure and remained unchanged up to 6 h of exposure. For c-*fos* and c-*myc*, a progressive increase in the induction of the mRNAs was observed. With the exception of c-*Jun* mRNA, the heart showed the strongest induction of the immediate early genes after CO exposure.

VI. SUMMARY AND CONCLUSION

The heart possesses a great capacity to produce CO because the substrate for CO production, heme, is readily available and localized in the vasculature and blood vessels.[60,61] The heme-catalyzing enzyme, heme oxygenase, is highly inducible in the heart. A several-fold induction of HO-1 was observed in the heart in response to ischemia/reperfusion and oxidative stress.[17,18] A significant number of studies demonstrate a role for CO signaling in the modulation of cardiovascular function.[62,63] CO is believed to function in the heart by activating soluble guanine cyclase, leading to the activation of cGMP, a second messenger responsible for the modulation of physiological function. The NO–CO signaling pathway plays a crucial role in the pathologic heart including ischemia/reperfusion, hypertension, and atherosclerosis.

CO shares some of the properties of NO, e.g., like NO, CO has the ability to bind to the iron atoms of the hemoproteins. The most important difference between NO and CO lies in the fact that NO, but not CO, undergoes redox signaling. Regulation of vascular tone by CO involves binding and dislocation of heme iron to induce a conformational change and activation of the catalytic site of guanylyl cyclase.[64] CO is believed to potentiate cardioprotection through NO-dependent and -independent mechanisms. NO contributes to myocardial preservation by both cGMP-dependent and -independent mechanisms; the former is modulated by CO signaling and the latter by virtue of its antioxidant mechanism.

ACKNOWLEDGMENT

This study was supported in part by grants from the National Institutes of Health (HL 22559, HL 33889, and HL 56803).

REFERENCES

1. Johnson, R.A. et al., A heme oxygenase product, presumably carbon monoxide, mediates a vasodepressor function in rats, *Hypertension*, 25, 166, 1995.
2. Morita, T. et al., Smooth muscle cell-derived carbon monoxide is a regulator of vascular cGMP, *Proc. Natl. Acad. Sci., U.S.A.*, 92, 1475, 1995.
3. Maines, M.D., Heme oxygenase: function, multiplicity, regulatory mechanisms, and clinical applications, *FASEB J.*, 2, 2557, 1988.
4. Fukushima, T. et al., Cyclic GMP formation in rat cerebellar slices is stimulated by endothelins via nitric oxide formation and by sarafotoxins via formation of carbon monoxide, *Biochemistry*, 25, 652, 1994.
5. Pozzoli, G. et al., Carbon monoxide as a novel neuroendocrine modulator: inhibition of stimulated cortocotrophin releasing hormone release from acute rat hypothalamic explants, *Endocrinology*, 135, 2314, 1994.
6. Hawkins, R.D., Zhuo, M., and Arancio, O., Nitric oxide and carbon monoxide as possible retrograde messengers in hippocampal long-term potentiation, *J. Neurobiol.*, 25, 652, 1994.
7. Graser, T., Vedernikov, Y.P., and Li, D.S., Study on the mechanism of carbon monoxide-induced endothelium-independent relaxation in porcine coronary artery and vein, *Biomed. Biochim. Acta*, 49, 293, 1990.
8. Lin, H. and McGrath, J.J., Vasodilating effects of carbon monoxide, *Drug Chem. Toxicol.*, 11, 371, 1988.
9. Murad, F. et al., The nitric oxide–cyclic GMP signal transduction system for intracellular and intercellular communications, in *Advances in Second Messenger and Phosphoprotein Research*, Brown, B.L. and Dobson, P.R.M., Eds., Raven Press, New York, 1991, 101.
10. Sato, K. et al., Carbon monoxide generated by heme oxygenase-1 suppresses the rejection of mouse-to-rat cardiac transplants, *J. Immunol.*, 166, 4185, 2001.
11. Woo, J. et al., Stress protein-induced immunosuppression: inhibition of cellular immune effector functions following overexpression of heme oxygenase (HSP 32), *Transpl. Immunol.*, 6, 84, 1998.
12. Reeve, V.E. and Tyrrell, R.M., Heme oxygenase induction mediates the photoimmunoprotective activity of UVA radiation in the mouse, *Proc. Natl. Acad. Sci. U.S.A.*, 96, 9317, 1999.
13. Liesuy, S.F. and Tomar, M.L., Heme oxygenase and oxidative stress. Evidence of involvement of bilirubin as physiological protector against oxidative damage, *Biochim. Biophys. Acta*, 1223, 9, 1994.

14. Poss, K.D. and Tonegawa, S., Reduced stress defense in heme oxygenase 1-deficient cells, *Proc. Natl. Acad. Sci. U.S.A.*, 94, 10925, 1997.
15. Shibahara, S., Muller, R.M., and Taguchi, H., Transcriptional control of the rat heme oxygenase by heat shock, *J. Biol. Chem.*, 262, 12889, 1987.
16. Keyse, S.M. and Tyrrell, R.M., Heme oxygenase is the major 32 Kda stress protein induced in human skin fibroblasts by UVA radiation, hydrogen peroxide and sodium arsenate, *Proc. Natl. Acad. Sci. U.S.A.*, 86, 99, 1989.
17. Maulik, N., Sharma, H.S., and Das, D.K., Induction of the heme oxygenase gene expression during the reperfusion of ischemic rat myocardium, *J. Mol. Cell. Cardiol.*, 28, 1261, 1996.
18. Sharma, H., Das, D.K., and Verdow, P.D., Enhanced expression and localization of heme oxygenase-1 during recovery phase of porcine stunned myocardium, *Mol. Cell. Biochem.*, 196, 133, 1999.
19. Seki, T. et al., Induction of heme oxygenase produces load-independent cardioprotective effects in hypertensive rats, *Life Sci.*, 65, 1077, 1999.
20. Raju, V.S. and Maines, M.D., Renal ischemia/reperfusion up-regulates heme oxygenase-1 (HSP 32) expression and increases cGMP in rat heart, *J. Pharmacol. Exp. Therap*, 277, 1814, 1996.
21. Katayose, D. et al., Separate regulation of heme oxygenase and heat shock protein 70 mRNA expression in rat heart by hemodynamic stress, *Biochem. Biophys. Res. Commun.*, 191, 587, 1993.
22. DaSilva, J.L. et al., Tin mediated heme oxygenase gene activation and cytochrome P450 arachidonate hydroxylase inhibition in spontaneously hypertensive rat, *Am. J. Med. Sci.*, 307, 173, 1994.
23. Levere, R.D. et al., Effect of heme arginate administration on blood pressure in spontaneously hypertensive rats, *J. Clin. Invest.*, 86, 213, 1990.
24. Johnson, R.A. et al., Heme oxygenase substrates acutely lower blood pressure in hypertensive rats, *Am. J. Physiol.*, 271, H1132, 1996.
25. Siow, R.C.M., Sato, H., and Mann, G.E., Heme oxygenase-carbon monoxide signaling pathway in atherosclerosis: anti-atherogenic actions of bilirubin and carbon monoxide, *Cardiovasc. Res.*, 41, 385, 1999.
26. Chinkers, M. and Garbers, D.L., Signal transduction by guanylyl cyclases, *Annu. Rev. Biochem.*, 60, 553, 1991.
27. Mancuso, C. et al., The role of carbon monoxide in the regulation of neuroendocrine function, *Neuroimmunomodulation,* 4, 225, 1998.
28. Liu, H., Song, D., and Lee, S.S., Role of heme oxygenase-carbon monoxide pathway in pathogenesis of cirrhotic cardiomyopathy in the rat, *Am. J. Physiol.* 280, G68, 2001.
29. Duke, H.N. and Killick, E.M., Pulmonary vasomotor responses of isolated perfused cat lungs to anoxia, *J. Physiol.*, 117, 303, 1952.
30. Sylvester, J.T. and McGowan, C., The effects of agents that bind to cytochrome P450 on hypoxic pulmonary vasoconstriction, *Circ. Res.*, 43, 429, 1978.
31. Marshall, C., Cooper, D.Y., and Marshall, B.E., Reduced availability of energy initiates pulmonary vasoconstriction, *Proc. Soc. Exp. Biol. Med.*, 187, 282, 1988;
32. Tamayo, L. et al., Carbon monoxide inhibits hypoxic pulmonary vasoconstriction in rats by a cGMP-independent mechanism, *Pflügers Arch.*, 434, 698, 1997.
33. Vassalli, F. et al., Inhibition of hypoxic pulmonary vasoconstriction by carbon monoxide in dogs, *Crit. Care Med.*, 29, 359, 2001.
34. Morita, T. and Kourembanas, S., Endothelial cell expression of vasoconstrictors and growth factors is regulated by smooth muscle cell-derived carbon monoxide, *J. Clin. Invest.*, 96, 2676, 1995.

35. Johnson, R.A. et al., Role of endogenous carbon monoxide in central regulation of arterial pressure, *Hypertension,* 30, 962, 1997.

36. Hartsfield, C.L. et al., Regulation of heme oxygenase-1 gene expression in vascular smooth muscle cells by nitric oxide, *Am. J. Physiol.,* 273, L980, 1997.

37. Durante, W. et al., Nitric oxide induces heme-oxygenase-1 gene expression and carbon monoxide production in vascular smooth muscle cells, *Circ. Res.,* 80, 557, 1997.

38. Denninger, J.W. and Marletta, M.A., Guanylate cyclase and the NO/cGMP signaling pathway, *Biochem. Biophys. Acta,* 1411, 334, 1999.

39. Verma, A. et al., Carbon monoxide: a putative neural messenger, *Science,* 259, 381–384, 1993.

40. Hansson, G.K. et al., Arterial smooth muscle cells express nitric oxide synthase in response to endothelial injury, *J. Exp. Med.,* 180, 733, 1994.

41. Beasley, D.J., Schwartz, J.H., and Brenner, B.M. Interleukin-1 induces prolonged L-arginine-dependent cyclic guanosine monophosphate and nitrite production in rat vascular smooth muscle cells, *J. Clin. Invest.,* 87, 602, 1991.

42. Verbeurin, T.J. et al., Evidence for the induction of nonendothelial NO synthase in aortas of cholesterol-fed rabbits, *J. Cardiovasc. Pharmacol.,* 21, 841, 1993.

43. Albakri, Q.A. and Stuehr, D.J. Intracellular assembly of inducible NO synthase is limited by nitric oxide-mediated changes in heme insertion and availability, *J. Biol. Chem.,* 271, 5414, 1996.

44. Padmanaban, G., Venkateswar, V., and Rangarajan, P., Haem as a multifunctional regulator, *Trends Biol. Sci.,* 14, 492, 1989.

45. Mathers, G. et al., Role of L-arginine-nitric oxide pathway in myocardial reoxygenation injury, *Am. J. Physiol.,* 288, H616, 1992.

46. Nathanson, J.A. et al., The cellular Na^+ pump as a site of action for glutamate: a mechanism for long-term modulation of cellular activity, *Neuron,* 14, 781, 1995.

47. Ingi, T. and Ronnett, G.V., Direct demonstration of a physiological role for carbon monoxide in olfactory tissue, *Neuroscience,* 31, 459, 1994.

48. Seki, T. et al., Roles of heme oxygenase carbon monoxide system in genetically hypertensive rats, *Biochem. Biophys. Res. Commun.,* 241, 574, 1997.

49. Ingi, T., Cheng, J., and Ronnettt, G., Carbon monoxide: an endogenous modulator of the nitric oxide-cyclic GMP signaling system, *Neuron,* 16, 835, 1996

50. Otterbein, L.E. et al., Carbon monoxide has antiinflammatory effects involving the mitogen-activated protein kinase activity, *Nature Med.,* 6, 422, 2000.

51. Christova, T., Diankova, Z., and Setchenska, M., Heme oxygenase-carbon monoxide signaling pathway: physiological regulator of vascular smooth muscle cells, *Acta Physiol. Pharmacol. Bulg.,* 25, 9, 2000.

52. Utz, J. and Ullrich, V., Carbon monoxide relaxes ileal smooth muscle through activation of gualylate cyclase, *Biochem. Pharmacol.,* 41, 1195, 1991.

53. Sammut, I. et al., Involvement of the heme oxygenase/carbon monoxide pathway in the suppression of acute pressor responses in rat aortic rings, *Br. J. Pharmacol.,* 122, 194, 1997.

54. Maulik, N. et al., Nitric oxide — a retrograde messenger for carbon monoxide signaling in ischemic heart, *Mol. Cell. Biochem.,* 157, 75, 1996.

55. Maulik, N. et al., Nitric oxide/carbon monoxide. A molecular switch for myocardial preservation during ischemia, *Circulation,* 94 (Suppl. 2), 398, 1996.

56. Sharma, H.S. et al., Coordinated expression of heme oxygenase-1 and ubiquitin in the porcine heart subjected to ischemia and reperfusion, *Mol. Cell. Biochem.,* 157, 111, 1996.

57. Hangaishi, M. et al., Induction of heme oxygenase-1 can act protectively against cardiac ischemia/reperfusion *in vivo*, *Biochem. Biophys. Res. Commun.*, 279, 582, 2000.
58. Beckman, J.S. et al., Apparent hydroxyl radical production by peroxynitrite: implications for endothelial injury from nitric oxide and superoxide, *Proc. Natl. Acad. Sci. U.S.A.*, 87, 1620, 1990.
59. Gess, B. et al., *In vivo* carbon monoxide exposure and hypoxic hypoxia stimulate immediate early gene expression, *Pflügers Arch.*, 434, 568, 1997.
60. Cook, M.N. et al., Heme oxygenase activity in the adult aorta and liver as measured by carbon monoxide formation, *Can. J. Physiol. Pharmacol.*, 73, 515, 1999.
61. Grundemar, L. et al., Heme oxygenase activity in blood vessel homogenates a measure by carbon monoxide production, *Acta Physiol. Scand.*, 153, 203, 1995.
62. Furchgott, R.F. and Jothianandan, D., Endothelium-dependent and -independent vasodilation involving cGMP: relaxation induced by NO, CO and light, *Blood Vessels*, 28, 52, 1991.
63. Kharitonov, V.G. et al., Basis of guanylate cyclase activities of carbon monoxide, *Proc. Natl. Acad. Sci., U.S.A.*, 92, 2568, 1995.
64. Marks, G. et al., Does carbon monoxide have a physiological function? *Trends Pharmacol. Sci.*, 12, 185, 1991.

Section 2

Carbon Monoxide and Pathophysiology of the Cardiovascular System

9 The Heme–Heme Oxygenase–Carbon Monoxide System and Hypertension

Robert A. Johnson and Fruzsina K. Johnson

CONTENTS

I. INTRODUCTION

Carbon monoxide (CO) is commonly recognized as an environmental toxin that arises from the incomplete combustion of fossil fuels.[1,2] However, the biological research community now recognizes that living systems also generate CO endogenously via heme metabolism in a reaction catalyzed by heme oxygenase (HO).[3] Endogenously formed CO is now gaining acceptance as a potentially important regulator of cardiovascular functions.[4-6]

During the 1960s, we learned that endogenously formed CO was associated with erythrocyte formation/degradation.[7] During the subsequent decades, HO was isolated

0-8493-1041-5/02/$0.00+$1.50

149

and extensively characterized as the enzyme that catalyzes the conversion of heme to biliverdin, iron, and CO.[3] This led to the identification of distinct isoforms and a multitude of associated HO mRNAs that could be correlated with numerous pathological conditions.[8] The endogenous formation of CO was seen eventually as a pathological marker for hemolysis[9] and means for clearance of spent porphyrin carbon.[8]

In 1991, Gerald Marks and colleagues stimulated the research community's interest in endogenously formed CO when they published a theoretical work[6] noting the ability of CO to activate soluble guanylate cyclase (sGC) to increase the formation of cGMP. Since cGMP was established as a second messenger that promotes relaxation of vascular smooth muscle, Marks et al. made the controversial suggestion that endogenously formed CO might stimulate the formation of cGMP to promote vasodilation. Accordingly, activation of the heme–HO–CO system might serve to lower blood pressure and the failure of this system might consequently remove a vasodilatory influence that promotes hypertension. Reports regarding regulation of HO expression accumulated, but only the most recent studies — those demonstrating that endogenous CO can be acutely manipulated to affect blood pressure — stimulated speculation that endogenous CO may be involved in the development of hypertension.[4,6]

II. HYPERTENSION: A FAILURE OF BLOOD PRESSURE REGULATION

Blood pressure is regulated in a manner that allows for sufficient perfusion of tissues while minimizing the risk for pressure-related organ damage. When arterial pressure rises to levels that significantly increase the risk of such damage, the condition is known as hypertension. Hypertension is not one disease *per se*, but rather a collection of disorders that share the trait of elevated blood pressure.

Current evidence suggests that the heme–HO–CO system may interact with blood pressure in two ways. First, it appears that the heme–HO–CO system may impact vascular tone, cardiac output, and water and electrolyte homeostasis to affect blood pressure.[4] Conversely, it appears that disorders of blood pressure regulation can lead to metabolic alterations that may have an impact on the heme–HO–CO cascade.[10,11] Alterations of the heme–HO–CO cascade may be either causes or results of hypertension.

III. THE HEME–HEME OXYGENASE–CARBON MONOXIDE SYSTEM AND REGULATION OF BLOOD PRESSURE

Endogenous formation of CO mainly arises from the metabolism of heme. Monomeric free heme is degraded to form equimolar amounts of iron, biliverdin, and CO in a reaction catalyzed by HO.[3,4,6,8] Zinc deuteroporphyrin 2,4 bis-glycol is a heme analogue that bears a zinc core (instead of iron) and a modified porphyrin ring.[12,13] Zinc deuteroporphyrin 2,4 bis-glycol is a powerful competitive inhibitor of HO-mediated conversion of heme to CO.[13] The modified porphyrin ring of zinc deuteroporphyrin 2,4 bis-glycol increases its solubility in water and permits it to effectively pass the blood–brain barrier.

In awake normotensive rat models, intraperitoneal administration of zinc deuteroporphyrin 2,4 bis-glycol systemically inhibits CO production and produces a rapid rise in arterial pressure.[14] This systemic blockade of HO activity that increases arterial pressure is accompanied by a decrease in cardiac output and paralleled by an increase in calculated total peripheral resistance.[14] In addition, other HO inhibitors have been shown to increase blood pressure[14] and exacerbate angiotensin-II-induced hypertension.[11] Thus it appears that some HO products play a vasodepressive role.

The iron and biliverdin products of HO do not appear to be vasodepressive.[14,15] In contrast, CO is an HO product and an established vasodepressant that can reverse zinc deuteroporphyrin 2,4 bis-glycol-induced increases in blood pressure.[16] Such evidence strongly suggests that the vasodepressive HO product is most likely CO.

Heme-L-lysinate is a highly soluble heme preparation[17] that provides monomeric free heme substrate to drive HO-mediated formation of CO. In the spontaneously hypertensive rat (SHR), a model of genetically transferable hypertension, heme-L-lysinate has been shown to produce a fall in blood pressure within minutes.[15] Heme-L-lysinate-induced decreases in arterial pressure can be blocked by pretreatment with an inhibitor of HO. Such observations suggest that heme preferentially lowers arterial pressure in hypertensive models via the generation of an HO product. Neither the iron nor the biliverdin product can account for the fall in blood pressure.[15] In contrast, intraperitoneal administration of CO has been shown to exert a vasodepressive action in this rat strain, while the same dose exerts little or no effect in normotensive animals.[1,15,18] This is the strongest functional evidence that endogenously formed CO is involved in the regulation of blood pressure.

IV. CARBON MONOXIDE AND NEURAL REGULATION OF BLOOD PRESSURE

The central nervous system (CNS) generates CO from the degradation of heme. HOs are abundant in the brain, but are discretely distributed in intensely dense patterns that resemble tracts.[19] Heme does not appear to pass the blood–brain barrier,[17,20] but the entire heme biosynthetic cascade has been identified in neural tissues.[4] Thus, it appears that CO formed in the CNS is locally contained and constitutes a biosynthetic system relatively isolated from that of the periphery.

Included in the first evidence that endogenously generated CO regulates cardiovascular functions is the demonstration that zinc deuteroporphyrin 2,4 bis-glycol, an inhibitor of HO shown to pass the blood–brain barrier, inhibits the heme–HO–CO cascade in the central nervous system and produces a reliable increase in arterial pressure.[12,14] Zinc deuteroporphyrin 2,4 bis-glycol-induced elevations in blood pressure can be prevented by inhibitors of alpha-1-adrenergic receptors or chemical blockade of ganglionic functions.[14] Such observations suggest that endogenously formed CO may suppress the sympathetic nervous system and that this influence is relayed through the ganglia. Zinc deuteroporphyrin 2,4 bis-glycol-induced increases in arterial pressure are not accompanied by reflex bradycardia, and that specifically suggests that HO may play a role in the baroreceptor reflex pathway.

The nucleus of the tractus solitarius is a medullary structure key to the integration of baroreceptor reflexes.[21] In response to elevated arterial pressure, increased stretching of baroreceptors in the carotid and aortic sinuses promotes increased firing of neural afferent tracts that terminate at the nucleus of the tractus solitarius. The nucleus uses L-glutamate as a transmitter to integrate appropriate responses including withdrawal of sympathetic influences and activation of a parasympathetic discharge. In this manner, increases in blood pressure are normally partially corrected by a slowing of the heart rate. HO inhibitors centrally affect baroreceptor function[16,22] and systemic administration of HO inhibitors leads to a marked attenuation of baroreceptor reflex functions.[16]

Carotid bodies are sensory organs that regulate heart rate by responding to alterations in blood gas levels. The carotid bodies sense changes in blood gas levels and regulate activity of the carotid sinus nerves that project to the nucleus of the tractus solitarius. An HO inhibitor has been shown to increase carotid body sensory activity in a manner that can be reversed by exogenously applied CO.[23] Such evidence suggests that endogenously formed CO may be a physiologic regulator of carotid body sensory activity.

Within the nucleus of the tractus solitarius, endogenously formed CO appears to interact with L-glutamatergic transmission to impact baroreceptor reflex and blood pressure functions. In transverse slices of rat dorsomedial subdivisions of the nucleus of the tractus solitarius, L-glutamate-induced monosynaptic excitatory postsynaptic currents can be blocked by an inhibitor of HO.[24] In awake rats, microinjections of L-glutamate into the nucleus of the tractus solitarius usually invoke increases in arterial pressure and decreases in heart rate.[25] These L-glutamate-induced changes in blood pressures and heart rate are blocked by microinjections of HO inhibitors.[22] Thus it appears that endogenously formed CO may interact with L-glutamate-mediated transmissions in the nucleus of the tractus solitarius.

Baroreceptor reflexes mediated via the nucleus of the tractus solitarius are also blocked by microinjections of HO inhibitors into the nucleus of the tractus solitarius.[22] The actions of these inhibitors do not appear to completely disrupt functions of the nucleus as they do not interfere with the chemoreceptor-mediated refexes that share this neural tract.[22] The selective nature of the neuromodulatory actions of HO inhibitors in the nucleus of the tractus solitarius indicate that the actions of CO on glutamatergic transmission can be complex.

Endogenously formed CO in the nucleus of the tractus solitarius appears to be a prominent acute regulator of arterial pressure. Microinjections of HO inhibitors into the nucleus can increase arterial blood pressure acutely,[16] similar to systemic blockade of CO production, and these effects can be rapidly reversed by microinjections of CO into the nucleus. The centrally mediated vasoregulatory effects of CO are so pronounced that nucleus microinjections of CO also rapidly normalize the elevated blood pressures produced by systemic blockade of HO activity.[16]

The central nervous system seems to play a vital role in CO-mediated regulation of blood pressure. Inhibitors of HO that cross the blood–brain barrier, such as zinc deuteroporphyrin 2,4 bis-glycol, cause rapid sustained increases in arterial pressures.[14] In contrast, HO inhibitors that can cause systemic inhibition of CO production but are unable to pass the blood–brain barrier appear to have little effect on blood pressure.[26] The actions of CO within the CNS, more specifically within the nucleus of the tractus solitarius, are likely to play a very important role in the regulation of blood pressure.

Early works suggest that the L-glutamate receptors of the nucleus of the tractus solitarius might be coupled to HO, so that activation of the glutamate receptors would stimulate the formation of CO.[24] In turn, L-glutamate-stimulated formation of CO would stimulate cGMP formation to affect the responsive tracts descending from the nucleus of the tractus solitarius. If CO were the second messenger generated from L-glutamate stimulation, then one would expect CO to mimic the actions of L-glutamate. However, microinjections of L-glutamate into the nucleus of the tractus solitarius of awake animals invoked a rapid pressor response, whereas microinjections of CO promoted a vasodepressor response.[16] Since the vasoregulatory effects generated by L-glutamate are in opposition to those generated by exogenous CO, it appears unlikely that CO is a second messenger for L-glutamate-induced activation of the nucleus of the tractus solitarius.

While the second messengers involved with the neuromodulatory actions of CO have not been clearly identified, it is clear that CO can centrally exert an influence on blood pressure. It appears that the central action of CO is to suppress the sympathetic activity, and that its regulatory actions likely arise both in the chemoreceptors and in the integrating tracts of the nucleus of the tractus solitarius. It also appears that the regulation of blood pressure, more specifically the development of hypertension, may potentially arise from aberrations in endogenous CO formation in the nucleus of the tractus solitarius.

V. ENDOGENOUSLY FORMED CARBON MONOXIDE AND THE REGULATION OF VASCULAR TONE

A. ENDOGENOUSLY FORMED CARBON MONOXIDE PROMOTES RELAXATION OF VASCULAR SMOOTH MUSCLE

The discovery that endogenously formed CO may contribute to vascular tone has ramifications for the pathological development and treatment of hypertension. If vascular smooth muscle normally generates CO sufficient to contribute to basal tone, then the removal of this vasodepressive agent should prompt vasoconstriction and encourage hypertension. From a therapeutic perspective, hypertensive disorders might potentially be treated by maneuvers that enhance vascular tissue production of CO.

The toxicology literature established CO as an activator of sGC[27,28] and an agent that relaxes vascular smooth muscle.[29] HO-2 is a constitutive isoform identified in arterial vascular smooth muscle.[30] CO production in vascular smooth muscle can be accelerated in response to heme and inhibited upon exposure to certain metalloporphyrins such as zinc deuteroporphyrin 2,4 bis-glycol or chromium mesoporphyrin.[13,31] In isolated vessel preparations, the introduction of heme can promote vasodilation.[32,33] Heme-induced dilation can be prevented by inhibitors of HO.[32] These features suggest that heme-induced dilation of vascular smooth muscle is the result of the generation of an HO product.

Biliverdin, iron, and CO are products of heme oxygenase that have been implicated as vasoactive substances.[34-36] Biliverdin is rapidly converted to bilirubin, a
primary antioxidant of mammalian systems.[35] It has been suggested that antioxidants
may buffer free radical oxygen species to prolong the actions of vasodilatory radicals
such as nitric oxide (NO). However, biliverdin does not seem to promote dilation
of isolated vascular preparations.[32] It has also been suggested that iron propagates
vasodilatory mechanisms.[36] However, heme-induced dilation of isolated vessel preparations is not sensitive to iron chelation by deferoxamine.[32] In contrast, CO has
consistently been shown to promote dilation of vascular smooth muscle,[29,32,33,37-39]
implying that CO is the HO product that promotes relaxation of vascular smooth
muscle.

Basal CO production in vascular smooth muscle is sufficient to provide a sustained relaxing influence. Inhibitors of HO produce powerful constriction in isolated
vessel preparations[38,40,41] and the constrictive actions of these metalloporphyrins are
also evident in vessel preparations that have been denuded of endothelium.[41] The
vasoconstrictive effects of HO inhibitors[40] seem to arise specifically from the inhibition of CO synthesis as they can be blocked by authentic CO, but not by other
vasodilators such as sodium nitroprusside. The specific mechanism underlying CO-
induced vasorelaxation is unclear. CO is an activator of sGC,[27,28] but CO-induced
dilation can occur independently of sGC activity.[39,40] Considerable evidence suggests
CO may confer blood pressure effects through interactions with potassium channels,[33,37] interference with P-450-mediated functions,[42] or by modulating endothelin
formation.[39,43,44]

Regardless of the specific messengers involved, the formation of CO in vascular
smooth muscle is apparently sufficient to contribute to resting tone of the vasculature.
The typical levels of HO-mediated formation of CO may be either increased or
decreased to promote vasodilation or vasoconstriction, respectively. This suggests
that endogenously formed CO qualifies as a physiological regulator of vascular tone.

B. CARBON MONOXIDE AS AN INHIBITOR OF NITRIC OXIDE SYNTHASE: ENDOTHELIUM-DEPENDENT VASOCONSTRICTION

While CO is commonly accepted to promote relaxation of vascular smooth muscle,
it can also indirectly promote vasoconstriction by inhibiting the production of another
powerful vasodilator, nitric oxide (NO). Endothelial cells possess nitric oxide synthase, an enzyme that catalyzes the conversion of L-arginine to NO.[45] Constant
endothelial generation of NO helps maintain blood pressure by providing a constant
vasodilatory influence on the vasculature. CO is a powerful inhibitor of nitric oxide
synthase,[46,47] which binds competitively with L-arginine to inhibit NO production.[46]
The endothelium of the arterial vasculature is a rich source of nitric oxide synthase,
but the endothelium also constitutively bears HO-2.[30,45] In addition, it has now been
shown that the levels of CO formed in the tissues[48] are sufficient to partially inhibit
nitric oxide synthase.[49]

Evidence suggests that endogenously formed CO may impair the activities of
the NO system.[4] For example, an inhibitor of endogenous CO formation, zinc
protoporphyrin IX, has been cited to relax pulmonary arterial rings in a manner

prevented by an inhibitor of nitric oxide synthesis.[50] In addition, *in vivo* studies established that an inhibitor of nitric oxide synthase, N^{ω}-nitro-L-arginine methyl ester (L-NAME), does not raise the blood pressure in rats in postoperative states of increased CO formation, unless they are pretreated with an inhibitor of HO.[51]

We have recently conducted original studies that strongly suggest that CO can inhibit nitric oxide synthase to promote vasoconstriction. Experiments were conducted on rat isolated pressurized first order gracilis arterioles superfused with oxygenated (14% O_2/5% CO_2 balanced with N_2), modified Krebs buffer ($CaCl_2$ 1.4 m*M*) using a previously published technique.[32,40]

In gracilis arterioles denuded of endothelium (Figure 9.1A), heme-L-lysinate, an HO substrate that drives endogenous CO formation, promotes *dilation*. In contrast (Figure 9.1B), heme-L-lysinate produces *constriction* in vessels with functionally intact endothelium. In similar vessels with intact endothelium, exogenous CO also elicits a vasoconstrictive response. Based on these observations, CO must either (1) stimulate the release of some endothelium-derived constricting factor or (2) inhibit the release of some endothelium-derived relaxing factor.

NO is a well established endothelium-derived relaxing factor,[45] and CO is a well established inhibitor of nitric oxide synthase.[46,47] To determine whether nitric synthase is involved in CO-induced constriction, the effects of heme-L-lysinate and exogenous CO were also examined in vessels with intact endothelium, but in the presence of L-NAME, an inhibitor of nitric oxide synthase. In the presence of L-NAME, vessels with intact endothelium dilate in response to heme-L-lysinate (Figure 9.1C). In order to inhibit nitric oxide synthase in the presence of L-NAME, similarly prepared vessels dilated in response to exogenously applied CO.

The fact that CO produces endothelium-dependent vasoconstriction only in the presence of a functional endothelium-derived nitric oxide system serves as compelling evidence that CO, even biologically generated CO, may exert a vasoconstrictive influence consequent to its inhibition of nitric oxide synthesis. If this is correct, then endogenously formed CO may be regarded as a physiological regulator of the NO system.

The idea that CO is a vasodilator that can simultaneously inhibit the production of another vasodilator may seem illogical (Figure 9.2). In many cases, the vascular effects resulting from changes in CO production may be completely masked. Even so, shifts between the CO and NO systems may have enormous consequences.

In response to increased shear forces within the vascular lumen, the adjacent endothelium quickly releases NO to promote local vasodilation and partially restore vessel diameter.[45] In this manner, the effects of vasoconstrictors, such as angiotensin-II or endothelin, can be buffered via shear force-mediated production of NO. While shear force-mediated release of nitric oxide is rapid, HO-mediated generation of CO appears to be insensitive to acute changes in shear forces. Consequently, enhanced production of CO would compromise shear force-mediated generation of NO and heighten the responsiveness of the adjacent vasculature.

Hyper-responsiveness is a vascular property displayed in various forms of hypertension. Of potential diagnostic and therapeutic importance, hyper-responsiveness often precedes essential hypertension.[52] Hyper-responsiveness may be the result of multiple factors that promote hypertension or it may arise consequent to hypertension. As endogenously formed CO appears to interfere with the vasodilatory actions

A) Arterioles Denuded of Endothelium

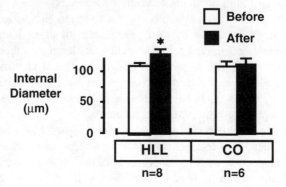

B) Arterioles with Intact Endothelium

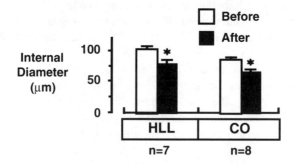

C) Arterioles Pretreated with L-NAME

FIGURE 9.1 Maximal effects of the HO substrate, 10 µM heme-L-lysinate, and 50 µM exogenous CO on internal diameters of first order gracilis arterioles isolated from male Sprague–Dawley rats denuded of endothelium (A), with intact endothelium (B), or pretreated with 1 mM N$^{\omega}$-nitro-L-arginine methyl ester (L-NAME) to maximally inhibit nitric oxide synthesis (C). Data expressed as mean ± SEM; * indicates p < 0.05.

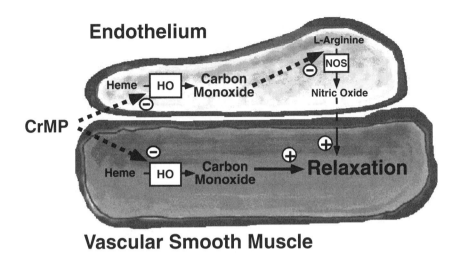

FIGURE 9.2 A working model of heme-derived CO-promoting vascular relaxation in the smooth muscle, while competing with L-arginine binding to nitric oxide synthase. The use of heme to drive CO synthesis would promote endothelium-independent dilation and endothelium-dependent L-NAME-sensitive constriction. The use of an HO inhibitor, such as chromium mesoporphyrin (CrMP), would promote endothelium-independent constriction that would be buffered in the presence of endothelium.

of the NO system and potentially promote hyper-responsiveness, the heme–HO–CO system may play an important role in the development of hypertension.

Dahl/Rapp salt-sensitive rats are vulnerable to the hypertensive effects of high salt diets.[53] When fed an 8% NaCl-supplemented diet, these rats rapidly develop hypertension. However, when fed a low salt diet (0.3% NaCl), these rats remain normotensive.[53] Salt-induced hypertension is accompanied by an increase in total peripheral resistance.[54] Aortic rings isolated from hypertensive Dahl/Rapp salt-sensitive rats display impaired endothelium-dependent vasodilation with a resulting increase in responsiveness to vasoconstrictors.[55] The basis of decreased NO formation displayed in this hypertensive model remains controversial. While L-arginine substrate levels are normal in hypertensive Dahl/Rapp salt-sensitive rats, the development of salt-induced hypertension can be prevented by administration of L-arginine.[53] This trait suggests that a competitive inhibitor of nitric oxide synthase may influence NO production in this hypertensive model.

CO is a competitive inhibitor of nitric oxide synthase-mediated conversion of L-arginine to L-citrulline.[46] If enhanced production of CO compromises nitric oxide synthase activity in hypertensive Dahl/Rapp salt-sensitive rats, then it only follows that metalloporphyrins should restore the ability of nitric oxide synthase to promote vasodilation. We conducted a simple study to determine whether endogenously formed CO might contribute to impaired endothelium-dependent vasodilation.

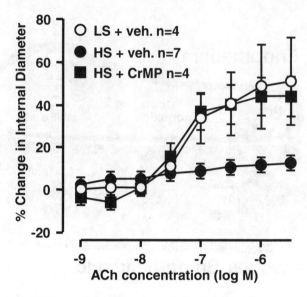

FIGURE 9.3 Acetylcholine (ACh)-induced (1 nM to 3 μM) concentration-dependent changes in internal diameters of first order gracillis arterioles isolated from Dahl/Rapp salt-sensitive rats after 4 weeks of high salt (HS, 8% NaCl) diet pretreated with 15 μM chromium meso-porphyrin, an inhibitor of endogenous CO production (HS + CrMP); high salt diet with vehicle (HS + veh.); or low salt (0.3% NaCl) diet pretreated with vehicle (LS + veh.).

　　Under conditions described above, gracilis arterioles with intact endothelium isolated from Dahl/Rapp salt-sensitive rats after 4 weeks of high (8% NaCl) or low salt (0.3% NaCl) diets were exposed to increasing concentrations of an endothelium-dependent vasodilator, acetylcholine. Acetylcholine promoted a robust dilatory response in vessels isolated from the low salt normotensive animals (Figure 9.3), but had little effect on vessels isolated from the high salt hypertensive group. In other vessels isolated from high salt hypertensive animals, the inclusion of chromium mesoporphyrin restores the vasodilatory actions of acetylcholine. Since chromium mesoporphyrin is a powerful inhibitor of HO-mediated formation of CO, and since chromium mesoporphyrin restored nitric oxide synthase-mediated dilation, endog-enously formed CO may underlie the impaired endothelium-dependent vasodilation displayed in hypertensive Dahl/Rapp salt-sensitive rats.

　　In summary, it appears that CO can serve dual vascular roles. Endogenous CO can promote vasodilation through its effects on vascular smooth muscle. In contrast, CO can inhibit nitric oxide synthase and promote vasoconstriction. While the vas-oconstrictive properties of CO may exacerbate the debilitating actions of vasocon-strictors, the heme–HO–CO system may constitute an alternative vasorelaxing influ-ence that confers protection in conditions in which the endothelium is destroyed. In addition, regulation of the CO and NO systems may potentially be orchestrated to set a suitable level of resting vascular tone without compromising vascular reactivity. Imbalances of these two gaseous systems could potentially produce hypertension and/or vascular hyper-responsiveness.

VI. CARBON MONOXIDE AND RENAL FUNCTION DURING HYPERTENSION

Hypertension is associated with abnormal renal functions. Normally, increases in renal perfusion pressure promote renal sodium/water excretion to decrease circulating blood volume and suppress the vasoconstrictive- and sodium/water-retaining influences of the renin–angiotensin–aldosterone system.[56] Increases in arterial pressure are corrected through renal-mediated adjustments in sodium/water balance and vascular tone. For this reason, sustained increases in arterial pressure are clear indications that renal-mediated adjustments in water/electrolyte and hormonal functions have been compromised. It has been well established that the kidney is a rich source of HOs. Even so, little is known about the specific roles of HO-derived CO in the regulation of renal functions.

Renal levels of constitutive type HO-2 mRNA are significantly increased in stroke-prone SHRs as compared with Wistar Kyoto rats.[57] That suggests that endogenously formed CO may modify renal functions in some genetically transmittable forms of hypertension. Administration of heme substrate lowers blood pressure in SHRs,[15,42] and increases renal HO mRNA and HO activity.[42]

It has been suggested that medullary blood flow is important to the long-term control of arterial blood pressure.[58] The levels of HO-1 and HO-2 in the renal medulla are higher than those expressed in the renal cortex.[59] Interstitial infusion of an inhibitor of HO-mediated formation of CO decreases renal medullary blood flow and lowers local concentrations of cGMP. Such findings are initial evidence that the heme–HO–CO system may serve an antihypertensive role by maintaining the constancy of renal medullary blood flow.

HO-1 has been suggested to regulate renal excretory functions in angiotensin-II-dependent hypertension.[11] In kidneys taken from normotensive rats, HO-1 was expressed primarily in the basal sides of the renal tubules. Angiotensin-II infusion shifts HO-1 expression to be dispersed in the tubular epithelial cells. In rats made chronically hypertensive by angiotensin-II infusions, administration of hemin protects against angiotensin-induced decreases in glomerular filtration rates and decreases urinary protein excretion. In contrast, administration of the HO inhibitor, zinc protoporphyrin, further aggravates angiotensin-induced decreases in glomerular filtration rates and exacerbates proteinuria. These data suggest that up-regulation of HO may locally exert renoprotection during angiotensin-II-induced hypertension.

The renin–angiotensin–aldosterone system is of paramount importance in hypertension. Decreases in renal perfusion pressure and increases in renal sympathetic nerve activity stimulate the renal release of renin.[56] Renin, in turn, drives the formation of angiotensin-II and aldosterone which promote vasoconstriction and sodium/water retention, respectively. While little work has been done on the roles of endogenously formed CO in the regulation of the renin–angiotensin–aldosterone system, toxicological studies may provide clues to its potential actions.

CO has been shown to increase plasma renin activity, but it also inhibits the formation and release of aldosterone.[2] If these properties are also displayed under physiological conditions, then endogenously formed CO could potentially promote vasoconstriction by driving the formation of angiotensin-II, while simultaneously

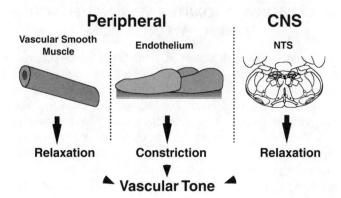

FIGURE 9.4 Culmination of local and central influences of CO on vascular tone. Endogenously formed CO relaxes vascular smooth muscle and appears to inhibit endothelial nitric oxide synthase. *In vivo*, endogenously formed CO appears to suppress sympathetic tone of the vasculature.

interfering with sodium/water retention consequent to formation of aldosterone. Conversely, suppression of the heme–HO–CO system may promote hyperaldosteronism in the face of relatively normal levels of renin and angiotensin. The pathological and physiological consequences of such uncoupling of aldosterone formation from renin release are unclear, but we speculate that endogenously formed CO might be important in establishing aldosterone release in response to angiotensin formation.

VII. SUMMARY

The initial proposal that endogenously formed CO plays a role in the regulation of blood pressure is truly unconventional, but the information gathered from creative studies is compelling. It appears that endogenously formed CO is a neuromodulator that acts in the nucleus of the tractus solitarius to suppress sympathetic discharge. In the periphery, endogenously formed CO arising within the vascular smooth muscle serves to decrease vascular tone (Figure 9.4). In addition, endogenously formed CO appears to interfere with the vasodilatory properties of the endothelial NO system, which, in turn, may affect vascular responsiveness. Initial reports suggest that the heme–HO–CO system may contribute to renal functions.

Since heme-derived CO seems to contribute to cardiovascular functions under basal conditions, changes in CO formation would ultimately change central, vascular, or renal functions and, in turn, impact blood pressure regulation. While this highly novel area of research is in its infancy, initial progress has been striking. Aberrations in CO production can initiate and exacerbate hypertension. The over-production of CO may help lower blood pressure, but it may come at the cost of increased vascular responsiveness which may contribute to stroke. In addition, it is unclear whether the renoprotective actions of the heme–HO–CO system constitute normal physiological responses, or serve as last ditch efforts to minimize kidney damage when all other systems have failed. Regardless, the increasing interest in the heme–HO–CO system as it applies to the establishment of blood pressure and its adjustments during hypertension serves as an impetus for exploring novel roles for endogenously formed CO as a regulator of cardiovascular functions.

ACKNOWLEDGMENTS

R.A.J. is supported by a grant from the National Heart, Blood, and Lung Institute of the National Institutes of Health (1RO1HL64577-01). F.K.J. receives support from a fellowship provided by the Southeast Affiliate of the American Heart Association (0020335B) and from the Solvay Pharmaceuticals Hypertension Yearly Grants Program–2000. The authors also wish to acknowledge Dr. Alberto Nasjletti for his enthusiasm and most gracious support in the seminal years of this project.

REFERENCES

1. Penney, D.G. and Robinson, M.C., Effects of verapamil and carbon monoxide on blood pressure and heart mass in the spontaneously hypertensive rat, *Eur. J. Pharmacol.*, 182, 29, 1990.
2. Penney, D.G., Acute carbon monoxide poisoning: animal models: a review, *Toxicology*, 62, 123, 1990
3. Tenhunen, R., Marver, H.S., and Schmid, R., Microsomal heme oxygenase. Characterization of the enzyme, *J.Biol.Chem.*, 244, 6388, 1969.
4. Johnson, R.A., Kozma, F., and Colombari, E., Carbon monoxide: from toxin to endogenous modulator of cardiovascular functions, *Braz. J. Med. Biol. Res.*, 32, 1, 1999.
5. Wang, R., Resurgence of carbon monoxide: an endogenous gaseous vasorelaxing factor, *Can. J. Physiol. Pharmacol.*, 76, 1, 1998.
6. Marks, G.S. et al., Does carbon monoxide have a physiological function? *Trends Pharmacol. Sci.,* 12, 185, 1991.
7. Coburn, R.F., The production of carbon monoxide from hemoglobin *in vivo*, *J. Clin. Invest.*, 46, 346, 1967.
8. Maines, M.D., The heme oxygenase system: a regulator of second messenger gases, *Annu. Rev. Pharmacol. Toxicol.*, 37, 517, 1997.
9. Stevenson, D.K. et al., Bilirubin production in healthy term infants as measured by carbon monoxide in breath, *Clin. Chem.*, 40, 1934, 1994.
10. Ishizaka, N. et al., Angiotensin II-induced hypertension increases heme oxygenase-1 expression in rat aorta, *Circulation*, 96, 1923, 1997.
11. Aizawa, T. et al., Heme oxygenase-1 is up-regulated in the kidney of angiotensin II-induced hypertensive rats: possible role in renoprotection. *Hypertension*, 35, 800, 2000.
12. Chernick, R.J. et al., Sensitivity of human tissue heme oxygenase to a new synthetic metalloporphyrin, *Hepatology*, 10, 365, 1989.
13. Vreman, H.J., Ekstrand, B.C., and Stevenson, D.K., Selection of metalloporphyrin heme oxygenase inhibitors based on potency and photoreactivity, *Pediatr. Res.*, 33, 195, 1993.
14. Johnson, R.A. et al., A heme oxygenase product, presumably carbon monoxide, mediates a vasodepressor function in rats, *Hypertension*, 25, 166, 1995.
15. Johnson, R.A. et al., Heme oxygenase substrates acutely lower blood pressure in hypertensive rats, *Am. J. Physiol.*, 271, H1132, 1996.

16. Johnson, R.A. et al., Role of endogenous carbon monoxide in central regulation of arterial pressure, *Hypertension,* 30, 962, 1997.
17. Tenhunen, R., Tokola, O., and Linden, I.B., Haem arginate: a new stable haem compound, *J. Pharm. Pharmacol.,* 39, 780, 1987.
18. Penney, D.G. and Skikun, R.M., Hypertension is not exacerbated by chronic carbon monoxide exposure, with or without added salt, in the borderline hypertensive rat, *Arch. Toxicol. Suppl.,* 14, 118, 1991.
19. Verma, A. et al., Carbon monoxide: a putative neural messenger, *Science,* 15, 259, 381, 1993.
20. Linden, I.B. et al., Fate of haem after parenteral administration of haem arginate to rabbits, *J. Pharm. Pharmacol.,* 39, 96, 1987.
21. Talman, W.T., Glutamatergic transmission in the nucleus tractus solitarii: from server to peripherals in the cardiovascular information superhighway, *Braz. J. Med. Biol. Res.,* 30, 1, 1977.
22. Silva, C.C. et al., Role of carbon monoxide in L-glutamate-induced cardiovascular responses in nucleus tractus solitarius of conscious rats, *Brain Res.,* 824, 147, 1999.
23. Prabhakar, N.R. et al., Carbon monoxide: a role in carotid body chemoreception. *Proc. Natl. Acad. Sci. U.S.A.,* 92,1994, 1995.
24. Glaum, S.R. and Miller, R.J., Zinc protoporphyrin-IX blocks the effects of metabotropic glutamate receptor activation in the rat nucleus tractus solitarii, *Mol. Pharmacol.,* 43, 965, 1993.
25. Colombari, E., Menani, J.V., and Talman, W.T., Commissural NTS contributes to pressor responses to glutamate injected into the medial NTS of awake rats, *Am. J. Physiol.,* 270, R1220, 1996.
26. Johnson, F.K. et al., L-NAME, but not phenylephrine, enhances the effects of endogenous carbon monoxide on vascular tone *in vivo* and *in vitro, Hypertension,* 36, 678, 2000.
27. Karlsson, J.O., Axelsson, K.L., and Andersson, R.G., Effects of hydroxyl radical scavengers KCN and CO on ultraviolet light-induced activation of crude soluble guanylate cyclase, *J. Cyclic Nucleotide Protein Phosphor. Res.,*10, 309, 1985.
28. Kharitonov, V.G. et al., Basis of guanylate cyclase activation by carbon monoxide, *Proc. Natl. Acad. Sci. U.S.A.,* 92, 2568, 1995.
29. Furchgott, R.F. and Jothianandan, D., Endothelium-dependent and -independent vasodilation involving cyclic GMP: relaxation induced by nitric oxide, carbon monoxide and light, *Blood Vessels,* 28, 52, 1991.
30. Grozdanovic, Z. and Gossrau, R., Expression of heme oxygenase-2 (HO-2)-like immunoreactivity in rat tissues, *Acta Histochim.,* 98, 203, 1996.
31. Cook, M.N. et al., Heme oxygenase activity in the adult rat aorta and liver as measured by carbon monoxide formation, *Can. J. Physiol. Pharmacol.,* 73, 515, 1995.
32. Kozma, F., Johnson, R.A., and Nasjletti, A., Role of carbon monoxide in heme-induced vasodilation, *Eur .J. Pharmacol.,* 323, R1, 1997.
33. Wang, R., Wang, Z., and Wu, L., Carbon monoxide-induced vasorelaxation and the underlying mechanisms, *Br. J. Pharmacol.,* 121, 927, 1997.
34. Kutty, R.K. and Maines, M.D., Hepatic heme metabolism: possible role of biliverdin in the regulation of heme oxygenase activity, *Biochem. Biophys. Res. Commun.,* 122, 40, 1984.
35. Stocker, R. et al., Antioxidant activities of bile pigments: biliverdin and bilirubin, *Methods Enzymol.,* 186, 301, 1990.
36. Balla, J. et al., Ferriporphyrins and endothelium: a 2-edged sword promotion of oxidation and induction of cytoprotectants, *Blood,* 95, 3442, 2000.

37. Wang, R., Wu, L., and Wang, Z., The direct effect of carbon monoxide on K_{Ca} channels in vascular smooth muscle cells, *Pflügers Arch.*, 434, 285, 1997.

38. Coceani, F. et al., Carbon monoxide formation in the ductus arteriosus in the lamb: implications for the regulation of muscle tone, *Br. J. Pharmacol.*, 120, 599, 1997.

39. Coceani, F., Kelsey, L., and Seidlitz, E., Carbon monoxide-induced relaxation of the ductus arteriosus in the lamb: evidence against the prime role of guanylyl cyclase, *Br. J. Pharmacol.*, 118, 1689, 1996.

40. Kozma, F. et al., Contribution of endogenous carbon monoxide to regulation of diameter in resistance vessels, *Am. J. Physiol.*, 276, R1087, 1999.

41. Johnson, F.K. et al., Vascular effects of endogenous carbon monoxide are enhanced in the absence of endothelium-derived nitric oxide, *Acta Haematol.*, 103, 72, 2000.

42. Martasek, P. et al., Hemin and L-arginine regulation of blood pressure in spontaneous hypertensive rats, *J. Am. Soc. Nephrol.*, 2, 1078, 1991.

43. Coceani, F., Carbon monoxide in vasoregulation: the promise and the challenge, *Circ. Res.*, 86, 1184, 2000.

44. Morita, T. and Kourembanas, S., Endothelial cell expression of vasoconstrictors and growth factors is regulated by smooth muscle cell-derived carbon monoxide, *J. Clin. Invest.*, 96, 2676, 1995.

45. Moncada, S., Palmer, R.M., and Higgs, E.A., Nitric oxide: physiology, pathophysiology, and pharmacology, *Pharmacol. Rev.*, 43, 109, 1991.

46. Matsuoka, A. et al., L-arginine and calmodulin regulation of the heme iron reactivity in neuronal nitric oxide synthase, *J. Biol. Chem.*, 269, 20335, 1994.

47. White, K.A. and Marletta, M.A., Nitric oxide synthase is a cytochrome P-450 type hemoprotein, *Biochemistry*, 31, 6627, 1992.

48. Vreman, H.J., Wong, R.J., and Stevenson, D.K., Carbon monoxide in breath, blood, and other tissues, in *Carbon Monoxide Toxicity*, Penney, D.G., Ed., CRC Press, Boca Raton, FL, 2000, chap. 2.

49. Thorup, C. et al., Carbon monoxide induces vasodilation and nitric oxide release but suppresses endothelial NOS, *Am. J. Physiol.*, 277, F882, 1999.

50. Zakhary, R. et al., Heme oxygenase 2: endothelial and neuronal localization and role in endothelium-dependent relaxation, *Proc. Natl. Acad. Sci. U.S.A*, 93, 795, 1996.

51. Motterlini, R. et al., Heme oxygenase-1-derived carbon monoxide contributes to the suppression of acute hypertensive responses *in vivo*, *Circ. Res.*, 83, 568, 1998.

52. Wells, A.M. et al., Pressor and vascular responsiveness in renal prehypertensive rabbits with a nonfiltering kidney, *Proc. Soc. Exp. Biol. Med.*, 180, 24, 1985.

53. Chen, P.Y. and Sanders, P.W., Role of nitric oxide synthesis in salt-sensitive hypertension in Dahl/Rapp rats, *Hypertension*, 22, 812, 1993.

54. Ganguli, M., Tobian, L., and Iwai, J., Cardiac output and peripheral resistance in strains of rats sensitive and resistant to NaCl hypertension, *Hypertension*, 1, 3, 1979.

55. Luscher, T.F., Raij, L., and Vanhoutte, P.M., Endothelium-dependent vascular responses in normotensive and hypertensive Dahl rats, *Hypertension*, 9, 157, 1987.

56. Hall, J.E., Brands, M.W., and Shek, E.W., Central role of the kidney and abnormal fluid volume control in hypertension, *J. Hum. Hypertens.*, 10, 633, 1996.

57. Seki, T. et al., Roles of heme oxygenase/carbon monoxide system in genetically hypertensive rats, *Biochem. Biophys. Res. Commun.*, 241, 574, 1997.

58. Cowley, A.W., Role of the renal medulla in volume and arterial pressure regulation, *Am. J. Physiol.*, 273, R1, 1997.

59. Zou, A.P., Billington, H., Su, N., and Cowley, A.W., Expression and actions of heme oxygenase in the renal medulla of rats, *Hypertension*, 35, 342, 2000.

10 Carbon Monoxide and Cardiovascular Inflammation

Joseph Fomusi Ndisang, Emanuela Masini, Pier Francesco Mannanoni, and Rui Wang

CONTENTS

I. GENERAL OVERVIEW

Profound physiological adaptations are triggered during the inflammatory process as an attempt to limit tissue damage and remove pathogenic insult. Such mechanisms include local and systemic vasodilation, pyrexia, and the activation of the immune system. These changes are regulated by a number of diverse mediators such as cytokines, bacterial products, (neuro)-peptides, and eicosanoids. Should the physiological responses be inadequate to counteract the inflammatory stimuli, more severe conditions such as anaphylactic shock and even death may ensue.

Generally speaking, immune processes that lead to the elimination of antigen go on without necessarily producing clinically detectable inflammation. Clinical inflammation does develop, however, when the immune system encounters an unusually large amount of antigen, an antigen in an unusual location, or an antigen that is difficult to digest. The immune system consists of many types of cells, each with different and important roles. For instance, lymphocytes determine the specificity of immunity. Other cells with immunologic functions are mast cells and basophils.

Tissue mast cells are strategically located around the blood vessels, releasing histamine and other vasoactive mediators in response to immunological and non-immunological stimuli. Mast cells and human basophils are also capable of generating carbon monoxide (CO), which exerts a negative feedback on histamine release.[1,2] Thus, mast cells can modulate vascular reactivity through the release of dilator and constrictor substances.[3-5]

Our understanding of the role of CO as an inter- and intracellular messenger molecule has been considerably advanced recently. Several metabolic reactions lead to the production of endogenous CO, and the best characterized reaction is the one catalyzed by heme oxygenase (HO).[6,7] HO is found in the endoplasmic reticulum (ER), mainly localized to the smooth ER fraction,[8] Three isoforms of HO have been identified to date. The 32-kDa inducible isoform (HO-1) was the first one isolated. HO-1 is not constitutively present in cells, and is expressed following exposure of cells to different stimuli. The regulation of HO-1 expression is complex, and the mechanisms by which CO modulates inflammatory processes are multi-faceted and might be protective or detrimental, depending upon its local concentrations. The release of CO from HO-1 is greater than that from the constitutive form (HO-2), a 36-kDa protein constitutively expressed in many organs under normal physiological conditions.[9] It is believed that HO-1 is the predominant source of CO during pathophysiological episodes. Not much is known about the third isoform (HO-3) that shares about 90% homology with HO-2, and has a molecular weight of 33 kDa.[10] Like HO-2, HO-3 is constitutively expressed in liver, spleen, brain, and kidney. The products of heme degradation possess important antivasoconstrictive, antiinflammatory, antiapoptotic, and antioxidant properties as well as the ability to down-regulate the immune response.[11,12]

II. CARBON MONOXIDE, ISCHEMIA, AND INFLAMMATION

In the post-ischemic heart, increased mRNA levels of HO have been reported[13] and it was proposed that the maintenance of healthy function of myocardium by nitric oxide (NO) might be modulated at least in part by CO signaling. Post-ischemic reperfusion is accompanied by the release of proinflammatory and fibrogenic mediators, an event that is meant to restore and promote tissue healing although it may subsequently lead to cardiac injury.[14] Coincidentally, reperfusion is accompanied by a decrease in venular shear forces and increases in neutrophil rolling, adhesion, and extravasation. All these conditions enhance neutrophil recruitment in tissues[15] and thus their migration to inflammatory sites.

Kubes[16] reported that in post-ischemic mesenteric microvasculature, maintaining the shear forces at control value did not affect rolling leukocytes but reduced the number of adherent cells. This observation suggests that the decreased shear force did not contribute to the initial neutrophil activation, but was a necessary component for neutrophil adhesion and extravasation in post-ischemic circulation.[15] The slow-flow reperfusion that characterizes post-ischemic hearts further enhances the accumulation of neutrophils in post-capillary vessels, causing a great obliteration of blood vessels, and thus obstructing blood flow. This phenomenon of impeded blood flow has some clinical implications[17] since it is associated with higher incidence of arrhythmias, difficult recovery of the contracted ventricle after the systole phase, and congestive heart failure in humans.[18] These problems associated with post-ischemic reperfusion may be addressed by reducing neutrophil adhesion and extravasation. CO has been shown to enhance neutrophil migration in a cGMP-dependent way.[19] Our previous studies also demonstrated that CO and hemin abated the immunological and non-immunological release of histamine from serosal mast cells and human basophils.[1,20] It is therefore postulated that CO may attenuate the proinflammatory and inflammatory mediators released during post-ischemic reperfusion. To participate effectively in the inflammatory process, neutrophils must leave the blood stream and migrate into the tissue. The ability of neutrophils to cross the vessel walls is fundamental because it allows them to rapidly reach the sites of inflammation where they exert their actions. Neutrophil adherence to the endothelium is also an important step of this migratory process,[21] which involves selectin and integrins. CO facilitates the migration of neutrophils.[19]

Post-ischemic reperfusion also leads to the overproduction of reactive free radicals. Excessive release of reactive oxygen and nitrogen species (ROS and RNS) has been demonstrated to be responsible for the tissue damage seen in ischemia/reperfusion and in inflammation. Moreover, increased cytosolic ROS and RNS concentrations can activate a number of transcription factors including NF-κB and AP-1.[22,23] The overproduced ROS and RNS can be counteracted by bilirubin, a product from the same metabolic pathway as CO, generally known for its antioxidative property.[24] Bilirubin also exerts anticomplement effects[25] and has been shown to increase the survival time of guinea pigs undergoing anaphylactic reactions. In this regard, the HO/CO system offers a dualistic and synergistic role in combatting reperfusion injury and may be considered an alternative avenue in designing therapeutic strategies against reperfusion injury.

III. CARBON MONOXIDE, ATHEROSCLEROSIS, AND INFLAMMATION

The antiinflammatory/antioxidative effect of the HO/CO system may have further applications for inflammation-related problems developed in atherosclerosis. The increased expression of HO-1 in human atherosclerotic lesions[26] and in vascular smooth muscles exposed to oxidized LDL[27] have been reported. Atherosclerotic lesions may represent a response of vascular cells to oxidative stress in an attempt to mount a self-defensive strategy.[22,23,28]

Glutathione is the primary defense mechanism against oxidative stress in mammalian cell systems.[29] It is induced in many cell types by oxygen-derived free radicals including oxidized LDL.[30,31] In conditions of reduced NO production associated with depleted glutathione in human endothelial cells, the impaired structures of vascular tissues may lead to atherosclerosis.[32,33] Lapenna et al.[34] demonstrated the existence of a diminished glutathione-related enzymatic antioxidant shield within human atherosclerotic lesions, which in turn induces HO-1 as an alternative defense mechanism. The induction of HO-1 results in enhanced production of bilirubin and CO. The latter may have two important functions. One is the vasodilatory action through the soluble guanylate cyclase/cyclic guanosine monophosphate (sGC/cGMP) pathway, and the other is the antiinflammatory effect[20] to attenuate inflammation that might result in atherosclerosis. Similarly, Hopkins et al.[35] reported increased HO-1 production during atherosclerosis. These studies indicate that the vasodilatory actions of CO may become more important in atherogenesis when endothelium-derived NO production is impaired.

Several mechanisms have been proposed for the relaxation of vascular smooth muscle cells (SMCs). Notable among them are the rise of intracellular levels of cGMP and the opening of big-conductance K_{Ca} channels,[36] which lead to a decrease in intracellular calcium concentration. Detailed discussions of this topic can be found in Chapters 2 and 5. An increase of intracellular calcium is the final event leading to either the contraction of vascular SMCs or the release of histamine from mast cells. In fact, an increase of cytosolic calcium triggers both the sliding of cross-bridges that supports the contraction of muscle fibres and the shortening of actin microfilaments that promotes the sequential exocytosis of mast cell granules. Assuming that mast cells react to CO in the same way as vascular SMCs, a decrease in cytosolic calcium can easily explain both the vasodilatation and the inhibition of mast cell secretion induced by CO. This vasodilatory and antiinflammatory property may underlie a beneficial role for CO in the pathogenesis of atherosclerosis.

IV. HEME OXYGENASE AND INFLAMMATION

Heme oxygenase (HO) is the rate-limiting enzyme in the conversion of heme to CO and bilirubin. The lack of the enzyme causes hyperbilirubinaemia, particularly in premature newborns.[8] HO-1, also called heat shock protein 32 (hsp32), can be induced by numerous stressors including elevated temperature, cytokines, UVA radiation, hydrogen peroxide, heavy metal ions, and its heme substrate.[37] Glutathione depletion is a powerful inducer of HO-1 and therefore the enzyme is more correctly termed a marker of redox imbalance.[38,39] The antirheumatic compound disodium aurothiomalate ("gold"),[40] lipid peroxidation products,[41] arachidonate,[42] and prostaglandins[43,44] also induce the expression of HO-1. Moreover, various non-steroidal antiinflammatory drugs have been reported to potentiate HO-1 expression in rat carrageenan pleurisy.[45]

The increased HO-1 activity and expression were associated with the resolution phase of both delayed (type IV) and immediate (type III) types of hypersensitivity.[46] For example, the application of hemin facilitated the resolution of acute inflammation induced by the injection of carrageenan into the pleural cavities of rats.[11] HO-1 induction through the administration of ferriprotoporphyrin (FePP) has also been shown to abate the influx of inflammatory cells in nephrotoxic nephritis.[47] The increased HO-1 activity and expression have been observed in lung inflammation induced by ozone[48] and influenza virus A/PR/8/34 (H1N1).[49]

Further evidence for the cytoprotective/antiinflammatory role of HO-1 has recently been presented using HO-1 knockout mice.[50,51] HO-1-deficient mice have increased ratios of CD^{4+}:CD^{8+} T lymphocytes, and develop progressive chronic inflammatory disease. This disease is manifested by the infiltration of inflammatory cells into the liver and increased adherence of monocytes to the vasculature, a pathology similar to autoimmune disease. How HO-1 exerts its cytoprotective/anti-inflammatory action is not yet clear, but several putative mechanisms should be considered: (1) increased CO production results in more CO binding to and inhibition of heme-containing enzymes involved in inflammatory reactions; (2) increased HO activity depletes the intracellular heme pool, thus inhibiting the activity of heme-dependent enzymes by preventing apoprotein complex formation — two such targets are cyclooxygenase-2 (COX-2) and inducible nitric oxide (*i*NOS); and (3) increased HO activity is associated with cytochrome P-450-dependent arachidonyl acid metab-olites. This mechanism has been elucidated in FePP-treated hypertensive rats[52] and in a model of corneal inflammations.[53]

V. CARDIAC ANAPHYLAXIS AS A MODEL OF HYPERSENSITIVITY REACTION

The exposure of humans or animals to a particular substance may result in sensiti-zation and subsequent re-exposure to the same antigen might lead to anaphylactic anaphylaxis. Symptoms and signs of this IgE-mediated reaction include cardiovas-cular collapse (shock), bronchospasm or laryngeal edema, and marked anxiety and apprehension. In severe cases, loss of consciousness, hypotension, and sudden death occur. Cardiac anaphylaxis is characterized by an increase in the rate and strength of cardiac contraction and the onset of arrhythmias in the heart in sensitized animals or individuals challenged with specific antigen. These changes in myocardial func-tions are caused by the release of histamine as the sole mediator,[54] or by histamine release coupled with the production and release of vasoactive products of arachidonic acid cascade.[55] Cardiac anaphylaxis is widely recognized as a type 1 hypersensitivity reaction in which the release of histamine from resident cardiac mast cells contributes to myocardial damage.[56]

Endogenous autacoids modulate cardiac anaphylaxis. In the isolated sensitized guinea pig heart, the levels of catecholamines and the availability of adrenoceptors regulate the release of histamine. Depletion of catecholamines and the blockade of β-receptors decrease the anaphylactic histamine release, which is otherwise enhanced by noradrenaline.[54] Histamine down-regulates cardiac anaphylaxis in guinea pig hearts in an autocrine feedback manner. The H_2-receptor agonists decrease, but cimetidine increases histamine release,[57] thus indicating an autoregu-latory effect of this receptor. Like NO,[14] CO also exerts antianaphylactic actions in guinea pig mast cells from actively sensitized animals.[2] We recently investigated the role of the HO/CO system in the modulation of inflammatory and immune processes in the cardiovascular system. Our novel observations are summarized below.

A. HEMIN, CO, AND BASOPHIL ACTIVATION

In our experiments, human basophils were preincubated with hemin for 30 min. This treatment served two purposes. One was to induce the expression of HO-1 and the other to provide more substrate for HO to produce CO. After the hemin treatment, human basophils were challenged with human anti-IgE. As shown in Figure 10.1,

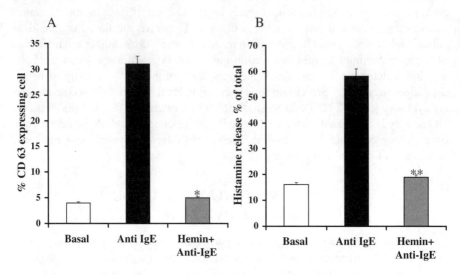

FIGURE 10.1 Effect of hemin on immunological activation and histamine release from human basophils pre-incubated with hemin for 30 min and challenged with human anti-IgE. The activation morphology was evaluated cytofluorimetrically by means of fluorescent antibodies to label membrane IgE and CD63 expression on activated cells (A). The release of histamine from the activated basophils (B). Data represent mean ± SE of six experiments in duplicate; * P <0.01; ** P <0.05.

the hemin treatment abated basophil activation (antigen-induced CD63 expression) and decreased the immunological histamine release from basophils.

These effects of hemin were mimicked by exogenous CO. The inhibition of basophil degranulation and activation afforded by CO could not be accounted for by hypoxia developed after 30-min exposure to CO. This conclusion was supported by our nitrogen control experiments.[58,59] Instead of treating human basophils with CO gas, nitrogen gas was introduced into the saline that bathed human basophils for 30 min. This nitrogen treatment did not reduce the immunological reactivity of human basophils to IgE stimulation. The experiment with nitrogen therefore disproved the possibility that the development after 30 min of hypoxia, a condition that stimulates HO-1,[28,60] was a sufficient stimulus to achieve basophil inhibition. However, we are aware of the fact that nitrogen does not bind to the heme moiety; it simply denies oxygen access. We cannot rule out an interaction between CO and cytochromes involved in electron transport. Thus, the inhibition of the immunological release of histamine elicited by CO could be explained mainly by the activation of the sGC/cGMP pathway.

B. HO, CO, AND CARDIAC ANAPHYLAXIS

The presence of HO-1 in human basophils has been previously shown.[1] To examine our hypothesis that the HO/CO system also operates in guinea pigs and that up-regulation of this system may have a protective role during anaphylaxis, experiments

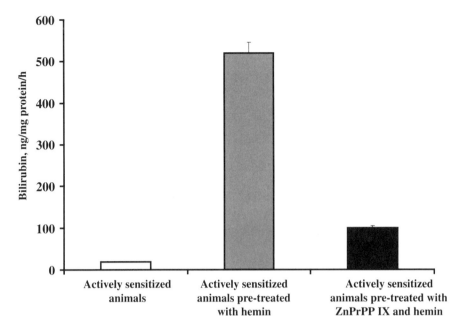

FIGURE 10.2 Evidence for the presence of HO-1 in guinea pig heart homogenates measured by the spectrophotometric assay of bilirubin in the presence of biliverdin reductase. Animals treated with hemin alone (4 mg/kg i.p. 18 h before anaphylaxis) showed significant increases in bilirubin production. The combined treatment with hemin and zinc protoporphyrin IX applied 6 h before hemin (50 μmol/kg i.p.) blocked the hemin-induced bilirubin production. $P < 0.01$.

were performed by pre-treating sensitized guinea pigs with hemin alone or hemin with zinc protoporphyrin IX, an HO inhibitor.

Our results demonstrated HO expression and activity in guinea pig hearts by showing small but detectable amounts of bilirubin in control hearts, which could represent the activity of HO-2 (Figure 10.2). Hearts pre-treated with hemin showed significant increases in the production of bilirubin (Figure 10.2), indicating the induction of HO-1. Pre-treatment of the animals with zinc protoporphyrin IX before hemin injection fully abrogated the increase in enzymatic activity (Figure 10.2).

Guinea pigs were sensitized by intraperitoneal and subcutaneous injections of egg albumin. Cardiac anaphylaxis was induced 20 to 25 days later by the antigenic challenge. These animals exhibited typical anaphylactic reactions including sinus tachycardia, severe arrhythmias, and an increase in the strength of contraction of Langendorff-perfused isolated guinea pig hearts (Figure 10.3A). The presence of large amounts of histamine and other autacoids released during anaphylaxis could account for these abnormalities.[5] The first phase of intense coronary constriction is followed by a second phase of less pronounced but lasting coronary constriction and diminution of coronary flow. We also noted a massive release of histamine throughout the 10-min period that immediately followed the onset of anaphylaxis (Figure 10.3B).

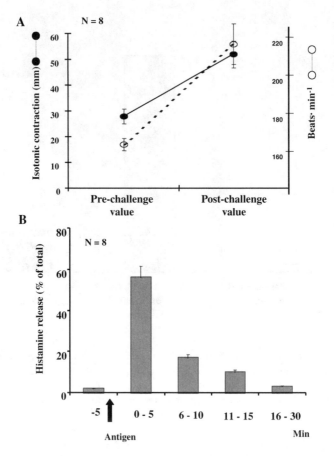

FIGURE 10.3 Effect of antigen challenge on isotonic contraction and heart rate (A) and histamine release (B) in Langendorff perfused guinea pig heart isolated from sensitized animals. Values represent mean ± SE of eight experiments. The measurements of cardiac parameters were taken at the peak of the anaphylactic response (5 min after antigen injection).

When egg albumin was injected via the aortic cannulae of sensitized guinea pig hearts 30 min after the perfusion of the hearts with a Tyrode solution saturated with CO, the inotropic and chronotropic responses to antigen challenge were fully abated (Figure 10.4). The same effect was observed when the anaphylactic reaction was evoked in hearts isolated from animals pre-treated with hemin; cardiac frequency and strength of contraction were not modified after the injection of specific antigen. It is interesting that the incidence of arrhythmias was much reduced in the hemin-treated animals (40%) compared to control animals (100%). The intense coronary constriction and the massive release of histamine following the onset of anaphylaxis were also significantly reduced by hemin treatment.

To understand whether the antianaphylactic effect of hemin was a result of HO-1 induction, the isolated guinea pig hearts were pre-treated with zinc protoporphyrin IX before the administration of hemin. Interestingly, under this condition, the antigenic

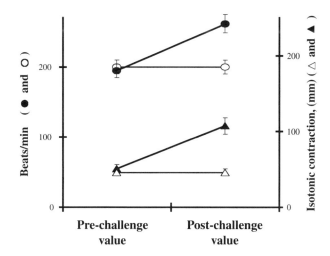

FIGURE 10.4 Effect of CO on cardiac anaphylaxis. The perfusion of the heart with Tyrode solution saturated with 100% CO (open symbols) decreased the chronotropic and inotropic responses to antigen (closed symbols).

challenge resulted in a complete recovery of the positive inotropic and chronotropic responses, accompanied by the same changes in the coronary outflow and release of histamine observed in control hearts.[57] We also directly measured the tissue level of cGMP — one of the major targets of CO. When actively sensitized guinea pig hearts were pre-treated with hemin and then challenged with specific antigen, a striking increase in cGMP levels accompanied by a significant reduction of calcium content occurred. These effects were reversed by zinc protoporphyrin IX.

Do the hemin-induced inhibition of the immunological activation and release of histamine from human basophils and the antianaphylactic action in sensitized guinea pig hearts result from a cromoglycate-like membrane stabilizing effect? We found that the inhibitory action of hemin on basophil activation was reversed after sGC was inhibited by 1H-[1,2,4]oxadiazolo[4,3-alpha]quinoxalin-1-one (ODQ)[61] or by the CO scavenger, oxyhaemoglobin. Since these maneuvers target downstream of CO action or the availability of CO, a direct effect of hemin on cell membranes is remote. Bilirubin is an effective antioxidant and a protective role for bilirubin in the immunological inflammation might be reasoned. However, the full reversion of the allergic activation of basophils afforded by ODQ and oxyhaemoglobin also excluded the involvement of bilirubin, one of the end products of the HO pathway.[24,62]

In our recent investigations, we also showed that hemin-treated hearts are capable of generating bilirubin in amounts many-fold higher than control hearts. Since both bilirubin and CO are the end products of heme metabolism, it is conceivable that the pre-treatment of sensitized guinea pigs with hemin would produce higher amounts of CO than control cells. The increased generation of endogenous CO could account for the inhibition of reduction of the pathophysiological responses evoked by antigen-challenge in sensitized guinea pig hearts. Our investigations further indicate that pre-treatment with hemin provides protection against cardiac anaphylaxis in that

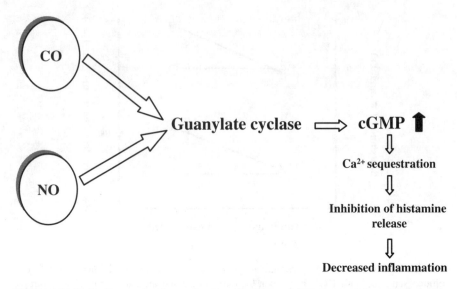

FIGURE 10.5 Similar mechanisms of action for CO and NO in regulating inflammatory reaction. Both stimulate soluble guanylyl cyclase, which causes a rise in the level of cGMP. cGMP may cause calcium sequestration, inhibit inositol triphosphate, or inhibit calcium influx. The result is a fall in intracellular calcium concentration and inhibition of histamine release.

the characteristic responses to antigen challenge were fully abated and the release of histamine was reduced.[63] We cannot rule out the possibilities that the antianaphylactic action of hemin is due to the blockade of H_1/H_2 receptors or to the direct inhibition of histamine secretion from repository cells. Even if this holds true, the increased HO activity and the end products of heme metabolism may still take major credit for the antianaphylactic action of hemin.

Our results demonstrate that CO may play an important role in the resolution of inflammation by providing protection against anaphylaxis as it does against oxidative stress.[64,65] In hemin-treated animals, antigen challenge evoked less sustained coronary constriction and more pronounced coronary dilatation than in saline-treated animals, thus consolidating the hypothesis that hemin-elicited CO may be considered a potential antianaphylactic substance.

Our findings also indicated that CO may modulate cell function in a similar fashion to NO (Figure 10.5).

The CO-induced increases in cGMP levels have been repeatedly described[60,66-69] in vascular SMCs and in the rat brain.[70] Our studies showed that hemin and CO are capable of increasing cGMP levels in human basophils and sensitized guinea pig hearts.[1] It has been suggested that the increase in cGMP is responsible for the inhibition of platelet aggregation and for the relaxation of smooth muscle afforded by both CO and NO.[66] It has been shown that CO, like NO, activates sGC by inducing the conformational changes in the catalytic site of the heme moiety,[71] which leads to an increase in intracellular concentrations of cGMP. It is interesting that HO-1 expression and protein activity in the liver can be stimulated by NO donors.[72,73] This could lead to enhanced production of CO and more pronounced antiinflammatory activity because both gases are thought to act through the sGC/cGMP-dependent pathway. Another note worth mentioning is that CO may exert a negative feedback on NO production by inhibiting iNOS activity.[74] Whether the interaction of CO and NO leads to the inhibition of inflammatory reactions depends on the delicate balance of the production and actions of these two gases.

VI. CONCLUSION

Our findings demonstrate that endogenously generated and exogenously applied CO is a powerful antianaphylactic agent at the cellular level (human basophils), tissue level (heart), and whole animal level (sensitized guinea pigs). That the administration of the sGC inhibitor ODQ completely reverses the inhibition of basophil degranulation and activation afforded by CO suggests that the inhibitory effect of CO on immunological histamine release may be attributed to the activation of sGC. The lack of antianaphylactic effect of nitrogen suggests a specific action of CO rather than hypoxic stunning. Our results are consistent with other studies showing CO-enhanced human neutrophil migration in a cGMP-dependent way[19] and HO-induced suppression of carrageenan pleurisy in the rat.[11] The reversion of the inhibitory effect of hemin when cells are pre-treated with HbO_2 indicates that CO is responsible for the antianaphylactic effect of hemin.

Other products of heme catabolism, biliverdin and bilirubin, may also contribute to the different aspects of the antioxidant effects of hemin.[75] Although CO synthesis by HO occurs in a large number of tissues, research concerning the role of CO in the immune system is new and very stimulating because substances capable of generating endogenous CO through the HO metabolic pathway present great potential as possible pharmacological armaments in the immune system.

During the inflammatory process, heme released by necrotic cells may promote the production of CO. CO can also be generated from basophils, endothelial cells, and other types of cells. The released CO could diffuse to neighboring basophils where the activation of sGC results in elevated intracellular cGMP levels, leading to the decrease of their immunological responsiveness in an autocrine/paracrine fashion. CO may also diffuse to adjacent vascular SMCs, leading to their relaxation through a similar sGC/cGMP-mediated effect.

In addition to the sGC/cGMP pathway, the inhibitory effect of CO on basophil activation may be mediated by a cGMP-independent modulation of cytosolic calcium levels. CO could directly augment K^+ currents through the activation of Ca^{2+}-dependent potassium channels, hyperpolarizing the membranes and inactivating the voltage-dependent Ca^{2+} channels. This would lower cytosolic Ca^{2+} levels, preventing anaphylactic degranulation.[76] A similar mechanism has been proposed to explain the sGC-independent vasodilatation actions of CO[77] and the inhibition of carotid body sensory activity by endogenous CO.[78] Our recent observations showing that CO and hemin significantly reduced the anti-IgE-induced rise of intracellular Ca^{2+} are supportive of this hypothesis.

Accumulating evidence indicates that the expression of HO-1 in vascular endothelial cells and SMCs is induced by a variety of agents encompassing oxidative stress: proinflammatory cytokines, tumor necrosis factor,[79] interferon-γ,[72] interleukin-1-β,[9] and peroxynitrite,[80] all of which are known to be involved in the pathogenesis of allergic inflammation. The induction of HO-1 activity provides an endogenous defense mechanism against proinflammatory and immunological stimuli. The CO produced binds and inhibits heme-containing enzymes involved in inflammatory reactions. Enzymes such as COX and NOS may be depleted by high activity of the HO/CO system and this may result in an antiinflammatory effect. This feedback mechanism may apply to the modulation of many type 1 hypersensitivity allergic reactions, and to the design of drugs capable of interfering with the endogenous generation of CO. It should be mentioned, however, that the overproduction of CO might depress the ability of a tissue to mount an adequate protective inflammatory response.

The antiinflammatory effect of the HO/CO system is beneficial to many cardiovascular disorders such as atherosclerosis and reperfusion injury after ischemia. Graft rejection in transplantation is another case in point. Since the HO/CO system is capable of abating the immune response, the enhancement of the activity of this system could conceivably reduce the incidence of immunorejections.

ACKNOWLEDGMENTS

J.F. Ndisang is supported by a post-doctoral fellowship award from the University of Saskatchewan. R. Wang is supported by a scientist award from the Canadian Institutes of Health Research.

REFERENCES

1. Mirabella, C. et al., Hemin and carbon monoxide modulate the immunological response of human basophils, *Int. Arch. Allergy Immunol.,* 118, 259, 1999.
2. Ndisang, J.F. et al., Modulation of the immunological response of guinea pig mast cells by carbon monoxide, *Immunopharmacology,* 43, 65, 1999.
3. Bydlowski, S.P., Mast cell: its mediators and effects on arterial wall metabolism, *Gen. Pharmacol.,* 17, 625, 1986.
4. Wasserman, S.I., The regulation of inflammatory mediator production by mast cell products, *Am. Rev. Resp. Dis.,* 135, S46, 1987.
5. Masini, E. et al., The role of nitric oxide in anaphylactic reaction of isolated guinea pig hearts and mast cells, in *Nitric Oxide: Brain and Immune System,* Moncada, S. et al., Eds., Portland Press, London, 1994, p. 277.
6. Tenhunen, R., Marver H.S., and Schmid R., Microsomal heme oxygenase. Characterization of the enzyme, *J. Biol. Chem.,* 244, 6388, 1969.
7. Maines, M.D. and Kappas A., Cobalt induction of hepatic heme oxygenase; with evidence that cytocrome P-450 is not essential for this enzyme activity, *Proc. Natl. Acad. Sci. U.S.A.,* 71, 4293, 1974.
8. Maines, M.D., Heme oxygenase: function, multiplicity regulatory mechanism and clinical applications, *FASEB J.,* 2, 2557, 1988.
9. Yet, S.F. et al., Induction of heme oxygenase-1 expression in vascular smooth muscle cells. A link to endotoxic shock, *J. Biol. Chem.,* 272, 4295, 1997.
10. McCoubrey, W.K., Huang, T.J., and Maines, M.D., Isolation and characterisation of a cDNA from the rat that encodes hemoprotein heme oxygenase-3, *Eur. J. Biochem.,* 247, 725, 1997.

11. Willis, D. et al., Heme oxygenase: a novel target for the modulation of the inflammatory response, *Nature Med.,* 2, 87, 1996.

12. Thom, S.R. et al., Adaptive response and apoptosis in endothelial cells exposed to carbon monoxide, *Proc. Natl. Acad. Sci. U.S.A.,* 97, 1305, 2000.

13. Maulik, N. et al., Nitric oxide/carbon monoxide. A molecular switch for myocardial preservation during ischemia, *Circulation,* 94, Suppl. II, 398, 1996.

14. Mazzoni, M.C. and Schmid–Schonbein, G.W., Mechanisms and consequences of cell activation in the microcirculation, *Cardiovasc. Res.,* 32, 709, 1996.

15. Tritto, I. and Ambrosio, G., Spotlight on microcirculation: an update, *Cardiovasc. Res.,* 600, 1999.

16. Kubes, P., The role of shear forces in ischemia/reperfusion-induced neutrophil rolling and adhesion, *J. Leukocyte Biol.,* 62, 458, 1997.

17. Ambrosio, G., Weisman, H.F., and Mannisi, J.A., Progressive impairment of regional myocardial perfusion after initial restoration of postischemic blood flow, *Circulation,* 80, 1846, 1989.

18. Ito, H. et al., Clinical implications of the "no reflow" phenomenon. A predictor of complications and left ventricular remodeling in reperfused anterior wall myocardial infarction, *Circulation,* 93, 223, 1996.

19. Vanuffelen, B.E. et al., Carbon monoxide enhances human neutrophil migration in a cyclic GMP-dependent way, *Biochem. Biophys. Res. Comm.,* 226, 21, 1996.

20. Di Bello, M.G. et al., A regulatory role for carbon monoxide in mast cell function, *Inflamm. Res.,* 47, Suppl 1, S7, 1998.

21. Ley, K., Molecular mechanisms of leukocyte recruitment in the inflammatory process, *Cardiovasc. Res.,* 32, 733, 1996.

22. Sen, C. and Packer, L., Antioxidant and redox-regulated transcription factors and inflammation, *Adv. Pharmacol.,* 38, 403, 1996.

23. Sen, C. and Packer, L., Antioxidant and redox regulation of the gene-transcription, *FASEB J.,* 10, 709, 1996.

24. Minetti, M. et al., Bilirubin is an effective antioxidant of peroxynitrite-mediated protein oxidation in human blood plasma, *Arch. Biochem. Biophys.,* 352, 165, 1998.

25. Nakagami, T. et al., A beneficial role of bile pigments as an endogenous tissue protector: anti-complement effects of biliverdin and conjugated bilirubin, *Biochem. Biophys. Acta,* 1158, 189, 1993.

26. Wang, L.J. et al., Expression of heme oxygenase-1 in atherosclerotic lesions, *Am. J. Pathol.,* 152, 711, 1998.

27. Ishikawa, K. et al., Induction of heme-oxygenase-1 inhibits the monocyte transmigration induced by mildly oxidised LDL, *J. Clin. Invest.,* 100, 1209, 1997.

28. Siow, R.C.M., Sato, H., and Mann, G.E., Heme oxygenase-carbon monoxide signaling pathway in atherosclerosis: anti-atherogenic actions of bilirubin and carbon monoxide? *Cardiovasc. Res.,* 41, 385, 1999.

29. Meister, A., Glutathione–ascorbic acid antioxidant system in animals, *J. Biol. Chem.,* 269, 9397, 1994.

30. Jomot, L. and Junod, A.F., Variable glutathione levels and expression of antioxidant enzymes in human endothelial cells, *Am. J. Physiol.,* 264, L482, 1993.

31. Siow, R.C.M. et al., Vitamin C protects human arterial smooth cells against atherogenic lipoproteins: effects of antioxidant vitamins on oxidised LDL-oxidised increases in cystine transport and glutathione, *Arterioscler. Thromb. Vasc. Biol.,* 18, 1662, 1998.

32. Ghigo, D. et al., Nitric oxide synthase is impaired in glutathione depleted human umbilical vein endothelium cells, *Am. J. Physiol.,* 256, C728, 1993.

33. Cox, D.A. and Cohen, M.L., Effects of oxidised low-density lipoproteins on vascular contraction and relaxation: clinical and pharmacological implications in artherosclerosis, *Pharmacol. Rev.,* 48, 3, 1996.
34. Lapenna, D. et al., Glutathione-related antioxidant defences in human atherosclerotic plaques. *Circulation,* 97, 1930, 1998.
35. Hopkins, P.N. et al., Higher serum bilirubin is associated with decreased risk for early familial coronary artery disease, *Artheroscler. Throm. Biol.,* 16, 250, 1996.
36. Wang, R., Resurgence of carbon monoxide: an endogenous gaseous vasorelaxing factor, *Can. J. Physiol. Pharmacol.,* 76, 1, 1998.
37. Keys, S.M. and Tyrrel, R.M., Heme oxygenase is the maior 32-Kda stress protein induced in human skin fibroblasts by UVA radiation, hydrogen peroxide and sodium arsenite, *Proc. Nati. Acad. Sci. U.S.A.,* 86, 99, 1989.
38. Applegate, LA., Luscher, P., and Tyrrel, R.M., Induction of heme oxygenase: a general response to oxidant stress in cultured mammalian cells, *Cancer Res.,* 5 1, 974, 1991.
39. Lautier, D., Luscher, P., and Tyrrel, R.M., Endogenous glutathione levels modulate both constitutive and UVA radiation/hydrogen peroxide inducible expression of the human heme oxygenase gene, *Carcinogenesis,* 13, 227, 1992.
40. Caltabiano, M.M., Poste, G., and Grieg, G., Induction of the 32-kD human stress protein by auranofin and related triethylphosphine gold analogues, *Biochem. Pharmacol.,* 37, 4089, 1986.
41. Basu–Modak, S., Luscher, P., and Tyrrel, R.M., Lipid metabolite involvement in the activation of the human heme oxygenase-1 gene, *Free Rad. Biol. Med.,* 20, 887, 1996.
42. Jurivich, D.A. et al., Arachidonate is a potent modulator of human heat shock gene transcription, *Proc. Nati. Acad. Sci. U.S.A.,* 91, 2280, 1994.
43. Koizumi, T., Neigishi, M., and Ichikawa, A., Induction of heme oxygenase by delta 12- prostaglandin J2 in porcine aortic endothelial cells, *Prostaglandins,* 43, 121, 1992.
44. Rossi, A. and Santoro, M.G., Induction of prostaglandin Al of heme oxygenase in myoblastic cells: an effect independent of expression of the 70-kDa heat shock protein, *Biochem. J.,* 308, 455, 1995.
45. Willis, D., Overview of HO-1 in inflammatory pathology, in *Inducible Enzymes in the Inflammatory Response,* Willoughby, D.A. and Tomlinson, A., Eds., Birkháuser Verlag, Basel, 1999, p. 55.
46. Moore, A.R. et al., Cyclooxygenase in rat pleural hypersensitivity reactions, *Adv. Prostaglandin Thromboxane Leukot. Res.,* 23, 349, 1995.
47. Mosely, K. et al., Heme-oxygenase is induced in nephrotoxic nephritis and hemin, a stimulator of heme-oxygenase synthesis, ameliorates disease, *Kidney Int.,* 53, 672, 1998.
48. Choi, A.M. et al., Oxidant stress responses in influenza virus: gene expression and transcription factor activation, *Am. J. Physiol.,* 271, L383, 1996.
49. Takahashi, Y. et al., Increases of MRNA levels of gamma-glutamyltransferase and heme oxygenase-1 in rat lung after ozone exposure, *Biochem. Pharmacol.,* 53, 1061, 1997.
50. Poss, K.D. and Tonegawa, S., Heme oxygenase-1 is required for mammalian iron reutilisation, *Proc. Natl. Acad. Sci. U.S.A.,* 14, 10919, 1997.
51. Poss, K.D. and Tonegawa, S., Reduced stress defence in heme oxygenase-deficient cells, *Proc. Natl. Acad. Sci. U.S.A.,* 14, 10925, 1997.
52. Martasek, P. et al., Hemin and L-arginine regulation of blood pressure in spontaneously hypertensive rats, *J. Am. Soc. Nephrol.,* 2, 1078, 1991.
53. Conners, M.S. et al., A close eye contact lens model of corneal inflammation. Part II: inhibition of cytochrome P450: arachidonic acid metabolism alleviates inflammation sequelae, *Invest. Ophthalmal. Vis. Sci.,* 36, 841, 1995.

54. Giotti, A. et al., The influences of andrenotropic drugs and noradrenaline on the histamine release in cardiac anaphylaxis *in vitro*, *J. Physiol. (Lond.)*, 184, 924, 1966.
55. Levi, R. et al., Acetyl glyceryl ether phosphorylcholine (AGEPC). A putative mediator of cardiac anaphylaxis in the guinea pig, *Circ. Res.*, 54, 117, 1984.
56. Capurro, N. and Levi R., The heart as a target organ in systemic allergic reactions, *Circ. Res.*, 36, 520, 1975.
57. Blandina, P. et al., The antianaphylactic action of histamine H2-receptor agonists in the guinea pig isolated heart, *Br. J. Pharmacol.*, 90, 459, 1987.
58. Lin, H. and McGrath, J.J., Vasodilating effects of carbon monoxide, *Drug Chem. Toxicol.*, 11, 371, 1988.
59. McFaul, S.J. and McGrath, J., Studies on the mechanism of carbon monoxide-induced vasodilation in the isolated perfused rat heart, *Toxicol. Appl. Pharmacol.*, 87, 464, 1987.
60. Morita, T. et al., Smooth muscle cell-derived carbon monoxide is a regulator of vascular cGMP, *Proc. Natl. Acad. Sci. U.S.A.*, 92, 1475, 1995.
61. Hussain, A.S. et al., The soluble guanylyl cyclase inhibitor 1H-[1,2,4]oxadiaz-olo[4,3-alpha]quinoxalin-1-one (ODQ) inhibits relaxation of rabbit aortic rings induced by carbon monoxide, nitric oxide, and glyceryl trinitrate, *Can. J. Physiol. Pharmacol.*, 75, 1034, 1997.
62. Stocker, R., Induction of heme oxygenase as a defence against oxidative stress, *Free Radical Res. Commun.*, 9, 101, 1990.
63. Ndisang, J.F. et al., Induction of heme oxygenase provides protection against cardiac anaphylaxis, *Inflamm. Res.*, 49, S76, 2000.
64. Otterbein, L.E. et al., Exogenous administration of heme oxygenase-1 by gene trans-fer provides protection against hyperoxia-induced lung injury, *J. Clin. Invest.*, 103, 1047, 1999.
65. Otterbein, L.E., Mantell, L.L., and Choi, A.M., Carbon monoxide provides protection against hyperoxic lung injury, *Am. J. Physiol.*, 276, L688, 1999.
66. Brüne, B. and Ullrich, V., Inhibition of platelet aggregation by carbon monoxide is mediated by activation of guanylate cyclase, *Mol. Pharmacol.*, 32, 497, 1987.
67. Utz, J. and Ullrich, V., Carbon monoxide relaxes ileal smooth muscle through acti-vation of guanylate cyclase, *Biochem. Pharmacol.*, 41, 1195, 1991.
68. Christodoulides, N. et al., Vascular smooth muscle cell heme oxygenases generate guanylyl cyclase-stimulatory carbon monoxide, *Circulation*, 91, 2306, 1995.
69. Sammut, I.A. et al., Carbon monoxide is a major contributor to the regulation of vascular tone in aortas expressing high levels of haem oxygenase-1, *Br. J. Pharmacol.*, 125, 1437, 1998.
70. Laitinen, K.S.M. et al., Regulation of cyclic GMP levels in the rat frontal cortex *in vivo*: effects of exogenous carbon monoxide and phosphodiesterase inhibition, *Brain Res.*, 755, 272, 1997.
71. Marks, G.S. et al., Does carbon monoxide have a physiological function? *Trends Pharmacol. Sci.*, 12, 185, 1991.
72. Motterlini, R. et al., NO-mediated activation of heme oxygenase: endogenous cyto-protection against oxidative stress to endothelium, *Am. J. Physiol.*, 270, H I 07, 1996.
73. Motterlini, R. et al., A precursor of the nitric oxide donor SIN-1 modulates the stress protein heme oxygenase-1 in rat liver, *Biochem. Biophys. Res. Commun.*, 225, 167, 1996.
74. White, K.A. and Marletta, M.A., Nitric oxide synthase is a cytocrome P450 type hemo-protein, *Biochemistry*, 31, 6627, 1992.
75. Llesuy, F.S. and Tomaro, M.L., Heme oxygenase and oxidative stress. Evidence of involvement of bilirubin as physiological protector against oxidative damage, *Biochem. Biophys. Acta*, 1223, 9, 1994.

76. Dvorak, A.M. et al., Comparative ultrastructural morphology of human basophils stimulated to release histamine by anti-IgE, recombinant IgE-dependent histamine-releasing factor, or monocyte chemotactic protein-1, *J. Allergy Clin. Immunol.*, 98, 355, 1996.
77. Wang, R. and Wu, L., The chemical modification of K_{Ca} channels by carbon monoxide in vascular smooth muscle cells, *J. Biol. Chem.,* 272, 8222-8226, 1997.
78. Prabhakar, N.R., Endogenous carbon monoxide in control of respiration, *Respir. Physiol.*, 114, 57, 1998.
79. Wagener, F. et al., Heme induces the expression of adhesion molecules ICAM-1, VCAM-I and E selectin in vascular endothelial cells, *Proc. Soc. Exp. Biol. Med.,* 216, 456, 1997.
80. Foresti, R. et al., Thiol compounds interact with nitric oxide in regulating heme oxygenase-1 induction in endothelial cells. Involvement of superoxide and peroxynitrite anions, *J. Biol. Chem.*, 272, 18411, 1997.

11 Human HO-1 Deficiency and Cardiovascular Dysfunction

A. Yachie, A. Kawashima, K. Ohta, Y. Saikawa, and S. Koizumi

CONTENTS

0-8493-1041-5/02/$0.00+$1.50
© 2002 by CRC Press LLC

I. OVERVIEW

A. INTRODUCTION

Heme oxygenases (HOs) are known to play critical roles in physiological iron homeostasis, antioxidant defense mechanisms, and carbon monoxide (CO) production.[1-6] In
addition to classical biochemical studies, recent observations in HO-targeted mice have
further confirmed the important physiological functions of HOs.[7-12] Our laboratory
recently reported the first case of human HO-1 deficiency.[13-15] The important role of
HO-1 in the human body was highlighted at the First International Symposium on
Heme Oxygenase (HO/CO) held in New York in July of 2000.[16]

   This chapter will place special emphasis on recent findings concerning the
biochemical and molecular properties of the HO system and the clinical aspects of
human HO-1 deficiency and other disease states.

B. HEME OXYGENASES (HOs)

HOs function as the initial and rate-limiting step in heme degradation.[1-6] HOs
catalyze the conversion of heme into biliverdin, which is subsequently reduced to
bilirubin by biliverdin reductase, free iron, and one molecule of CO. Biliverdin is
an antioxidant capable of scavenging peroxy radicals. Ferritin is an intracellular
repository for iron, and safely sequesters the unbound iron liberated during degradation of heme. Finally, CO, similar to nitric oxide (NO), has recently been recognized to exert vasodilatory effects, thereby contributing to the maintenance of the
microvascular circulation.[17,18]

   Oxidation of heme is carried out by two known isoforms, HO-1 and HO-2,[3,6]
which differ in their tissue expression patterns. HO-1 is expressed ubiquitously at
very low levels, and is rapidly induced not only by heme but also by other stresses,

TABLE 11.1
Characteristics of Heme Oxygenase Isoforms

Properties	HO-1	HO-2	HO-3
Cellular localization	Microsomes	Mitochondria	Unknown
Chromosome	22q12	16p13.3	Unknown
Molecular weight	~32 kD	~36 kD	~33 kD
Tissue distribution	Inducible in liver, spleen, pancreas, intestine, kidney, heart, retina, prostate, vascular smooth muscle cells, endothelium, lung, skin, brain, spinal cord	Constitutive in brain, spinal cord, testis, vascular smooth muscle cells, endothelium, pancreas, kidney, intestine	Constitutive in liver, spleen, kidney, heart, prostate, thymus, brain, testis
Regulation	Heme, hydrogen peroxide, cytokines, endotoxin, heavy metals, UV, NO and NO donors, oxidized LDL, shear stress, hyper-oxia, hypoxia, growth factors (PDGF, TGF-β)	Glucocorticoids	Unknown

Note: UV = ultraviolet; PDGF = platelet-derived growth factor; TGF-β = transforming growth factor-β.

including hypoxia, hyperthermia, oxidized lipoproteins, UV and visual light, metals, and inflammatory cytokines.[1,6,18] A second isoform is HO-2 which, in contrast, is constitutively expressed and widely distributed in the body, with higher concentrations in the brain and testes. Recently, McCoubery et al.[19] isolated and characterized a third isoform from rats and referred to it as HO-3 (Table 11.1). The amino acid structure of HO-3 differs from that of HO-1, and is closely related to that of HO-2. HO-3, like HO-2, is widely distributed in the body. This new protein species is suggested to have a regulatory role as a heme-dependent protein, but its role is not yet fully defined.[3]

C. HO-1 AND CLINICAL DISORDERS

HO-1 has been implicated in an increasing number of clinically relevant disease states, including cardiovascular disorders,[20-22] renal and hepatic diseases,[23,24] nervous system disorders,[17,25] and chronic inflammation.[26]

1. Cardiovascular Diseases

An abundance of HO-1 mRNA and protein was identified in human atherosclerotic plaques,[20] specifically induced by linoleyl hydroperoxide, a fatty acid component,[21] indicating the *in vivo* relevance of this enzyme in atherosclerosis. A correlation between angiotensin II-induced hypertension and increased HO-1 expression was shown in rat aorta.[22] According to this report, blood pressure may be subject to a CO-dependent pressure regulation mechanism. Suzuki et al. showed predominantly induced HO-1 mRNA in the basilar artery and modest amounts in brain tissue in a rat vasospasm model after aneurysmal subarachnoid hemorrhage.[25] A role for CO has been suggested in the cardiovascular and other systems. CO is believed to function as the activator of cGC, leading to generation of cGMP, which mediates various physiological functions.[1,18] As HO-2 is constitutively expressed in the endothelial and smooth muscle layers of blood vessels, and HO-1 is induced at high levels in the heart and blood vessels, the cardiovascular system has a high capacity to generate CO.

CO, similar to NO, appears to be involved in the maintenance of vascular tone in the aorta, medium-sized arteries, and even in capillaries and other small vessels. The relative potency of CO and NO varies widely according to organs and animal species.[27] Relaxation of blood vessels in response to exogenous CO has also been reported.

2. Renal and Hepatic Diseases

HO-1 is induced in the kidney in certain disease models of acute renal injury, including rhabdomyolysis, toxic nephropathy, acute glomerulonephritis, and cisplatin nephrotoxicity.[28,29] We identified tubular injury as a cardinal pathologic feature in human HO-1 deficiency as described in Section III.[14] In steatotic rat liver models of ischemia/reperfusion injury, up-regulation of HO-1 gene expression significantly improved portal venous flow, increased bile production, and decreased hepatocyte injury.[23] CO is involved in the regulation of various hepatobiliary functions. HO-1-derived CO has been shown to protect the hepatic microcirculation under stress conditions.[24]

3. Lung Injuries and Other Disorders

In the lung, HO-1 appears to be localized to the peribronchiolar epithelium and the endothelial cells of blood vessels.[1,4,5] However, the majority of HO activity is derived from HO-2. Exogenous administration of HO-1 by gene transfer was shown to provide protection against hyperoxia-induced lung injury.[30] Elevated expression of HO-1 and HO-2 in pregnant myometrium is involved in the limitation of uterine contractility and maintenance of the quiescent state of the uterus during pregnancy.[31]

D. HO-1 and HO-2-Targeted Mice

The important physiological function of HO-1 was demonstrated in HO-1-targeted mice.[7-12] Poss and Tonegawa of the Massachusetts Institute of Technology initially generated HO-1-targeted mice by deletion of exons 3 and 4 and a portion of exon 5 of the mouse HO-1 gene.[7,8] Prenatal deaths occurred. Adult mice were also smaller than the wild types. HO-1-targeted mice developed iron deficiency anemia combined with hepatic iron overload. Progressive chronic inflammation characterized by hepatosplenomegaly, lymphadenopathy, and leukocytosis was observed.

Cultured fibroblasts from HO-1-targeted mice were highly susceptible to heme- and hydrogen peroxide-mediated toxicity. In addition, exposure of these animals to endotoxin resulted in higher mortality from endotoxin shock as compared to control animals.

Another strain of HO-1-targeted mice was generated by Yet et al. at Harvard Medical School. They showed that severe right ventricular dilatation and infarction were significantly induced by hypoxia in HO-1-targeted mice.[9] These data suggest that, in the absence of HO-1, cardiomyocytes develop a maladaptive response to hypoxia and subsequent pulmonary hypertension.

HO-2-targeted mice were also generated by some investigators.[10-12] These mice showed moderate overexpression of HO-1, and demonstrated augmentation of lung iron and hemoprotein during hyperoxia. Another observation was ejaculatory abnormalities.[11] Because of the preponderance of HO-2 in neuronal structures, reflex activity of the bulbospongiosus muscle, which mediates ejaculatory function, appeared to be markedly diminished in HO-2-targeted mice, probably related to reduced production of CO.[2,17]

E. THE FIRST CASE OF HUMAN HO-1 DEFICIENCY

Yachie et al. described the first case of human HO-1 deficiency in 1999.[13] Several phenotypical similarities to the HO-1-targeted mice described earlier were noted, but different clinical aspects were also demonstrated (Table 11.2). The patient was 26 months old when medical advice was first sought at a hospital because of recurrent fever and generalized erythematous rash. His brother and sister were healthy. The mother had experienced two intrauterine fetal deaths. The patient was referred to our hospital when he was 3 years old. Growth retardation was apparent and marked hepatomegaly was noted. Asplenia was confirmed by abdominal ultrasonography and isotope image scanning; this finding was in marked contrast to those for HO-1-targeted mice.

The patient had suffered from persistent hemolytic anemia characterized by marked erythrocyte fragmentation, intravascular hemolysis, and red wine-colored serum. Paradoxically, serum haptoglobin was increased and birilubin concentrations were low. An abnormal coagulation/fibrinolysis system associated with elevated thrombomodulin and von Willebrand's factor indicated severe and persistent endothelial damage. However, the peripheral blood platelet count was significantly increased. Other notable laboratory findings were hypertriglyceridemia and hypercholesterolemia. Coombs' tests were consistently negative. Several serum cytokines including IL-2, IL-6, TNF-α, and IFN-γ were at low levels.

Kidney biopsy revealed mild mesangial proliferation. Electron microscopic examination of renal glomeruli showed detachment of endothelium, with subendothelial deposition of an unidentified material.[14] Liver biopsy showed mild inflammatory changes with minimal lymphocyte infiltration. Iron deposition was noted mainly in renal and hepatic tissues. No histopathological confirmation of presence in the spleen was made in conjuction with the biopsy.

The patient took oral steroids and various nonsteroidal antiinflammatory medications and underwent regular transfusions of erythrocytes. He died of intracranial hemorrhage at 6 years of age. An autopsy was performed. No significant macroscopic changes were noted in the endothelium of the aorta or medium-sized arterial and venous vessels. Detailed autopsy findings are described in Sections II and III.

TABLE 11.2
Comparison of Clinical Findings of HO-1
Deficient Human and HO-1 Knockout Mice

Finding	Human	Mice
Intrauterine death	Stillbirth, abortion	20% birth rate
Growth failure	+	+
Anemia	+	+
Fragmentation	+	Unknown
Iron-binding capacity	Increased	Increased
Ferritin	Elevated	Elevated
Iron deposition	+	+
Hepatomegaly	+	+
Splenonegaly	Asplenia	+
Lymph node swelling	+	+
Leukocytosis	+	+
Thrombocytosis	+	Unknown
Coagulation abnormality	+	Unknown
Endothelial injury	+	Unknown
Hyperlipidemia	+	Unknown

Note: HO = heme oxygenase.

Immunohistochemistry of hepatic tissue and immunoblotting of a cadmium-stimulated Epstein–Barr virus-transformed lymphoblastoid cell line (LCL) revealed complete absence of HO-1 production. An LCL derived from the patient was remarkably sensitive to hemin-induced cell injury.

Sequence analysis of the patient's HO-1 gene revealed that the maternal allele showed a complete loss of exon 2; the paternal allele had a two-nucleotide deletion within exon 3. The proband, therefore, was a compound heterozygote. Further analysis of the maternal chromosomal gene revealed a large genomic deletion (1730 bp) including the entire exon 2, possibly caused by homologous recombination associated with *Alu* elements.[15] Further details of the HO-1 gene mutations will be discussed in Section IV.

F. LESSONS LEARNED

Hemolysis, hypobilirubinemia, and *hyperhaptoglobulinemia* were three key words used for identification of the new disease. When we saw the patient, we again checked a metabolic map of heme and bilirubin in a textbook of biochemistry, and found that HO-1 was the most important rate-limiting enzyme (Figure 11.1). We therefore examined the expression of HO-1 protein to develop a diagnosis. The discovery of the first case of human HO-1 deficiency clearly addressed the physiologically crucial role of HO-1 in the body, although additional cases have not yet been reported.

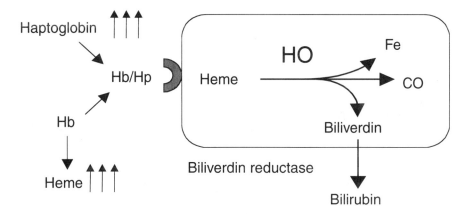

FIGURE 11.1 Role of heme oxygenase in the heme degradation pathway. Contradictory elevation of serum levels of haptoglobin and heme in contrast to intravascular hemolysis was shown in the human HO-1 deficiency.

One of the major differences in clinical findings in the comparison of the patient and the targeted mice was the presence of asplenia in the human patient. Whether asplenia contributed to modulating the clinical course of the patient is still controversial. Although asplenia without cardiac anomalies has never been reported, the HO-1 molecule may be involved in the growth of vascular vessels. Recently, an important role of HO-1 in angiogenesis, which is mediated by activation of macrophages in tumors, especially in malignant neoplasms, has been reported.[32]

HO-1 gene expression and protein production in normal peripheral blood mononuclear cell subsets were studied in our laboratory, and monocyte-specific HO-1 production was demonstrated as compared to lymphocyte population. Monocytes of our HO-1-deficient patient showed morphological abnormalities. Other findings suggest that the phagocytic function of the patient's monocytes was significantly reduced. Hyperlipidemia, with high cholesterol and triglyceride levels, may also be explained by functional impairment of his monocytes/macrophages. We tried to elucidate the mechanism of monocyte dysfunction seen in the HO-1-deficient patient in Section V.

To better understand the biological significance of the HO-1 molecule, a greater number of cases of HO-1 deficiency need to be identified. Peripheral blood monocytes may be useful and convenient target cells to check for HO-1 production and screen HO-1-deficient patients.

II. GENERAL PATHOLOGY

The HO-1-targeted mice generated by Poss and Tonegawa were characterized by both serum iron deficiency and pathological iron loading, indicating that HO-1 is crucial for the expulsion of iron from tissue stores.[7,8] The gene analysis, family pedigree, immunohistochemistry of biopsy specimens, immunoblotting, culture cell studies, and laboratory data of a human HO-1 deficiency case were cited earlier.[13] The autopsy findings of the 6-year-old boy are described in this section, with a focus on the difference between this case and HO-1-targeted mice.

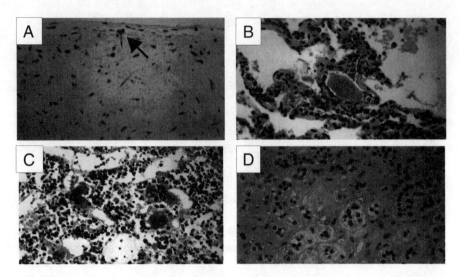

FIGURE 11.2 Histological findings of aorta, lung, bone marrow, and adrenal gland. (A) Thickened intima of the aorta. Immunohistochemical staining of CD68. Under the degenerated endothelial cells is a CD68-positive macrophage (arrow) infiltrating into the surface of the intima. Original magnification × 325. (B) High power view of the lung showing alveolitis characterized by interstitial cellular infiltrates with lymphocytes and neutrophils; a microthrombus is in the capillary. H&E stain. Original magnification × 325. (C) Histological findings of the bone marrow. H&E-stained microphotograph shows erythroid hyperplasia and slight megakaryocytic proliferation. Original magnification × 325. (D) Histological findings of the adrenal gland. H&E-stained microphotograph shows atrophy of cortical parenchymal cells and intercellular hyalinous deposits. Original magnification × 325.

A. PATHOLOGICAL FINDINGS

The body weight was 13 kg and height was 86.5 cm. Generalized edema, particularly in the face, was noted. No external anomalies were found. Bloody ascites (80 ml) was observed, but pleural and pericardial fluid were absent. No splenic tissue was identified at autopsy.

1. Cardiovascular System

The heart weighed 180 g and manifested left ventricular hypertrophy probably due to chronic hypertension and/or glomerulonephritis. No congenital heart disease, valvular disease, infarction, or myocarditis were found. No atherosclerotic lesions or embolisms were present in the coronary arteries. In the aorta, prominent atherosclerotic changes such as fatty streaks and fibrous plaques were noted. Such lesions have not been documented in HO-1-targeted mice. Microscopically, endothelial cells on the surfaces of fibrous plaques were often damaged. Fibrous plaques were characterized by the proliferation of smooth muscle cells and scarce macrophages (Figure 11.2A).

2. Lungs

The lungs weighed 70 g (left) and 95 g (right), and showed congestive edema. Microscopically, microthrombi were found in the arterioles and capillaries of the lungs along with focal alveolitis suggesting disseminated intravascular coagulation and septic state (Figure 11.2B). In HO-1-targeted mice, monocytes adhered to small vessel walls as in vasculitis and infiltrated into perivascular spaces. No definite vasculitis was noted in the human lung.

3. Hematopoietic and Lymphoid Systems

Bone marrow showed hypercellularity with reactive erythroid hyperplasia and mega-karyocytic proliferation (Figure 11.2C). Foamy macrophages were also seen in the bone marrow. Lymph nodes were atrophic rather than hyperplastic. No lymphadenopathy was present at autopsy, probably due to therapeutic steroid administration, although lymphadenopathy was seen in the neck when the patient was 2 years old. Extramedullary hematopoiesis was not found. In HO-1-targeted mice, splenomegaly with extramedullary hematopoiesis and follicular hyperplasia and lymphadenopathy were present.

4. Adrenal Glands

Adrenal glands have sinusoidal structures like those in the liver. At autopsy, parenchymal cells of the adrenal cortex were atrophic, and slight amyloid deposits were seen in the intercellular spaces (Figure 11.2D).

5. Liver

The liver was markedly enlarged, weighing 1150 g, and pale yellowish tan in color. Light microscopy showed amorphous substances deposited in the sinusoidal spaces, resulting in marked atrophy of hepatocytes (Figure 11.3A). On polarized microscopy, a Congo red-stained section revealed light green birefringence. Electron microscopic examination confirmed randomly arranged nonbranching amyloid filaments (Figure 11.3B). Immunohistochemical studies performed on formalin-fixed, paraffin-embedded tissue showed no positive staining of amyloid precursor proteins for antiserum AA, immunoglobulin light chain, transthyretin, α_2-microglobulin, apolipoprotein AI, gelsolin, lysozyme, cystatin C, Aβ protein precursor, prion, calcitonin, islet amyloid polypeptide, atrial natriuretic factor, prolactin, insulin, or lactoferrin. The nature of the amyloid protein is not clear, although haptoglobin or other proteins elevated in serum may be candidates for the β-pleated sheet structure. A review of the liver biopsy findings at 5 years of age revealed a moderate degree of fatty change of hepatocytes, and Kupffer cells and foamy macrophages scattered in sinusoids with many hemosiderin pigments (Figure 11.3C). No amyloid substances were deposited. Amyloidosis was not observed in HO-1-targeted mice.

6. Kidneys

The kidneys each weighed 70 g. The cut surface revealed urate infarcts in medullary rays. Microscopically, glomerular changes with mesangial proliferation and thickened

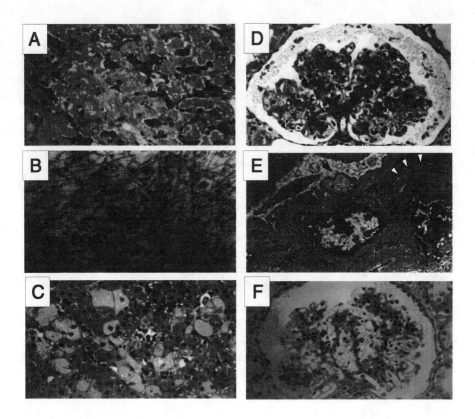

FIGURE 11.3 Histological findings of the liver and the kidney. (A) H&E-stained micropho-tograph shows marked atrophy of hepatocytes and intercellular hyalinous deposits at autopsy. (B) A dense network of nonbranching filaments is seen ultrastructurally. (C) H&E-stained microphotograph shows prominent Kupffer cells and foamy macrophages in the parenchyma at biopsy. (D) H&E-stained microphotograph of the kidney shows the significant increase of mesangial cells and splitting of the thickened basement membrane. (E) Ultrastructurally, a mesangial foot process is intervened within the thickened basement membrane (arrow). Basement membrane-like products are seen in the mesangial area (arrow heads). (F) Intense staining for collagen type IV is detected immunohistochemically in the mesangial areas. Original magnification × 325 (A, C, D, F); × 69,000 (B, E).

capillary loops were noted. Some of the capillary loops were split (Figure 11.3D). These findings are consistent with mesangial proliferative glomerulonephritis or focal membranoproliferative glomerulonephritis. Electron microscopic examination showed amorphous deposits between thickened basement membrane and endothe-lium. Basement membrane-like products were seen in the mesangial areas. Mesan-gial interpositions were occasionally seen in the basement membrane (Figure 11.3E). No immune complexes were found in the glomeruli. Immunohistochemically, intense staining of anti-collagen type IV was noted in the mesangial areas (Figure 11.3F). Severe tubulointerstitial injury with tubular atrophy, dilated Bowman's space, inter-stitial fibrosis, and inflammatory cell infiltration were observed. Foamy macrophages

TABLE 11.3
Comparison of Pathological Findings of HO-1 Deficient Human and HO-1 Knockout Mice

Finding	Human	Mice
Erythrocyte morphology	Fragmentation, anisocytosis	Anisocytosis
Hemosiderosis	+	+
Fatty streak, fibrous plaque	+	Not described
DIC, thrombus	+	Not described
Vasculitis	−	+
Amyloid deposition	+	Not described
Reticuloendothelial cells	Foam cells ++	Monocytes +
Spleen	Asplenia	Enlarged
Glomerulonephritis	+	+
Bone marrow hyperplasia	+	Not described

Note: DIC = Disseminated intravascular coagulation.

with iron pigments were scattered in the interstitium. No amyloid filaments were found in the glomeruli; slight amyloid deposits were observed in the interstitium.

7. Nervous System

The brain weighed 830 g. Except for subdural hemorrhage, no malformations or destructive lesions such as cerebral hemorrhage, infarction, or inflammation of the central nervous system were found. Central nervous system findings in HO-1-targeted mice were not described in the literature.

8. Other Organs

Mild acute pancreatitis with parenchymal necrosis and neutrophilic infiltration was seen. No amyloid deposit was noted in the pancreas. Patchy hemorrhages were present in the intestinal tracts. No abnormalities of the endocrine system or musculoskeletal system were found.

B. Discussion

The human patient exhibited similar clinical features to those noted in the HO-1-targeted mice. However, from a pathological view, some differences were noted at autopsy (Table 11.3). Marked amyloid deposition was observed in spite of the patient's youth, whereas no amyloidosis was present in senile HO-1-targeted mice. The exact pathogenesis of the amyloidosis is not clear, but injury to the sinusoidal endothelium and macrophage dysfunction may lead to deposition of an amyloid precursor protein of unknown nature.

Many foam cells were present in the liver and generalized reticuloendothelial tissue. The irregular distribution of foam cells as represented by Kupffer cells in the

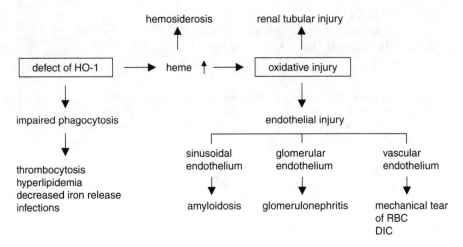

FIGURE 11.4 Putative scheme of pathological mechanism of heme oxygenase (HO)-1 deficiency. RBCs = red blood cells; DIC = disseminated intravascular coagulation.

sinusoidal space was unusual. Some dysfunction of the macrophages may be associated with HO-1 deficiency, since HO-1 is a cytoprotective protein up-regulated in phagocytosis.[33]

Another problem was the hyperlipidemia. The prominent atherosclerotic changes such as fatty streaks and fibrous plaques were not documented in the HO-1-targeted mice. Fatty streaks of the aorta at 6 years of age may be explained by hyperlipidemia-accelerating atherosclerosis. Fibrous plaques were characterized by the proliferation of smooth muscle cells and scarce foamy macrophages. Carbon monoxide produced by vascular smooth muscle cells, one of the products derived from the HO reaction, is known to indirectly suppress the gene expression of vasoconstrictors such as endothelin-1 and platelet-derived growth factor-B in endothelial cells and subsequently inhibit the proliferation of smooth muscle cells.[34]

In the microenvironment of the fatty streak, proliferation signals of smooth muscle cells may not be regulated and may be up-regulated due to the functional loss of this cytoprotective enzyme. In HO-1-targeted mice, monocytes adhered to small vessel walls as in vasculitis and infiltrated perivascular spaces in the lungs, not the intima of the aorta.

The HO-1-deficient patient showed asplenia. It is possible that cell and tissue damage induced by oxidative stress is more seriously manifested in endothelial cells due to asplenia because of the absence of the splenic filtering function. Based on pathology and clinical findings, the human case of HO-1 deficiency was more severely affected by oxidative stressors than the targeted mice, as summarized in the scheme of HO-1-deficient tissue injury shown in Figure 11.4. Erythrocyte fragmentation and hemolysis, disseminated intravascular coagulation, and membrano-proliferative glomerular changes all seem to have resulted from endothelial injury and reticuloendothelial dysfunction.

III. RENAL PATHOLOGY

A. CLINICAL FEATURES ASSOCIATED WITH KIDNEY ABNORMALITY IN THE HO-1-DEFICIENT PATIENT

The HO-1-deficient patient consistently manifested both hematuria and pro-teinuria. The hematuria showed a glomerular pattern, because the red blood cells (RBCs) in the urine were dysmorphic, and RBC casts and/or granular casts were always present in the urine. The concentration of urinary protein was about 30 to 100 mg/dl. Urinary levels of N-acetyl-β-D-glucosaminidase (NAG) and β_2-micro-globulin (β_2-mg) were very high. Urinary NAG was about 100 to 200 IU/g crea-tinine (normal range in our hospital is below 7 IU/g creatinine). Urinary β_2-mg was about 5000 μg/g creatinine (normal range in our hospital is below 400 μg/g creatinine). Blood pressure (90 to 100/40 to 50 mmHg), total renal function, as estimated by serum creatinine (0.2 to 0.3 mg/dl), blood urea nitrogen (10 to 20 mg/dl), and 24-hour creatinine clearance (100 to 120 ml/min/1.73 m^2) remained nearly normal throughout the illness. These findings indicated the patient had glomerular and/or interstitial nephritis.

B. RENAL PATHOLOGY OF THE HO-1-DEFICIENT PATIENT

Three renal specimens, two from renal biopsies and a third obtained at autopsy, were examined. The renal biopsies were performed at 2 years and 5 years of age. In the initial biopsy specimen, mesangial proliferation and thickening of the capillary wall were mild. Narrowing of the capillary lumina was not severe. No crescent formation or glomerular adhesion to Bowman's capsule was found. Tubulo-interstitial damage was limited to a small part of the specimen. No peculiar staining pattern was observed on immunofluorescence. Fibrinogen was only weakly positive. IgG, IgA, IgM, C3, and C4 were very faintly detectable, and C1q was negative.

On electron microscopy, endothelial swelling and detachment were prominent throughout the glomerular capillary loop. Unidentifiable materials were deposited between the detached endothelium and glomerular basement membrane. These mate-rials were not amyloids. The histological diagnosis at the initial biopsy was diffuse mild mesangial proliferative glomerulonephritis with some vasculitis, the etiology of which was unknown.[13] Similar glomerular findings were observed in the second biopsy and in the autopsy samples, but the size of each glomerulus, mesangial proliferation, and thickening of the capillary wall increased. Bowman's capsules dilated progressively, in parallel with the accelerated collapses of the atrophic tubuli. It was striking how the tubulo-interstitial damage including tubular dilatation and/or atrophy, interstitial fibrosis, and inflammatory cell infiltration, advanced progres-sively. The area of tubulo-interstitial injury occupied 0.7% of the specimen at the first biopsy, 17.4% at the second, and 40.2% at autopsy (Figure 11.5A).[14]

Multiple foci of iron deposition were observed within the kidney. The basolateral site of the proximal tubular epithelium was the major site of iron deposition. In contrast, iron deposition was very rare within the glomeruli. Furthermore, we did not find iron deposition in samples from other glomerular diseases.[13] A urine sample

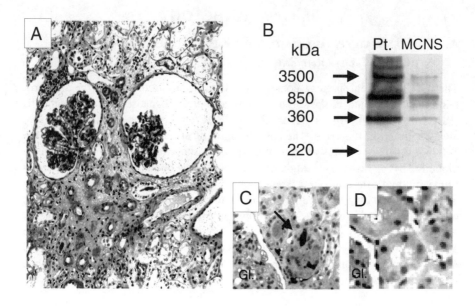

FIGURE 11.5 Renal pathological findings in the concentrated urine specimen of the HO-1-deficient patient at autopsy. (A) H&E staining. (B) Immunoblotting of haptoglobin in the urine samples. MCNS indicates minimal change nephrotic syndrome (MCNS) in the acute phase as control. The urine sample revealed a significant amount of type 2-2 haptoglobin. All bands show type 2-2 haptoglobins. Immunohistochemical examination revealed haptoglobin within the proximal tubular epithelium of the patient (C, arrow), but no MCNS (D). Gl. = glomerulus.

from the patient revealed a significant amount of type 2-2 haptoglobin. In contrast, the control sample exhibited only a trace level of haptoglobin, although urinary protein concentrations of the two samples were comparable. Sizes of the ladder bands did not change after preincubation of the urine sample with free hemoglobin, indicating that most of the haptoglobin had been already conjugated with hemoglobin (Figure 11.5B).[14] Intense staining of haptoglobin was observed within the proximal tubular epithelium of the HO-1-deficient patient (Figure 11.5C). In marked contrast, haptoglobin was virtually absent within the tubular cells of a control kidney (Figure 11.5D). The absence of a functional spleen had a significant effect on heme metabolism. The tubular epithelial cells became the sites of haptoglobin uptake and hemoglobin metabolism, leading to heavy iron overload and accumulation of haptoglobin within these cells.

C. Renal Pathology of the HO-1-Targeted Mouse

Contrary to the findings in the human HO-1-deficient case, the glomeruli seemed more vulnerable than the tubular structures in HO-1-targeted mice, with widespread injury noted.[7] The reason for such marked differences in the pathological findings of human HO-1 deficiency and HO-1-targeted mice is not yet clear. Two fundamental differences may be the environment and the total duration of stress exposures. HO-1-targeted mice were presumably bred in a sterile, pathogen-free environment, without the danger of ubiquitous infectious agents, and the mice survived for a long period. Their renal lesions are, therefore, the results of long-standing, low level stress to the kidney. The HO-1-deficient patient was exposed to unremitting waves of infectious agents, starting shortly after birth.

This hypothesis was supported by two reports on renal injury in the HO-1-targeted mouse. Nath et al.[35] observed a significant reduction of renal function with severe tubular injury accompanied by 100% mortality in HO-1-targeted (–/–) mice exposed to glycerol. In sharp contrast, renal dysfunction was mild and reversible and not fatal in HO-1 +/+ mice. Hemoglobin also induced rapid renal damage in both young and old HO-1-targeted mice, but had little effect on normal mice. Immunohistochemistry studies showed that the principal sites of HO-1 production after glycerol challenge were the proximal tubuli, not the glomeruli. Our HO-1-deficient case suffered from systemic vascular endothelial cell injury, with massive intravascular hemolysis. His serum was loaded with heme, and a large amount of heme-conjugated haptoglobin and a high concentration of haptoglobin were detectable in urine too (Figures 11.5B through D). As a result, tubular epithelial cells became the sites of active haptoglobin uptake and hemoglobin metabolism, leading to accumulation of haptoglobin within these cells. Consequently, the renal tubular epithelium in this patient was consistently exposed to high concentrations of heme and severe tubular damage ensued.[13] Shiraishi et al.[36] reported that HO-1-targeted mice develop more severe renal damage and have significant renal tubular injuries (apoptosis and necrosis) compared with wild-type mice treated with cisplatin. They again showed *in vitro* that significant HO-1 production was inducible in proximal tubular cells. These results strongly indicate that renal tubular epithelial cells are constantly exposed to various oxidative stresses *in vivo*, and are therefore vulnerable to injury whenever the levels of the insults become overwhelming. Selective HO-1 production within these cells will thus play an important protective role in preserving renal functions.

D. Localization of HO-1 in Various Renal Diseases

HO-1 staining was observed within tubular epithelial cells, especially within distal tubuli, in all of the renal diseases including nephrotic syndrome in the complete remission stage, in which no apparent tubular and/or glomerular damage is usually seen (Figures 11.6A and B).[14] In contrast, HO-1 was not detected within intrinsic glomerular cells in any of these diseases. Distal tubuli showed no significant correlation between the intensity of HO-1 staining and degree of hematuria or proteinuria. HO-1 staining within proximal tubuli tended to be more intense, with greater degrees of hematuria, proteinuria, and tubulo-interstitial damage (Morimoto, K. et al., Kidney, Inc., in press). These results suggest that HO-1 plays important roles in protecting renal tubuli from oxidative injuries where these cells are constantly exposed to various oxidative stresses.

The reason for significant differences in the expression patterns of HO-1 between proximal and distal tubular epithelial cells are not clear. Recent studies reported low levels of constitutive expression of HO-1 in the renal inner medulla, where it may

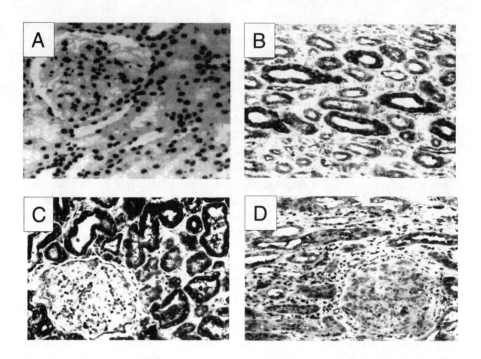

FIGURE 11.6 Immunohistochemical demonstration of HO-1 and carboxymethyllysine (CML). HO-1 was not detected in the renal specimen of the HO-1-deficient case (A), but was detectable in various renal diseases, including MCNS in complete remission (B). In the HO-1-deficient case, very intense immunostainings of CML (C) were observed within proximal and distal tubuli. In contrast, CML was only faintly detectable within epithelial cells of the proximal tubuli and glomeruli in renal tissues from patients with IgA nephropathy (D).

contribute to the maintenance of renal medullary circulation.[37] It is possible that the constant level of HO-1 expression seen in various renal diseases indicates that HO-1 expression *in vivo* contributes to the maintenance of renal circulation, in addition to the protection of tubular cells from oxidative injury. Liang et al. reported the differential induction of HO-1 in a renal proximal tubular cell line and a renal distal tubular cell line. They concluded that the renal expression of HO-1 was regulated in a tubule segment-specific and/or species-specific fashion and that such regional heterogeneity in the expression of HO-1 may be relevant to the different functions HO-1 plays in renal injury.[38]

E. OTHER OXIDATIVE STRESS MARKERS IN THE KIDNEY

We evaluated carboxymethyllysine (CML) and pentosidine in the kidney as surrogate markers of oxidative stress. Both compounds are formed under oxidative stress by carbonyl amine chemistry between protein amino groups and carbonyl compounds, and have been suggested as integrative biomarkers of cumulative oxidative stress in various tissues including kidney.[39] Several studies have shown that CML and pentosidine are accumulated within the kidney.[40-42] They have been identified within the expanded mesangial matrix and nodular lesions in diabetic nephropathy and in the interstitium of unilateral ureteral obstruction, which is a well-established experimental model of renal injury leading to interstitial fibrosis.

In renal tissues from patients with various renal diseases, immunostaining of CML and pentosidine was detected, but was faint in both glomeruli and tubuli. In contrast, intense immunostaining was observed within the renal tubular epithelial cells in renal tissue from the HO-1-deficient case (Figures 11.6C and D). These results clearly indicate that the tubular epithelial cells in HO-1 deficiency had been exposed to persistent, severe oxidative stress, which was markedly potentiated by the absence of HO-1. In contrast, progressive accumulation of oxidative stress is attenuated in HO-1-positive individuals by the potent cytoprotective effect of HO-1, which is rapidly induced within tubular cells in response to environmental insults.

IV. MOLECULAR PATHOLOGY

A. THE MRNA AND GENOMIC STRUCTURE OF HO-1

In the mammalian HO system, three isoforms of HO that catalyze the degradation of heme (Fe-protoporphyrin IX), designated HO-1, HO-2,[43] and HO-3,[19] have been identified. The genes for human HO-1 and HO-2 have been isolated and their chromosomal organizations were mapped on 22q13.1[44,45] and 16p13.3,[44] respectively. The HO-3 cDNA has been isolated in rats, and shows 90% amino acid identity with rat HO-2.[19] However, the human homologue to HO-3 has not yet been identified. The human HO-1 gene produces a single transcript of approximately 1.5 kb encoding 288 amino acids with a molecular mass of 32,800 Da.[46] The homologies in amino acid sequences of human HO-1 to rat and mouse HO-1 are 80% and 82%, respectively.

The human HO-1 gene is about 14 kb long and organized into five exons.[47] Exon 1 contains the start codon and exons 2 through 5 consist of 121 bp, 492 bp, 100 bp, and 734 bp sequences, respectively. At least two functionally active regulatory elements have been identified in this gene. The proximal elements within 121 bp of the sequence upstream of the mRNA cap site respond to various agents such as sodium arsenite, hydrogen peroxide, hemin, and cadmium chloride.[48] A 10-bp *cis*-acting element about 4 kb upstream from the transcription initiation site is responsible for cadmium-mediated induction as a distal enhancer.[49]

B. MUTATIONAL ANALYSES OF HO-1 MRNA IN THE PROBAND AND FAMILY MEMBERS

A complete defect of HO-1 induction after stimulation with several stress-inducing factors was documented in the proband.[13] Lymphoblastoid cell lines (LCLs) from the proband, family members, and normal controls were established under informed consent. LCLs were preincubated with 10 μM of cadmium chloride for induction of HO-1 gene transcripts and subjected to molecular analysis of HO-1 mRNA. Reverse transcriptase (RT) PCR was performed to amplify the entire open reading frame with coordinates 81/947 (numbers from the human HO-1 mRNA reference sequence X06985 from the GenBank).

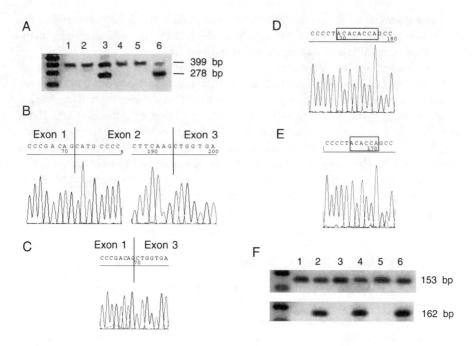

FIGURE 11.7 HO-1 gene mutations. Analysis of the maternal mutation (A through C). RT PCR amplification of the fragment containing exon 2. (A) Lanes 1 through 6 represent control, father, mother, sister, brother, and proband, respectively. (B) Sequence analysis of normal control and (C) maternal allele. Analysis of the paternal mutation (D through F). (D) Sequence analysis of normal control allele and (E) paternal allele. (F) Upper panel: RT PCR amplification of the fragment containing exon 3. Lanes 1 through 6 represent control, father, mother, sister, brother, and proband, respectively. Lower panel: mutation-specific PCR of genomic DNA.

Using the primer pairs to amplify the fragments containing exon 2, RT PCR products from the proband and his mother contained an extra, shorter fragment (278 bp) in addition to a normal-sized HO-1 mRNA fragment (399 bp). A single size of HO-1 mRNA fragment (399 bp) was amplified in the father, sister, and brother (Figure 11.7A). Direct sequencing of the shorter fragment observed in the proband and mother showed a complete loss of exon 2 (Figures 11.7B and C). Loss of exon 2 led to a frame shift and created a premature termination codon at the 10th residue. Analysis of the paternal PCR product revealed a two-nucleotide (AC) deletion within exon 3 (Figures 11.7D and E). Genomic amplification by mutation-specific PCR using synthesized mutation-specific primers confirmed the mutation in the proband, his father, and his sister (Figure 11.7F). The AC deletion led to a frame shift, resulting in a premature termination codon at the 131st residue. Dinucleotide tandem repeats (ACACAC) were observed at the deletion site of exon 3. This structural feature suggests slipped strand mispairing for the mechanism of AC deletion in exon 3.[50]

In summary, the proband was a compound heterozygote for a complete deletion of exon 2 from the maternal allele and a two-nucleotide deletion within exon 3 from the paternal allele. Both maternal and paternal mutations led to a frame shift and created a premature termination codon into the HO 1mRNA. The parents and the sister carrying the paternal mutation were shown to be heterozygotes, providing evidence for autosomal recessive inheritance.

C. MECHANISM OF EXON 2 DELETION IN THE HO-1 GENE

There are at least two possibilities for the molecular mechanisms of the exon 2 deletion mutation in HO-1 mRNA from the maternal allele: exon skipping due to alternative splicing or genomic deletion. We examined the nucleotide sequences flanking splice junctions for exons 1, 2, and 3 to investigate the former possibility. The approximately 200-bp genomic regions surrounding each of the exons were amplified from the genomic DNA of the family members. Sequence analysis of the PCR products revealed no substitution at the splice acceptor or donor sites of the indicated exons in the proband or mother (data not shown).

We next considered a large deletion or genomic rearrangement involving exon 2 rather than the exon-skipping mutation. Genomic fragments spanning exons 1 through 3 of the human HO-1 gene were amplified using primers PreExon1 and Exon3R (Figure 11.8A). The genomic PCR products from the proband (lane 4, Figure 11.8B) and his mother (lane 3, Figure 11.8B) contained an extra 4.3-kb fragment in addition to a normal 6.0 kb-fragment (lanes 2 through 6, Figure 11.8B) from the intact allele. The sequences of this shorter fragment from the proband and mother were identical and demonstrated the deletion of 1730-bp sequences that contained complete sequences of exon 2 (121 bp) and flanking intron sequences (1609 bp).

PCR amplification using PreExon1 and Exon3R primers successfully discriminated between the affected and intact alleles. To further confirm this genomic deletion in the maternal allele, Southern blot analysis was performed using PCR-generated genomic probes (530 bp) as indicated in Figure 11.8A. The probe was hybridized with 3.8-kb and approximately 8-kb HincII-restriction fragments in the genomic DNA from all of the family members and normal controls (lanes 2 through 8, Figure 11.8C). Since the 8-kb HincII-restriction fragment was consistently observed in all the DNA samples, the fragment may represent a pseudogene or gene family rather than the result of incomplete digestion of the genomic DNA.

An additional 4.4-kb genomic fragment resulting in loss of a HincII site was detected in the proband (lane 5, Figure 11.8C) and mother (lane 4, Figure 11.8C), confirming the genomic deletion.[15] The deletion junction contained sequences homologous to a consensus *Alu* element. Characteristically, *Alu* elements are composed of a tandem repeat of two highly homologous sequences separated by a short A-rich region and are 300 bp long.[51] As illustrated in Figure 11.8D, a number of *Alu* subfamily sequences[52-54] were identified in the human HO-1 gene by searching the database. The flanking sequences of exon 2 contained a tandem repeat of two *Alu-Sx* (*Sx*-1 and *Sx*-2) elements in intron 1 and an *Alu-Sq* element in intron 2. Analysis of the deletion junction sequence revealed fusion of a 133-bp 5′ *Sx*-1 element with a 169-bp 3′ *Sq* element (Figure 11.8E). In addition, the sequences with high homology (22/26) to the 26-bp *Alu* "core" sequence (CCTGTAATCCCAGCACTTTGG-GAGGC) considered to be a recombinogenic hotspot[55] were present in the deletion joint (Figure 11.8E).

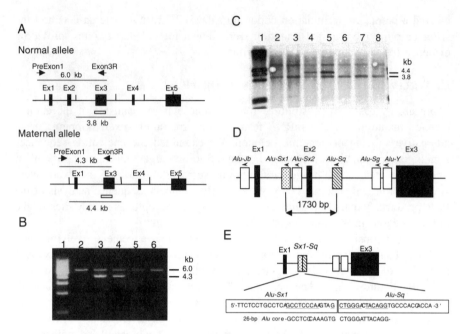

FIGURE 11.8 Analyses of the maternal allele. (A) Restriction map of the HO-1 gene. HincII sites are shown with vertical lines. The loss of a HincII site accompanied by the genomic deletion of exon 2 is illustrated as maternal allele. The primers and the genomic probe are indicated as arrows and an open rectangle, respectively. (B) Genomic PCR amplification of DNA fragments containing exons 1 through 3. Lane 1: DNA size markers; lanes 2 through 6: father, mother, proband, brother, and sister, respectively. (C) Southern blot analysis using the genomic probe. Lane 1: DNA size markers; lanes 2 though 8: control 1, control 2, mother, proband, father, brother, and sister, respectively. (D) Diagrammatic representation of *Alu* elements present in the HO-1 gene (exons 1 through 3 only). The locations of *Alu* family sequences are shown by open boxes. The arrow heads above the open boxes indicate the 5′ to 3′ directions of the *Alu* sequences. (E) Alignment of *Alu-Sx1* and *Alu-Sq* sequences results in a 1730-bp genomic deletion encompassing exon 2 in the maternal allele. The junction contains the sequences (underlined) with homology to 26-bp *Alu* "core" sequences.

Alu elements have been evolutionarily conserved in primates and are known to be involved in gene arrangements, including deletions, insertions, and partial tandem duplications in several different genes.[51] For example, recombination between two existing *Alu* elements resulting in loss of coding sequences has been reported in genetic disorders such as adenosine deaminase deficiency,[56] hypobetalipoproteine- mia,[57] maple syrup urine disease,[58] and glycogen storage disease type II,[59] and in cancers such as retinoblastoma,[60] breast,[61] and colon cancer.[62] Several mechanisms for *Alu*-mediated gene deletion have been proposed based on homologous recom- bination that occurs imperfectly or is associated with unequal crossing-over in meiotic cells.[50] These structural features of the HO-1 gene with respect to *Alu* elements and the deletion joint sequences led us to support the hypothesis that the recombination event between homologous *Alu* sequences encompassing exon 2 may be the mechanism responsible for genetic deletion in the case with this defect.

D. FUTURE DIRECTIONS

We described the molecular characterization of the human HO-1 gene in an inheritable phenotype of HO-1 deficiency. Population-based experimental data such as the frequency of HO-1 gene polymorphisms and/or genomic deletions involving these *Alu* sequences are required to understand the significance of *Alu*-mediated recombination. The single family presented here may simply represent an extremely rare genetic event.

Yamada et al. demonstrated the correlation between length polymorphism of the (GT)n dinucleotide repeat in the 5′ flanking region of the human HO-1 gene and susceptibility to chronic pulmonary emphysema.[63] Since we have no naturally occurring animal models or other families with this disease, no solid data are available at present. Further accumulation of typical and atypical cases will provide insight into the frequency of the HO-1 gene mutation, including polymorphisms of this disease, association between clinical expression and types of mutations, further understanding of the roles of HO-1 *in vivo*, and clarification of the molecular basis for gene therapy.

V. FUNCTIONAL ROLES OF HO-1 *IN VIVO*

A. FUNCTIONAL SIGNIFICANCE OF HO-1 DEFICIENCY

As summarized in the general pathology section, direct consequences of HO-1 deficiency are either extensive cell injury induced by lack of the enzyme or the induction of cell dysfunction, in particular, impaired phagocytic functions of macrophages (Figure 11.2A). Although it is extremely difficult to prove that these are the general phenomena observed in every HO-1-deficient patient, we tried to analyze the functional significance of HO-1 deficiency by two different experimental strategies. First, LCL from the patient was transfected with a retroviral vector containing normal HO-1 gene. HO-1 protein expression and sensitivity to hemin exposure of the HO-1-transfected LCL and non-transfected LCL from the same patient were compared. Second, the effects of exposure of monocytes to high heme environment were tested to see whether the result had any relevance to the observed morphological characteristics and the functional disturbances of the patient monocytes and the apparently impaired phagocytic function.

B. MECHANISM OF HEMIN-INDUCED INJURY OF HO-1-DEFICIENT CELLS

LCL derived from the HO-1-deficient patient was extremely sensitive to hemin-induced cell injury. When the cell injury was determined by decreased forward light scatter and annexin-V surface binding, significant cell injury was induced in patient LCL after 24 h (Figure 11.9A). As little as 20 μM of added hemin induced significant cell injury, whereas no significant cell injury was induced in control LCL even at 100 μM.[13] In accord with the sensitivity to hemin-induced cell injury, patient LCL did not produce a detectable level of HO-1 even at 100 μM of hemin (Figure 11.9B). In contrast, a low level of HO-1 production was already detectable in control LCL without stimulation, and the level increased in a dose-dependent fashion with added hemin (Figure 11.9C).

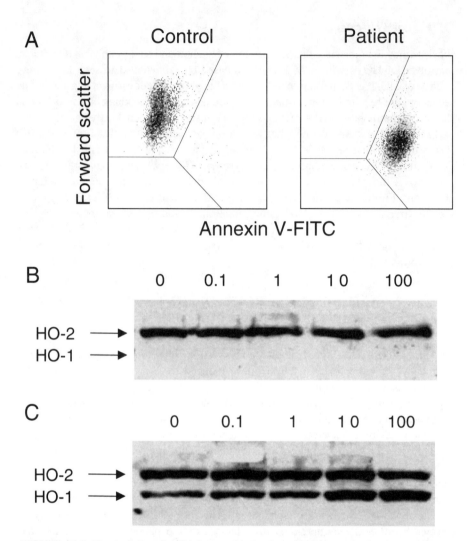

FIGURE 11.9 Hemin-induced cell injury and induction of HO-1 production in lymphoblastoid cell lines (LCLs). For hemin-induced injury, LCLs from the control and the HO-1-deficient patient were cultured in the presence of $100\,\mu M$ hemin for 24 h. Apoptotic cells were identified by decreased forward light scatter and FITC-conjugated annexin V binding (A) Immunoblotting analysis of HOs induced by variable concentrations of hemin. LCLs from the HO-1-deficient patient (B) and the control (C) were cultured with increasing concentrations of hemin for 8 h. Production of HO-1 and HO-2 was examined simultaneously by immunoblotting. LCLs established by transformation of peripheral blood B lymphocytes by Epstein–Barr virus were used.

HO-2 was produced constitutively by both control and patient LCLs. The patient serum consistently contained more than $400\,\mu M$ of heme. It is plausible to assume that the cells exposed to this high heme concentration were invariably vulnerable to cell injury in the absence of adequate production of heme-degrading enzyme HO-1.[13]

Extreme sensitivity of HO-1-deficient LCL to hemin stimulation was not reversed by the addition of apoferritin or bilirubin to the hemin stimulated cultures. Furthermore, ferritin production by HO-1-deficient LCL was comparable with normal control LCL with or without added hemin (data not shown). Although ferritin and bilirubin may act as antioxidants in certain situations, they do not contribute much to protect cells from hemin-induced cell injury, at least at high hemin concentrations.[64-68] Rather, direct degradation of heme by HO-1 was thought to play a significant role in protecting cells from high concentrations of hemin.

C. Effect of HO-1 Gene Transfer on Hemin-Induced Cell Injury

We next tried to explain the direct role of HO-1 in the protection of cells from hemin-induced cell injury by transfecting HO-1 gene into patient LCL using a retrovirus vector pGCsam. The vector pGCsam is a plasmid containing the Moloney murine leukemia virus, which has the encephalomyocarditis (EMC) virus internal ribosomal entry site (IRES) cloned upstream of the bacterial neomycin phosphotransferase (*neo*) gene. The human HO-1 cDNA was cloned into pGCsam so that the HO-1 translational start site was positioned precisely at the env translational initiation site in the wild type virus (Figure 11.10A).

A total of 15 µg of pGCsamENHO-1 or pGCsamEN without HO-1 DNA was transfected into an ecotropic packaging cell line, GP+E86, by calcium phosphate co-precipitation. Culture supernatant from these transfected cells was harvested and used to infect an amphotropic packaging cell line, PG13 cells in the presence of protamine sulfate.[69] The PG13/pGCsamEN producer cells were selected by the neomycin-analog G418. Culture supernatant from these producer cells was harvested, filtered, and transfected into LCLs using RetroNectin-precoated plates. LCLs successfully transfected with pGCsamEN were selected by G418.

To see if HO-1 gene is effectively transfected, LCLs were stained for HO-1 expression and evaluated by a flow cytometry using an anti-rat HO-1 mAb, GTS-1 (kindly provided by Dr. M. Suematsu). HO-1 expression was confirmed in patient LCL transfected with HO-1 gene by a flow cytometry and by immunohistochemistry. HO-1-transfected LCLs expressed HO-1 constitutively, without any stimulation. The level of HO-1 protein did not increase even after stimulation. Patient LCL transfected with *neo* control vector did not produce HO-1. HO-1 protein expression was further confirmed by immunoblotting assay (Figure 11.10B). When LCLs transfected with pGCsamENHO-1 were cultured with different concentrations of hemin, significant inhibition of cell injury was observed. LCLs transfected with pGCsamEN without HO-1 gene were injured dose dependently, like the patient's original LCL (Figures 11.10C and D). These results support the contention that degradation of heme by HO-1 is directly responsible for the reversal of hemin-induced cell injury.

D. Effect of Hemin Exposure on Macrophage Phagocytic Function

The most characteristic pathological findings were observed in the kidney and liver, as shown in Sections II.A.5 and 6.[14] Peculiar cell injury seen in the proximal tubular epithelium and glomerular endothelium is thought to reflect the vulnerability of these

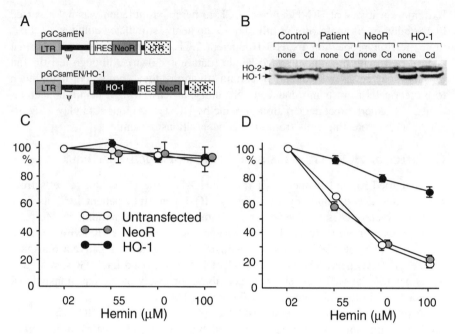

FIGURE 11.10 HO-1 gene transfection and reversal of hemin-induced cell injury. (A) Structures of retroviral vectors pGCsamEN (NeoR) and pGCsamEN cloned with HO-1 gene (HO-1). (B) LCLs from the control and the HO-1-deficient patient, HO-1-deficient LCL transfected with NeoR, and HO-1-deficient LCL transfected with HO-1 were cultured alone or with 20 μM of cadmium for 6 h. HO-1 and HO-2 expression was evaluated by immunoblotting. Both control LCL (C) and the patient LCL (D) were transfected with NeoR or HO-1. Untransfected LCL, LCL transfected with NeoR, and LCL transfected with HO-1 were cultured in the presence of various concentrations of hemin for 24 h. Cell injury was evaluated by flow cytometry.

cells to high concentrations of heme. Extremely high concentrations of circulating heme *in vivo* might have caused extensive injury, because endothelial cells and renal tubular epithelial cells are the target cells constantly exposed to high levels of heme *in vivo*. Extensive amyloidosis observed in the liver at autopsy may have resulted from injury to the sinusoidal endothelium.

In addition to the injury to the resident macrophages, the patient exhibited unusual findings indicating disturbed macrophage phagocytic function. Lack of a spleen certainly contributed significantly to the reduced phagocytic function resulting in overload of the other reticuloendothelial systems, including circulating macrophages and the hepatic Kupffer cells. The patient's peripheral blood monocytes exhibited some morphological characteristics, including prominent vacuolation and basophilic cytoplasm. These changes may reflect persistent, systemic inflammatory reaction.

In addition to the morphological changes, the surface antigen expression by these monocytes was abnormal. Expressions of HLA-DR and CD36 were significantly reduced as compared with normal monocytes (Figure 11.11). CD14 expression was comparable to that of the controls. The reduction in the expression of these

A

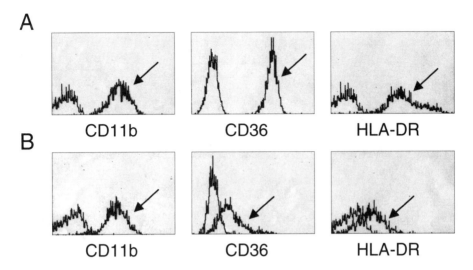

B

CD11b   CD36   HLA-DR

CD11b   CD36   HLA-DR

FIGURE 11.11 Surface expression of monocyte antigens. Monocytes from the control (A) and the HO-1-deficient patient (B) were evaluated for surface expression of CD11b, CD36, and HLA-DR by flow cytometry. Arrows indicate the profiles obtained by relevant monoclonal antibodies. Unmarked lines indicate the profiles obtained by isotype-matched control antibodies.

antigens was consistently observed after repeated examinations, indicating that these changes reflected abnormal monocyte functions.

To see whether exposure to a high concentration of heme induces down-regulation of monocyte antigens, isolated monocytes from peripheral blood were cultured for several hours in the presence of variable concentrations of hemin. Expressions of CD36, HLA-DR, CD16, and CD11b were rapidly down-regulated afer the culture, whereas CD45 expression did not change. These surface antigens are all thought to be involved in receptor-mediated phagocytosis by monocytes.[70-74] In parallel with the surface molecule changes, monocyte phagocytic functions were impaired dramatically.

Although phagocytosis of fluorescence-labeled latex beads did not change significantly (Figures 11.12A and B), phagocytosis of opsonized erythrocytes was virtually abolished (Figures 11.12C and D). The results indicated that hemin exposure and the subsequent reduction of surface molecules are directly related to the abolishment of receptor-mediated phagocytosis of opsonized erythrocytes by monocytes. Various hematological and biochemical abnormalities seen in the HO-1-deficient patient, including increased haptoglobin concentration, abundance of fragmented erythrocytes, thrombocytosis, and hyperlipidemia, may all be explained by the reduced scavenging functions of phagocytes secondary to heme exposure. Unlike HO-1 knocknout mice, our patient exhibited little monocyte infiltration within the atherosclerotic lesion of the aorta, as described in Section II. Macrophages are known to play pivotal roles in the pathogenesis of atherosclerotic lesions in the presence of major risk factors including hypercholesterolemia and endothelial injury.[75-77]

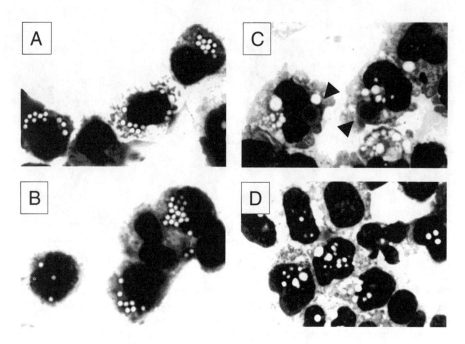

FIGURE 11.12 Effect of exposure to hemin on macrophage phagocytosis. Monocytes were cultured alone (A and C) or with 100 μM hemin (B and D) for 6 h. Cultured monocytes were incubated for 1 h with latex beads (A and B) or human erythrocytes opsonized with anti-RhD antibody (C and D). Cytospin preparations were made, and fractions of cells undergoing phagocytosis were evaluated under a microscope. Opsonized RBCs were phagocytized by untreated monocytes (arrows), but not by hemin-treated monocytes.

Dysfunction of macrophages may also explain why the patient exhibited paradoxically little atherosclerotic change of the aorta in the presence of endothelial injury and sustained hypercholesterolemia.

VI. CONCLUDING REMARKS

It is clear from the number of published studies and our experience with the HO-1-deficient patient that the HO/CO system plays pivotal roles in modulating cardiovascular functions and regulating defense against various stresses. HO-1, in particular, is a cardinal enzyme in the HO/CO system because it is vigorously induced upon stimulation. The majority of HO activity derives from HO-1 under oxidative stresses. Our experience with a single case of HO-1 deficiency contributed to understanding of the physiological roles of HO-1 *in vivo*. Although the experience is too limited to enable us to fully understand the complex pathophysiology of the illness and we need to analyze many cases to elucidate the precise role of HO-1 in the context of the whole HO/CO system, several important issues have been addressed. We would like to propose that HO-1 deficiency constitutes a new form of vasculitis that requires special attention and treatment modality because of its unique pathogenesis.

A. A New Vasculitis Syndrome

Iron metabolism was impaired in the HO-1-deficient patient. We do not think that impairment is the principal feature of HO-1 deficiency because iron deposition within the kidney and liver was not progressive and was not detectable at the time of autopsy. The most notable finding was the endothelial damage identified in the glomerular capillaries. In contrast to usual forms of systemic vasculitis, we did not see significant cell infiltration, fibrosis, or necrotic changes of major vessels. Laboratory data and pathological findings indicated that the prominent changes in the vessels were confined to the endothelium and not to the vessel walls.

We need to carefully evaluate the effects of asplenia, monocyte dysfunction, and the secondary accumulation of intravascular heme as the positive regulators of endothelial damage. HO-1 deficiency may constitute a new form of vasculitis or an endothelial cell injury syndrome encompassing a wide variety of clinical manifestations. The syndrome is also associated with undue susceptibility to oxidative stresses. Intense inflammatory reactions and monocyte dysfunction may further characterize the complicated clinical features. Accumulation of fragmented erythrocytes, non-functioning platelets, heme, and lipids may all be explained by the impaired monocyte functions. Screening of suspected cases for HO-1 deficiency is necessary to reveal the clinical spectrum of the illness. Monocyte HO-1 production will provide a useful diagnostic tool for this purpose.

B. Treatment Options

In addition to the use of several antiinflammatory agents, alone or in combination, several other treatment options are available. Attempts to remove unwanted materials from the circulation by plasma exchange failed because uncontrollable hypertension occurred. This resulted in intracranial bleeding followed by progressive deterioration of the patient's condition. It is possible that the homeostasis of vascular function had been delicately controlled by narrow margins. Removal of one factor might have resulted in the rapid destruction of the balance among the regulatory mechanisms of the vascular tonus.

Bone marrow transplantation may become the treatment of choice for future patients. Monocyte dysfunction will be corrected by successful transplantation of hematopoietic stem cells. Our concern is that acquisition of normal monocyte function may further complicate the clinical features of HO-1 deficiency if HO-1 expressions in other vulnerable cells are not corrected simultaneously. Normal monocyte function may lead to the development of vigorous inflammatory reactions within the kidneys or the vessel walls. Development of atheromatous plaques will be seen at the injured intima. Impaired regulation of cytokine production will be another problem. Monocytes may push cytokines toward unwanted directions in response to exogenous insults.

Gene therapy, if targeted to appropriate cells, may be promising. Local HO-1 gene transfer has already been performed for the purpose of preventing tissue injuries of various organs. Transpulmonary HO-1 gene transfer protected the lungs from hyperoxia-induced injury in a rat model.[30] Active up-regulation of HO-1 protects against ischemia/reperfusion injury of the liver.[78] These results indicate that local, transient up-regulation of HO-1 may certainly prevent the development of deleterious organ dysfunction.

However, gene therapy may not be simple for the treatment of HO-1-deficient patients. HO-1 gene transfections into endothelial cells and monocytes are required for successful therapy. We need to consider that HO-1 is an inducible enzyme that is not produced constitutively *in vivo*. It is not yet known whether overexpression or sustained expression of HO-1 within cells produces detrimental effects. Our preliminary experiments suggest that overexpression of HO-1 may alter the growth rates of certain cell types. Constitutive expression of HO-1 may also alter variable cell functions. Therefore, targeting gene transfection and application of certain regulatory machinery of HO-1 gene expression seem to be mandatory for successful gene therapy.[79] Despite these difficulties, we hope that the accumulation of basic data and clinical experiences will lead to the achievement of HO-1 gene therapy in the near future.

ACKNOWLEDGMENTS

We are grateful to the contributors in this study. Among them, special thanks are given to Dr. M. Suematsu for helpful discussion, Drs. Y. Niida, T. Toma, K. Maruhashi, K. Fujimoto, T. Wada, Y. Kasahara, H. Kaneda, S. Shimura, R. Sumita, and N. Igarashi for their active collaboration and patient care.

REFERENCES

1. Abraham, N.G. et al., The biological significance and physiological role of heme oxygenase, *Cell. Physiol. Biochem.*, 6, 129, 1996.
2. Dennery, P.A., Regulation and role of heme oxygenase in oxidative injury, *Current Topics Cell. Reg.*, 36, 181, 2000.
3. Elbirt, K.K. and Bonkovsky H.L., Heme oxygenase: recent advances in understanding its regulation and role, *Proc. Assoc. Am. Phys.*, 111, 438, 1999.
4. Otterbein, L.E. and Choi, A.M.K., Heme oxygenase: colors of defence against cellular stress, *Am. J. Physiol. Lung Cell Mol. Physiol.*, 279, L1029, 2000.
5. Choi, A.M.K. and Alam, J., Heme oxygense-1: function, regulation, and implication of a novel stress-inducible protein in oxidant-induced lung injury, *Am. J. Respir. Cell. Mol. Biol.*, 15, 9, 1996.
6. Maines, M.D., Heme oxygenase: function, multiplicity, regulatory mechanisms, and clinical applications, *FASEB J.*, 2, 2557, 1988.
7. Poss, K.D. and Tonegawa, S., Heme oxygenase 1 is required for mammalian iron reutilization, *Proc. Natl. Acad. Sci. U.S.A.*, 94, 10919, 1997.
8. Poss, K.D. and Tonegawa, S., Reduced stress defense in heme oxygenase 1-deficient cells, *Proc. Natl. Acad. Sci. U.S.A.*, 94, 10925, 1997.
9. Yet, S.F. et al., Hypoxia induces severe right ventricular dilatation and infarction in heme oxygenase-1 null mice, *J. Clin. Invest.*, 103, R23, 1999.
10. Dennery, P.A. et al., Oxygen toxicity and iron accumulation in the lungs of mice lacking heme oxygenase-2, *J. Clin. Invest.*, 101, 1001, 1998.

11. Burnett, A.L. et al., Ejaculatory abnormalities in mice with targeted disruption of the gene for heme oxygenase-2, *Nature Med.*, 4, 84, 1998.
12. Zakhary, R. et al., Targeted gene deletion of heme oxygenase 2 reveals neural role for carbon monoxide, *Proc. Natl. Acad. Sci. U.S.A.*, 94, 14848, 1997.
13. Yachie, A. et al., Oxidative stress causes enhanced endothelial cell injury in human heme oxygenase-1 deficiency, *J. Clin. Invest.*, 103, 129, 1999.
14. Ohta, K. et al., Tubular injury as a cardinal pathologic feature in human heme oxygenase-1 deficiency, *Am. J. Kidney Dis.*, 35, 863, 2000.
15. Saikawa, Y. et al., Structural evidence of genomic exon-deletion mediated by *Alu–Alu* recombination in a human case with heme oxygenase-1 deficiency, *Human Mut.*, 16, 178, 2000.
16. Abstracts of First International Symposium on Heme Oxygenase (HO/CO), *Acta Haematol.*, 103 (Suppl. 1), 2000.
17. Maines, M.D., The heme oxygenase system and its functions in the brain, *Cell. Mol. Biol.* 46, 573, 2000.
18. Maines, M.D., The heme oxygenase system: a regulator of second messenger gases, *Annu. Rev. Pharmacol. Toxicol.*, 37, 517, 1997.
19. McCoubrey, W.K. Jr., Huang, T.J., and Maines, M.D., Isolation and characterization of a cDNA from the rat brain that encodes hemoprotein heme oxygenase-3, *Eur. J. Biochem.*, 247, 725, 1997.
20. Wang, L.J. et al., Expression of heme oxygenase-1 in atherosclerotic lesions, *Am. J. Pathol.*, 152, 711, 1998.
21. Agarwal, A. et al., Linoleyl hydroperoxide transcriptionally up-regulates heme oxygenase-1 gene expression in human renal epithelial and aortic endothelial cells, *J. Am. Soc. Nephrol.*, 9, 1990, 1998.
22. Ishizaka, N. et al., Angiotensin II-induced hypertension increases heme oxygenase-1 expression in rat aorta, *Circulation*, 96, 1923, 1997.
23. Amersi, F. et al., Upregulation of heme oxygenase-1 protects genetically fat Zucker rat livers from ischemia/reperfusion injury, *J. Clin. Invest.*, 104, 1631, 1999.
24. Suematsu, M. and Ishimura, Y., The heme oxygenase–carbon monoxide system: a regulator of hepatobiliary function, *Hepatology*, 31, 3, 2000.
25. Suzuki, H. et al., Heme oxygenase-1 gene induction as an intrinsic regulation against delayed cerebral vasospasm in rats, *J. Clin. Invest.*, 104, 59, 1999.
26. Willis, D. et al., Heme oxygenase: a novel target for the modulation of the inflammatory response, *Nature Med.*, 2, 87, 1996.
27. Goda, N. et al., Distribution of heme oxygenase isoforms in rat liver, *J. Clin. Invest.*, 101, 6042, 1998.
28. Agarwal, A. and Nick, H.S., Renal response to tissue injury: lessons from heme oxygenase-1 gene ablation and expression, *J. Am. Soc. Nephrol.*, 11, 965, 2000.
29. Nath, K.A. et al., Induction of heme oxygenase is a rapid, protective response in rhabdomyolysis in the rat, *J. Clin. Invest.*, 90, 267, 1992.
30. Otterbein, L.E. et al., Exogenous administration of heme oxygenase-1 by gene transfer provides protection against hyperoxia-induced lung injury, *J. Clin. Invest.*, 103, 1047, 1999.
31. Acevedo, C.H. and Ahmed, A., Heme oxygenase-1 inhibits human myometrial contractility via carbon monoxide and is up-regulated by progesterone during pregnancy, *J. Lab. Clin. Invest.*, 101, 949, 1998.
32. Torisu–Itakura, H. et al., Co-expression of thymidine phosphorylase and heme oxygenase-1 in macrophages in human malignant vertical growth melanomas, *Jpn. J. Cancer Res.*, 91, 906, 2000.

33. Clerget, M. and Polla, B.S., Erythrophagocytosis induces heat shock protein synthesis by human monocytes–macrophages, *Proc. Natl. Acad. Sci. U.S.A.,* 87, 1081, 1990.

34. Morita, T. and Kourembanas, S., Endothelial cell expression of vasoconstrictors and growth factors is regulated by smooth muscle cell-derived carbon monoxide, *J. Clin. Invest.,* 96, 2676, 1995.

35. Nath, K.A. et al., The indispensability of heme oxygenase-1 (HO-1) in protecting against acute heme protein-induced toxicity *in vivo, Am. J. Pathol.,* 156, 1527, 2000.

36. Shiraishi, F. et al., Heme oxygenase-1 gene ablation or overexpression modulates cisplatin-induced renal tubular apoptosis and necrosis, *Am. J. Physiol.,* 278, F726, 2000.

37. Zou, A.P. et al., Expression and actions of heme oxygenase in the renal medulla of rats, *Hypertension,* 35, 342, 2000.

38. Liang, L. et al., Differential induction of heme oxygenase-1 (HO-1) in renal tubular epithelial cells, *J. Am. Soc. Nephrol.,* 11, 604A, 2000.

39. Anderson, M.M. et al., The myeloperoxidase system of human phagocytes generates N^ε-(carboxymethyl) lysine on proteins: a mechanism for producing advanced glycation end products at sites of inflammation, *J. Clin. Invest.,* 104, 103, 1999.

40. Kawada, N. et al., Increased oxidative stress in mouse kidneys with unilateral ureteral obstruction, *Kidney Int.,* 56, 1004, 1999.

41. Horie, K. et al., Immunohistochemical colocalization of glycoxidation products and lipid peroxidation products in diabetic renal glomerular lesions, *J. Clin. Invest.,* 100, 2995, 1997.

42. Suzuki, D. et al., Immunohistochemical evidence for an increased oxidative stress and carbonyl modification of proteins in diabetic glomerular lesions, *J. Am. Soc. Nephrol.,* 10, 822, 1999.

43. Maines, M.D., Trakshel, G.M., and Kutty, R.K., Characterization of two constitutive forms of rat liver microsomal heme oxygenase: only one molecular species of the enzyme is inducible, *J. Biol. Chem.,* 261, 411, 1986.

44. Kutty, R.K. et al., Chromosomal localization of the human heme oxygenase genes: heme oxygenase-1 (HMOX1) maps to chromosome 22q12 and heme oxygenase-2 (HMOX2) maps to chromosome 16p13.3, *Genomics,* 50, 513, 1993.

45. Seroussi, E. et al., TOM1 genes map to human chromosome 22q13.1 and mouse chromosome 8C1 and encode proteins similar to the endosomal proteins HGS and STAM, *Genomics,* 57, 380, 1999.

46. Yoshida, T. et al., Human heme oxygenase cDNA and induction of its mRNA by hemin, *Eur. J. Biochem.,* 171, 457, 1988.

47. Shibahara, S. et al., Structural organization of the human heme oxygenase gene and the function of its promoter, *Eur. J. Biochem.,* 179, 557, 1989.

48. Tyrrell, R.M., Applegate, L.A., and Tromvoukis, Y., The proximal promoter region of the human heme oxygenase gene contains elements involved in stimulation of transcriptional activity by a variety of agents including oxidants, *Carcinogenesis,* 14, 761, 1993.

49. Takeda, K. et al., Identification of a *cis*-acting element that is responsible for cadmium-mediated induction of the human heme oxygenase gene, *J. Biol. Chem.,* 269, 22858, 1994.

50. Cooper, D.N., Krawczak, M., and Antonarakis, S.E., The nature and mechanisms of human gene mutation, in *The Metabolic and Molecular Bases of Inherited Disease,* 7th ed., Scriver, C.R. et al., Eds., McGraw-Hill, New York, 1995, p. 259.

51. Miki, Y., Retrotransposal integration of mobile genetic elements in human disease, *J. Hum. Genet.,* 43, 77, 1998.

52. Schmid, C.W. and Jelinek, W.R., The *Alu* family of dispersed repetitive sequences, *Science*, 216, 1065, 1982.
53. Jurka, J. and Smith, T., A fundamental division in the *Alu* family of repeated sequence, *Proc. Natl. Acad. Sci, U.S.A.*, 85, 4775, 1998.
54. Jurka, J. and Milosavljevic, A., Reconstruction and analysis of human *Alu* genes, *J. Mol. Evol.*, 32, 105, 1991.
55. Rudiger, N.S., Gregersen, N., and Kielland–Brandt, M.C., One short well conserved region of *Alu* sequences is involved in human gene rearrangements and has homology with prokaryotic chi, *Nucleic Acid Res.*, 23, 256, 1995.
56. Markert, M.L. et al., Adenosine deaminase (ADA) deficiency due to deletion of the ADA gene promoter and first exon by homologous recombination between two *Alu* elements, *J. Clin. Invest.*, 81, 1323, 1998.
57. Huang, L. et al., Hypobetalipoproteinemia due to an apolipoprotein B gene exon 21 deletion derived *Alu–Alu* recombination, *J. Biol. Chem.*, 264, 11394, 1989.
58. Herring, W.J. et al., Branched chain acyltransferase absence due to an *Alu*-based genomic deletion allele and an exon skipping allele in a compound heterozygote proband expressing maple syrup urine disease, *Biochim. Biophys. Acta*, 1138, 236, 1992.
59. Huie, M.L. et al., A large *Alu*-mediated deletion, identified by PCR, as the molecular basis for glycogen storage disease type II (GSDII), *Hum. Genet.*, 104, 94, 1999.
60. Rothberg, P.G. et al., A deletion polymorphism due to *Alu–Alu* recombination in intron 2 of the retinoblastoma gene: association with human gliomas, *Mol. Carcinogen.*, 19, 69, 1997.
61. Puget, N. et al., A 1-kb *Alu*-mediated germ-line deletion removing BRCA1 exon 17, *Cancer Res.*, 57, 828, 1997.
62. Nystrom–Lahti, M. et al., Founding mutations and *Alu*-mediated recombination in hereditary colon cancer, *Nat. Med.*, 1, 1203, 1995.
63. Yamada, N. et al., Microsatellite polymorphism in the heme oxygenase-1 gene promoter is associated with susceptibility to emphysema, *Am. J. Hum. Genet.*, 66, 187, 2000.
64. Balla, J. et al., Endothelial cell heme oxygenase and ferritin induction by heme proteins: a possible mechanism limiting shock damage, *Trans. Assoc. Am. Physicians*, 105, 1, 1992.
65. Balla, G. et al., Ferritin: a cytoprotective antioxidant strategem of endothelium, *J. Biol. Chem.*, 267, 18148, 1992.
66. Stocker, R., Glazer, A.N., and Ames, B.N., Antioxidant activity of albumin-bound bilirubin, *Proc. Natl. Acad. Sci. U.S.A.*, 84, 5918, 1987.
67. Frei, B., Stocker, R., and Ames, B.N., Antioxidant defences and lipid peroxidation in human blood plasma, *Proc. Natl. Acad. Sci. U.S.A.*, 85, 9748, 1988.
68. Neuzil, J. and Stocker, R., Free and albumin-bound bilirubin are efficient co-antioxidants for α-tocopherol, inhibiting plasma and low density lipoprotein lipid peroxidation, *J. Biol. Chem.*, 269, 167712, 1994.
69. Onodera, M. et al., A simple and reliable method for screening retroviral producer clones without selectable markers, *Hum. Gene Ther.*, 8, 1189, 1997.
70. Schiff, D.E. et al., Increased phagocyte FcγRI expression and improved Fcγ-receptor-mediated phagocytosis after *in vivo* recombinant human interferon-γ treatment of normal human subjects, *Blood*, 90, 3187, 1997.
71. Wright, S.D., Ramos, R.A., and Tobias, P.S., CD14, a receptor for complexes of lipopolysaccharide (LPS) and LPS binding protein, *Science*, 249, 1431, 1990.
72. Wirthueller, U., Kurosaki, T., and Murakami, M.S., Signal transduction by FcγRIII (CD16) is mediated through the γ chain, *J. Exp. Med.*, 175, 1381, 1992.

73. Wiener, E. et al., Role of Fc gamma RIIα (CD32) in IgG anti-RhD-mediated red cell phagocytosis *in vitro*, *Transfus. Med.*, 6, 235, 1996.
74. Yesner, L.M. et al., Regulation of monocyte CD36 and thrombospondin-1 expression by soluble mediators, *Arterioscler. Thromb. Vasc. Biol.*, 16, 1019, 1996.
75. Han, J. et al., Native and modified low density lipoproteins increase the functional expression of the macrophage class B scavenger receptor, CD36, *J. Biol. Chem.*, 272, 21654, 1997.
76. Maxeiner, H. et al., Complementary roles for scavenger receptor A and CD36 of human monocyte-derived macrophages in adhesion to surfaces coated with oxidized low-density lipoproteins and in secretion of H_2O_2, *J. Exp. Med.*, 188, 2257, 1998.
77. Nozaki, S. et al., Reduced uptake of oxidized low density lipoproteins in monocyte-derived macrophages from CD36-deficient subjects, *J. Clin. Invest.*, 96, 1859, 1995.
78. Amersi, F. et al., Upregulation of heme oxygenase-1 protects genetically fat Zucker rat livers from ischemia/reperfusion injury, *J. Clin. Invest.*, 104, 1631, 1999.
79. Immenschuh, S. et al., Gene regulation of heme oxygenase-1 as a therapeutic target, *Biochem. Pharmacol.*, 60, 1121, 2000.

12 The Roles of Carbon Monoxide in the Pathogenesis of Diabetes and Its Vascular Complications

Lingyun Wu and Rui Wang

CONTENTS

I. INTRODUCTION

The blood glucose level is precisely controlled under physiological conditions. An elevation of plasma glucose concentration that occurs after dietary intake triggers the release of insulin from pancreatic islet β cells. Insulin facilitates glucose storage in the liver and stimulates glucose uptake from the blood into adipocytes and muscle cells. This chain reaction keeps the fluctuated circulating glucose level within a physiological range. Should this glucose homeostasis be disturbed by lack of insulin or loss of target sensitivity to insulin, diabetes mellitus (DM) ensues.

DM is manifested by hyperglycemia, polyuria, polydipsia, nocturia, polyphagia, etc. Juvenile-onset DM with idiopathic and autoimmune etiology is called type I DM. Patients of this subgroup are insulin-deficient and prone to ketoacidosis. Patients of type II DM have abnormal insulin secretion and increased insulin resistance in target tissues and are prone to hyperosmolar coma. Hypertension and hyperlipidemia are more often associated with type II DM. Most complications of type I and type II involve the vascular system. Vascular complications can be classified as macroangiopathy and microangiopathy. Inadequate control of hypertension, hyperglycemia, and cholesterol aggravates the vascular complications of diabetes.

Carbon monoxide (CO) plays an important role in the pathogenesis of diabetes and in the development of its vascular complications. Abnormal CO metabolism, including the expression and function of the CO-generating enzyme, heme oxygenase (HO), and altered vascular effects of CO have been documented. However, these observations in human and experimental animal diabetes have not been correlated in an effort to prevent, diagnose, and manage diabetic vascular complications. This chapter summarizes many pioneer discoveries in the involvement of CO in diabetes pathophysiology in an attempt to advance our understanding of the pathogenesis of diabetes and, ultimately, achieve better management of the vascular complications of diabetes.

II. CARBON MONOXIDE PRODUCTION IN DIABETES

A. EXHALED CARBON MONOXIDE LEVELS IN DIABETES

Endogenously produced CO can diffuse out of cells and bind to the hemoglobin of circulating erythrocytes to form carboxyhemoglobin which dissociates in the lungs where CO is excreted in breath.[1] Exhaled CO level has been used as an index for bilirubin production in human infants.[2,3] Less known is the diagnostic value of exhaled CO level in the management of diabetes.

As early as 1972, Nikberg et al.[4] reported elevated exhaled CO levels in diabetic patients. This observation was recently confirmed in a clinic survey showing that exhaled CO levels were significantly higher in type I and type II diabetic patients (4 to 5 ppm) than in healthy people (2.9 ppm).[5] Higher exhaled CO levels were positively correlated with the level of hyperglycemia and the duration of diabetes.

Increased exhaled CO may be due to the increased expression of the inducible HO-1 isoform of heme oxygenase (HO) and/or the modified activity of HO by direct effects of glucose or advanced glycation end products (AGEs) that oxidize HO. The increased CO production in diabetes may also be due to the stimulation of non-HO-related CO production, such as the auto-oxidation of L-dopa[6] and lipid peroxidation. In addition, a reduced binding affinity of CO to circulating hemoglobin may also elevate exhaled CO levels.

Glycosylation of hemoglobin may ameliorate the CO uptake by red blood cells across the lung due to the increased oxygen affinity of glycosylated hemoglobin

(HbA$_{1C}$), present in diabetics.[7] Paredi et al.[5] showed that acute elevation of blood glucose level less than 5 min after oral glucose uptake induced a phasic increase in exhaled CO levels. Clearly, this fast reaction mode does not involve HO induction or the formation of AGEs or HbA$_{1C}$. Rather, a direct effect of glucose on the existing CO generation pathway is indicated.

Can HO be activated directly by glucose? What is the underlying mechanism and what types of HO are activated by glucose? No answers are readily available for these questions. Does high glucose level generate oxidative stress, which in turn activates HO? This reaction is possible. High glucose can rapidly increase oxidative stress by the auto-oxidation and non-enzymatic glycation of unsaturated lipids and membrane proteins. The reduced antioxidant properties of albumin in the presence of hyperglycemia also contribute to the increased oxidative stress.[8] Moreover, the increased exhaled CO levels were not correlated to the blood levels of HbA$_{1C}$.[5] Does this mean that the glycation process for HO activation is not as important as high glucose level? For one thing, the CO levels in blood or in exhaled air may fluctuate but the HbA$_{1C}$ level is relatively stable.

Variation in exhaled CO levels can also be coupled to events other than hyperglycemia. In a study by Horvath et al.,[9] exhaled CO was significantly increased from 2.9 ppm to 5.8 ppm in untreated asthmatic patients. The increased exhaled CO levels in asthmatic patients coincided with increased HO-1 expression levels in airway macrophages. Furthermore, 4 h after inhalation of a hemin solution (2 ml of 0.1 mM), the exhaled CO level increased. The acute hemin action cannot to be explained by the induced HO-1 expression. More likely, hemin provides more substrates to enable the existing constitutive isoform of HO (HO-2) to generate more CO.

These lines of evidence seem to support the idea that increased HO activity leads to increased exhaled CO. Whether the inhalation of HO inhibitors, such as zinc protoporphyrin-IX (Zn PPIX) suppresses the exhaled CO level and whether the same conclusion from asthmatic patients can be applied to diabetic patients are not known. Although both asthma and diabetes are characterized by increased oxidative stress, the specific oxygen reactive species and the cells (more specifically, airway macrophages in asthma) that generate CO may be different. While the exhaled CO levels from asthmatic patients were increased by hemin inhalation, the exhaled NO levels were concomitantly decreased.[9] The underlying mechanisms for this differential change are not clear.

Steroid inhalation inhibited the enhanced expression of HO-1 and returned the exhaled CO levels to normal in asthmatic patients. This may be due to a direct inhibitory effect of the steroid on HO-1 expression or to the control of inflammation of the asthmatic airways. Unfortunately, the alterations of HO-2 level in asthmatic patients were not studied.

B. Circulating Carbon Monoxide Levels in Diabetes

Increased exhaled CO level has been suggested as a marker of diabetes and a monitor of disease progression and/or regression. If this higher exhaled CO level were all due to increased endogenous CO production, one may wonder what happened to the blood carboxyhemoglobin (COHb) concentrations in diabetics. Enhanced blood

COHb levels in diabetes patients were reported in several cases,[10,11] although the origin of the increased CO in the blood was unclear.

These results were confirmed in experimental animal diabetes models. Using diabetic rats induced by alloxan, Takano et al.[12] found that blood COHb levels were significantly increased. In contrast, Desoille et al.[13] did not observe changes in blood COHb levels of 47 diabetic patients. In one diabetic patient with a blood glucose level of 560 mg/100 ml, COHb level reached 44.8%.[14] A careful re-examination revealed that this was a false result. The patient's high serum lipid level interfered with the spectrophotometric method for measuring COHb.[14]

The lesson to be learned is that blood COHb levels of diabetes mellitus patients may vary, depending on the type and severity of diabetes. Furthermore, the method and instrument used to measure COHb level should be carefully evaluated and chosen. The reported COHb levels in diabetes may vary, but the increased production of CO reflected by higher exhaled CO levels and the potentially reduced diffusion capacity for CO[15] are well documented. The latter constitutes a risk factor for cardiovascular complications.

C. Expression of Heme Oxygenase (HO) in Diabetes

CO is endogenously produced mainly via the cleavage of the heme rings in hemo-proteins by HO.[16] At least two distinct forms of HO, inducible HO-1 and constitutive HO-2, have been characterized and their functions defined. Levels of HO-1 are increased by its substrate heme and hemoglobin, a variety of transition and heavy metals, oxidant stress, heat shock, xenobiotics, and cyclic adenosine monophosphate (cAMP).[16] Increased CO levels in exhaled air and circulating blood can be ascribed to increased HO activity, increased expression of HO, and/or increased substrates of HO.

Nishio et al.[17] showed that the mRNA content of HO-1 was significantly increased in the cardiac tissues of diabetic rats 4 to 24 weeks after streptozotocin (STZ) injection as compared with control rats. We recently examined the expression levels of HO in vascular tissues from diabetic rats using Western blot assay.[18] The expression of HO-1 proteins was hardly detected in normal rat vascular tissues, but visible in rat spleen. In 1-month diabetic rats, the expression of HO-1 proteins was significantly induced in all vascular tissues tested. In contrast, no differences in the levels of HO-1 proteins in normal and diabetic spleen tissues were seen. These results demonstrated that the induced HO-1 protein expression was a specific phe-nomenon for diabetic vascular tissues. Since HO-1 is a stress protein, its increased expression is expected because elevated oxidative stress is encountered in diabetic hyperglycemia, which induces the non-enzymatic glycosylation or glycation of proteins. Similar increases in HO-1 protein levels were also found via immunohistochemistry assays of retinal endothelial cells and glial cells of STZ-diabetic male Lewis rats[19] and in gingival vasculatures from diabetic patients and STZ-diabetic mice.[20]

Inconsistent results have been reported on the altered expression of HO-1 pro-teins in diabetes. For instance, in diabetic patients, the HO-1 mRNA expression in retinal pigment epithelium was significantly decreased.[21] This result was derived from an incomplete study, as the authors indicated. Decreased HO activity and elevated basal levels of heme and cytochrome P-450 were also reported in hepatic tissues from STZ-induced diabetic female Sprague-Dawley rats.[22,23]

Some of these conflicting reports on HO expression and activity in diabetic subjects may be related to the types of models, durations of studies, gender differences, tissue type variations, and focus on HO-1 or HO-2. HO-2 has a different expression pattern from HO-1. HO-2 proteins were detected in all rat tissues examined in our study.[18] More interestingly, the expression levels of HO-2 proteins were not altered in all vascular tissues from STZ-induced diabetic rats.

In summary, previous studies, including our own results, showed that the expression of HO-1, but not HO-2, proteins may be significantly altered in diabetic vascular tissues. Altered HO-1 expression and/or HO activity will lead to altered heme metabolism, thus modulating cellular production of CO.

III. CARBON MONOXIDE AND INSULIN SECRETION

Both CO and nitric oxide (NO) have been implicated in insulin secretion, but they may have opposing functions. NO inhibits glucose-induced insulin release and stimulates glucagon release from pancreatic islet cells of rats[24] and mice.[25] CO, on the other hand, may stimulate the secretion of both insulin and glucagon. Henningsson et al.[26] reported that Zn PPIX dose dependently inhibited, whereas hemin enhanced, both insulin and glucagon secretion from glucose-stimulated mice pancreatic islets.

The anatomic basis for the effects of these HO modulators is derived from a study of Alm et al.,[24] in which the immunoreactivity of HO in rat islets of Langerhans, including insulin-immunoreactive beta cells, was demonstrated. After treatment with alloxan to induce diabetes, the immunoreactivity virtually disappeared. Thus, one pathophysiological role of the HO/CO system in the development of insulin-dependent diabetes mellitus appears to be the modulation of islet hormone secretion. Confocal microscopy study showed the co-localization of HO-2, insulin, glucagon, somatostatin, and pancreatic polypeptide in mice islet cells,[26] adding another piece of evidence to support the interaction of CO and insulin release.

In normal rat pancreatic islets, constitutive NO synthase (cNOS) and HO-2 were co-expressed, but induced NO synthase (iNOS) and HO-1 were not documented.[24] After the introduction of endotoxin, iNOS was induced and HO-1 was still not detectable. Alloxan treatment of rats for 5 days produced hyperglycemia and diabetes, and this treatment also eliminated the expression of cNOS and HO-2 in rat pancreatic beta cells. It is believed that rat islet tissues produced a great amount of CO through HO-2 activation, and the generated CO enhanced insulin and glucagon release from islets.[27] Furthermore, both CO production and insulin/glucagon secretion were inhibited by Zn PPIX and stimulated by hemin.[27] If hemin can promote CO production and insulin secretion, the existing HO-2 would have enhanced activity or a new HO-1 would be induced. The induction of HO-1 in rat pancreatic beta cells was not examined in these studies. Other studies clearly demonstrated the expression of HO-1 induced by cytokines in rat pancreatic islets.[28-30] The sensitivities of the HO-1 expression assay and different inducers for HO-1 in these studies may explain the discrepancy in the detected expression levels of HO-1.

In the endocrine, but not exocrine, pancreas of mice, the expression of cNOS and HO-2 was confirmed by immunocytochemistry and Western blot. Again, HO-1 was not detectable in these mice islet cells.[26] Zn PPIX concentration dependently inhibited CO production from mice islet homogenates. When the homogenates were cultured *in vitro* for 60 min with CO-saturated incubation buffer, insulin secretion significantly increased. However, hypoxia and potential pH change brought about by the use of the CO-saturated solution may have complicated the interpretation of the results. Also, the CO-saturated solution had a CO concentration of approximately 1 mM, far over the physiological concentration range. Therefore, the insulin release from mice pancreatic islets may represent a toxic pathophysiological effect of CO.

The effect of CO on insulin release is also potentially affected by glucose concentration. When the concentration of glucose in incubation media was increased from 1 mM to 20 mM, CO production in islet homogenates prepared from intact islets incubated for 60 min almost doubled.[26] A further 30% increase in CO production was observed when 0.1 mM hemin was added to the 20 mM glucose incubation medium. The increased CO production by high glucose is putatively due to the stimulation of HO-2 since (1) Zn PPIX inhibited the secretion of insulin induced by high glucose (20 mM) in a concentration-dependent manner; (2) a 60-min incubation is not long enough to induce new HO-1 protein; and (3) the secretion of insulin in the presence of 1 mM glucose was not affected by Zn PPIX.

Elevated glucose concentration will stimulate insulin release in two different ways. First, high glucose increases cellular ATP production, which in turn closes ATP-sensitive K$^+$ channels in the membranes of beta cells. The subsequent membrane depolarization opens voltage-gated Ca^{2+} channels and promotes calcium influx. Increased intracellular calcium concentration stimulates the exocytosis of insulin. Second, high glucose may increase CO production, and CO increases insulin release. How high glucose concentration stimulates HO-2 activity and whether hyperosmolality also stimulates HO-2 activity remain to be investigated.

What are the intermediate steps between high glucose concentration stimulation and CO-induced insulin release? One hypothesis is that high glucose-stimulated CO production may directly stimulate cGMP pathways, leading to insulin release. The following lines of experimental evidence support this hypothesis:

1. High concentration of glucose (20 mM) induced a greater increase in cGMP levels in islet tissues as compared with 1 mM glucose.
2. Cellular cGMP levels correlated well with the extent of insulin release.
3. Zn PPIX decreased both the cGMP level and insulin release enhanced by 20 mM glucose.
4. Exogenous CO directly increased cGMP and insulin release.
5. The blockade of the cGMP pathway with ODQ (1H-[1,24]oxadiazolo[4,3,-a]quinoxalin-1-one) partially inhibited the 20 mM glucose-induced insulin release, but more significantly suppressed exogenous CO or hemin-induced insulin release.

ODQ is a specific inhibitor of soluble guanylyl cyclase (sGC).[31,32] This evidence suggests that CO-induced insulin release may largely result from an elevated cellular cGMP level, and the high concentration of glucose-induced insulin release may involve both the CO pathway and other mechanisms. The CO-induced insulin release may also be due to the inhibitory effect of CO on NOS activity in the presence of high glucose concentration.

Including hemin in the incubation medium markedly suppressed L-arginine-induced neuronal NO production.[33] Furthermore, NOS activity in islet tissues increased almost three-fold in the presence of high glucose concentration compared with low glucose concentration. Because NO is an inhibitor of insulin release and high glucose concentration increases NOS activity, a reduced insulin release in this situation would be expected. However, in the presence of a high concentration of glucose, CO level was simultaneously elevated and the inhibition of NOS by CO decreased NO production. This would lift the inhibitory effect of NO on insulin release. To strengthen this argument, it was shown that the hemin-derived CO significantly inhibited the high glucose-stimulated NOS activity.[26] On the other hand, the inhibition of NOS activity by administration of N^{ω} nitro-Langinine methyl ester (L-NAME) evoked the iNOS-derived NO production in mouse pancreatic islets and up-regulated CO production and HO-2 expression,[25] thus counteracting the inhibitory effect of NO on insulin release.

The high concentration of glucose-induced CO production and CO-induced insulin release define the important role of CO in the modulation of insulin release. An extrapolation of these observations is that decreased CO production may constitute a pathogenic factor of reduced insulin secretion in diabetes. By the same token, in established diabetes CO levels are elevated as a compensatory reaction.

Takano et al.[34] treated rats with intraperitoneal alloxan (300 mg/kg) to induce diabetes. They found that the endogenous production of CO in these diabetic rats was increased as compared to normal rats. The increase in endogenous CO (the sum of excreted pulmonary CO and CO in blood, V_{CO}) occurred as early as 2 days after alloxan injection and maintained for over 5 days of the monitoring period. The diabetic rats maintaining high blood sugar levels for over 120 hours had three-fold higher V_{CO} levels than control. The duration of the increase in blood glucose levels in these rats was not stated. Based on our own experience, blood glucose levels should start to increase after 2 days of alloxan injections, thus synchronizing with the increase in CO level. The putative mechanisms of CO-modulated insulin secretion under physiological conditions and in diabetes are schematically illustrated in Figure 12.1.

An additional comment on the role of the HO/CO system in the regulation of insulin release is directed to the differences in the insulin-producing cells from different species. The sensitivities of human pancreatic islets to many insults, including alloxan, STZ, nitroprusside, and cytokines, are much lower than those of mouse and rat islets. STZ induced apoptosis in rat, but not in human, islet cells. Similarly, the expression of HO was up-regulated in cultured rat islets upon stimulation, but not in human islets.[35] To comprehend the role of the HO/CO system in the pathogenesis of human diabetes, it is imperative to study the expression patterns of HO-1 and HO-2, the production of CO, the influence of CO on insulin release, and the glucose-regulated HO/CO system in human pancreatic islets. Such studies are lacking at the present time.

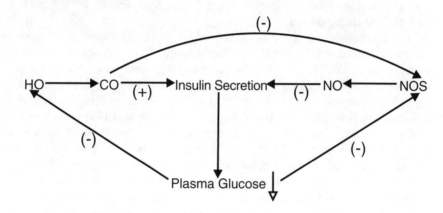

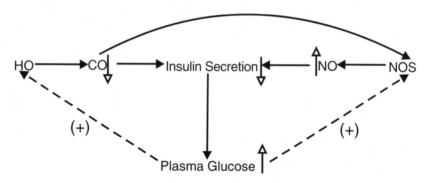

FIGURE 12.1 The role of CO in the regulation of insulin release. (A) The interaction among CO, NO, and glucose affects the insulin release from normal pancreatic islets. (B) Decreased CO production in pancreatic islets may account for the reduced insulin release in diabetes. Dashed lines denote the putative compensatory mechanisms in diabetes with established hyperglycemia.

IV. PUTATIVE MECHANISMS FOR THE VASCULAR COMPLICATIONS OF DIABETES

One fingerprint of diabetes is the hyperglycemia that is also the primary etiologic factor for vascular and other complications. Several mechanisms have been put forward to explain the etiology and progression of hyperglycemia-related vascular complications.

Glycation of circulating and immobilized proteins within the vascular wall damages vascular structure and function. Progressive glycation of proteins results

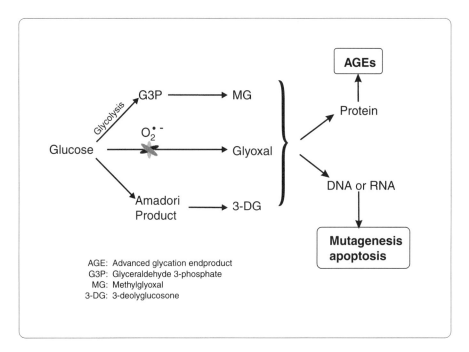

FIGURE 12.2 Different pathways for the formation of AGEs in the presence of hyperglycemia. AGEs can be formed via glyoxal generated from metal-catalyzed autoxidation of glucose, methylglyoxal generated from non-enzymatic fragmentation of triose phophates, and Amadori product.

from the attachment of glucose to the amino group of the exposed lysine side chain, leading to the formation of reversible Schiff's bases and Amadori products. These complex molecular rearrangements eventually generate irreversible advanced glycated end products (AGEs).[36] AGEs can also be formed from other pathways as shown in Figure 12.2. AGEs are responsible for many cellular abnormalities associated with diabetes mellitus.[37] Whether the activity of HO will be affected by hyperglycemia-induced glycation remains unknown.

Hyperglycemia induces oxidative structural changes of circulating proteins and cellular components via the action of free radicals. Glucose produces oxygen-reactive species and protein-reactive aldehydes either in solution (glucose auto-oxidation) or after attaching to protein (glycoxydation). Glycated proteins in the presence of metal ions will generate free radicals. AGEs can also produce reactive oxygen intermediates by interacting with their surface binding sites and generating malondialdehyde determinants in the vessel walls and thiobarbituric acid-reactive substances in the tissues and by inducing nuclear factor-kB.[5] AGE-induced oxidative stress significantly activated HO-1.[38] Increased oxidative stress resulting from auto-oxidation of proteins or AGEs increased expression level of HO-1, and the development of cardiovascular complications are correlated in diabetes.[39] The HO-mediated heme degradation to CO, biliverdin, and free iron has been regarded as an effective endogenous antioxidant pathway. Heme is a pro-oxidant existing in many intracellular proteins. Biliverdin is converted to bilirubin in a reaction catalyzed by biliverdin reductase. Bilirubin is an efficient antioxidant that scavenges hydroxyl radicals.[40,41] Although free iron catalyzes the formation of free radicals, this oxidative burden of the cells may be compensated by the free iron-induced expression of ferritin that limits the participation of free irons in the Fenton reaction.[42,43]

Hyperglycemia may deplete cellular myoinositol and inhibit the activity of Na^+/K^+ ATPase.[44] However, this mechanism has been mainly implicated in the pathogenesis of diabetic neuropathy. Whether a similar event occurs in vascular walls in diabetes has not been reported.

Protein kinase C (PKC) activity and diacylglycerol levels in vascular cells may be increased by hyperglycemia as reported both in diabetic vascular tissues, cultured vascular smooth muscle cells (SMCs), and endothelial cells.[45,46] The increased PKC activity might contribute to the altered membrane receptor turnover, neovascularization, and cell proliferation.

Calcium handling of vascular SMCs may be altered by hyperglycemia, leading to altered intracellular calcium levels and abnormal calcium sensitivity of the contractile machinery in diabetic SMCs. In STZ-induced diabetic rats with moderate hyperglycemia, videomicroscopic measurement showed that the contractile responses of afferent arterioles to Bay K8644, an opener of voltage-gated Ca^{2+} channels, decreased by 100-fold. The contraction induced by high concentration of KCl in diabetic arterioles was also reduced compared to the arterioles from normal rats.[47] KCl (40 mM) evoked a lesser increase in intracellular calcium concentration in diabetic afferent arterioles isolated by microdissection and loaded with Fura 2, compared to normal arterioles. Decreasing bath glucose concentration from 20 mM to 5 mM normalized this suppressed calcium response.[47]

A functional defect in afferent arteriolar L-type Ca^{2+} channels exists in diabetes, which may explain the suppressed afferent arteriolar vasoconstrictor responsiveness. In agreement with these tissue studies, we recently found that in tail artery SMCs isolated from STZ-induced diabetic rats, voltage-gated L-type Ca^{2+} channels exhibited reduced current density and altered sensitivity to dihydropyridines.[48] This reduced calcium entry was mirrored by an altered pattern of KCl-induced changes in intracellular free calcium concentrations.[49] Studies of cultured bovine retinal pericytes also demonstrated reduced function of L-type Ca^{2+} channels after culture with 25 mM glucose.[50] In addition, hyperglycemia significantly suppressed intracellular calcium release from cultured rat aortic SMCs and the capacitative Ca^{2+} influx through the plasma membrane.[51]

Among all these mechanisms for the vascular complications of diabetes, an altered HO/CO system is likely involved in the glycation and oxidation damage of vascular walls. Limited data from our previous study[16] showed that CO does not directly affect the intracellular free calcium concentrations of vascular SMCs. However, whether the CO-induced activation of the cGMP pathway indirectly affects the calcium handling of vascular SMCs under normal conditions or in diabetes has not been addressed.

V. CARBON MONOXIDE AND VASCULAR COMPLICATIONS OF DIABETES

The major cause of death in type II diabetes mellitus is macroangiography, e.g., coronary artery disease, stroke, hypertension,[52,53] and peripheral vessel occlusion, mainly resulting from accelerated atherosclerosis. Microangiography is associated with types I and II diabetes mellitus.[54] Among the best known vascular complications, retinopathy presents in 50% of patients with more than 10 years' diabetic history. While nephropathy is more often associated with type I diabetes, neuropathy is common in both types.

Retinopathy and nephropathy-related renal failure are the leading causes of blindness in North America. The vascular complications of diabetes are closely related to the toxic effects of AGEs and to increased oxidative stress, i.e., glycation-mediated and free radical-mediated cellular damages. Although the altered metabolism of CO in diabetes and the modulation of insulin secretion by CO are relatively well known, the vasoactive effects of CO in diabetes have not been fully explored. Recent studies in our laboratory provide insight into the altered vascular effects of CO in diabetes, and emphasize the important contribution of the altered vascular effect of CO to the etiology and progress of diabetes and its vascular complications.

A. VASORELAXANT EFFECTS OF CO ARE REDUCED

Altered vascular sensitivity to different vasoconstricting substances such as bradykinin,[55] changed properties of ion channels,[48] and abnormal calcium handling in diabetic vascular SMCs[49] are potentially related to the vascular complications of diabetes. We recently reported that the vasorelaxing effects of CO might change in diabetes, constituting a novel mechanism for diabetic vascular complications.[18]

We induced diabetes in adult male Sprague–Dawley rats by a single injection of STZ via the lateral tail vein or penis vein (60 mg/kg body weight). Age-matched control rats were injected with equal volumes of vehicle (sodium citrate buffer). STZ-induced experimental diabetes is a well established animal model of diabetes mellitus characterized by hyperglycemia and hypoinsulinemia.[48,49,55] One month after the induction of diabetes, rat tail arteries were isolated and cut into helical strips. These strips were mechanically stretched to achieve a basal tension of approximately 0.7 g, and allowed to equilibrate for 1 h before the start of experiments. CO-saturated saline was diluted and directly applied to these isolated tissues at the desired concentrations. Severe diabetes developed in the STZ-treated rats. Compared to normal control rats, diabetic rats lost body weight, had glycosuria, and developed hyperglycemia, with fasting glucose concentrations of plasma elevated to 32.2 ± 2.2 mM. The vasorelaxant effect of CO on the endothelium-free tail artery tissues of diabetic rats was significantly reduced compared to non-diabetic normal vascular tissues. The EC_{50} of the vasorelaxant effect of CO was 58 ± 24 µM in normal tissues but 131 ± 38 µM in diabetic tissues (p <0.05).

Whether the vascular responses to the endogenous CO were altered in diabetic vascular tissues was further studied. Tail artery tissues were pre-incubated in the dark for 6 h with hemin (20 µM). Hemin acts as an inducer for the expression of inducible HO (HO-1) and as a substrate of HO to promote endogenous CO production from vascular tissues, thus decreasing phenylephrine-induced vasoconstriction.[56] In agreement with our previous study,[56] 6 h incubation (without hemim) of tail artery tissues from normal rats and diabetic rats did not alter resting tension level or phenylephrine-induced concentration-dependent vasoconstriction. The concentration-dependent vasoconstriction of normal tissues induced by phenylephrine was significantly inhibited by hemin incubation. The EC_{50} of phenylephrine effects was $0.24 \pm 0.03 \mu M$ or $1.19 \pm 0.12 \mu M$ without or with hemin incubation, respectively (p <0.05). In contrast, the vasoconstrictive effect of phenylephrine on diabetic tail artery tissues was not affected by 6-h hemin (20 μM) incubation, indicating that the vasorelaxant potency of endogenously generated CO is greatly suppressed in diabetes.

B. CO-INDUCED cGMP PRODUCTION IN DIABETIC VASCULAR SMCs IS DECREASED

The elevation of cellular cGMP levels and the opening of plasma membrane K^+ channels are the main mechanisms proposed to explain the vascular effects of CO. CO may increase cGMP content via its stimulatory interaction with the heme in the regulatory subunit of guanylyl cyclase. Increased cGMP would consequently decrease $[Ca^{2+}]_i$ in SMCs through the inhibition of IP_3 formation, the activation of Ca^{2+}-ATPase, and the inhibition of Ca^{2+} channels. The opening of K^+ channels leads to membrane hyperpolarization, which in turn inhibits the agonist-induced increase in IP_3, reduces Ca^{2+} sensitivity and resting Ca^{2+} level, and relaxes SMCs.[57]

To explore the mechanisms underlying the reduced vasorelaxant effect of CO in diabetes, the effect of CO on cGMP levels was determined in normal and diabetic rat tail artery tissues. CO and sodium nitroprusside (SNP, an NO donor) significantly enhanced the levels of cGMP in both normal and diabetic vascular tissues. However, the effect of CO on cGMP levels was significantly reduced in diabetic vascular tissues. CO elevated the tissue level of cGMP by about 310% (taking the basal level as 100%) in normal tissues but only by about 130% in diabetic tissues (n = 8, p <0.05) (unpublished observation).

Whether the reduced production of cGMP fully accounted for the decreased CO effect on diabetic vascular tissues was examined by incubating vascular tissues with 10 μM ODQ, a specific inhibitor of soluble guanylyl cyclase. Without pretreating vascular tissues with ODQ, CO (300 μM) induced a $60 \pm 7\%$ relaxation of normal vascular tissues. In the presence of ODQ, CO only induced a $38 \pm 8\%$ relaxation of normal vascular tissues. This represents a 63% inhibition of CO effect by ODQ. In contrast, incubation of diabetic tail artery tissues with 10 μM ODQ completely abolished the vasorelaxant effect of CO. It appears that the vasorelaxant effect of CO in diabetes is solely mediated by cGMP. The remaining question is, what happens to the GMP-independent vascular effect of CO in diabetes?

C. THE EFFECTS OF CO ON K_{CA} CHANNELS IN VASCULAR SMCs ARE DECREASED IN DIABETES

Besides its effect on the cGMP pathway, CO directly enhanced the activity of the big-conductance calcium-activated K^+ (K_{Ca}) channels in rat tail artery SMCs via a cGMP-independent mechanism.[58,59] Therefore, we further investigated the characteristics of K_{Ca} channels and their modulation by CO in diabetic tail artery SMCs.[18]

Alterations in voltage-dependent K^+ channels in cardiac myocytes[60-62] or K_{ATP} channels in pancreatic islets[63] in diabetes have been reported. Whether the structures and functions of K_{Ca} channels are altered in diabetes is less known. In our study, with symmetric KCl (145 mM) on both sides of a patch membrane, single channel conductances of K_{Ca} channels were 239 ± 8 pS (n = 8) in normal tail artery SMCs, and 230 ± 6 pS (n = 6) in diabetic SMCs (p >0.05). The open probability (NPo) of K_{Ca} channels was decreased by ChTX (100 nM) and iberiotoxin (100 nM), but not by apamin (100 nM) in both normal and diabetic tail artery SMCs. ChTX and iberiotoxin are specific blockers for the high-conductance K_{Ca} channels whereas apamin is for the small-conductance K_{Ca} channels.

However, other differences in the electrophysiological behaviors of K_{Ca} channels were noticed between normal SMCs and diabetic SMCs. Instead of a relatively evenly spaced opening pattern of individual channels as observed in normal SMCs, clustered openings of single K_{Ca} channels were observed in diabetic SMCs. Frequent single-channel openings occurred in groups within short periods of time to form a series of clusters separated by long closing periods. CO significantly increased the NPo levels of K_{Ca} channels in normal tail artery SMCs in a concentration-dependent manner (3 to 30 μM) in both outside-out and inside-out patches. This stimulatory effect of CO was greatly reduced in diabetic artery SMCs.[18] For instance, CO (10 μM) increased the mean NPo by $81 \pm 24\%$ in normal SMCs, but had no effect on the mean NPo of K_{Ca} channels in diabetic SMCs.

D. The Relationship between Altered Effects of CO on K_{CA} Channels in Diabetes and the Glycation of K_{CA} Channel Proteins, Increased Glucose Metabolism, and Hyperosmolality

Our study demonstrated that decreased K_{Ca} channel sensitivity to CO may be induced by the hyperglycemia-related glycation of K_{Ca} channel proteins. We cultured tail artery SMCs from normal rats *in vitro* for 8 days with 5 mM glucose in the culture medium. This treatment did not change the single-channel conductance or the sensitivity to ChTX or iberiotoxin of high-conductance K_{Ca} channels recorded in the cell-free patches as compared to the freshly isolated normal SMCs. CO (10 μM) increased the mean NPo of the single K_{Ca} channels by $95 \pm 23\%$ in long-term cultured normal SMCs.

In another group of experiments, SMCs were isolated from diabetic rats and cultured for 8 days with 25 mM glucose in the culture medium. The high-conductance K_{Ca} channels in these long-term cultured cells had characteristics similar to those of freshly isolated diabetic SMCs. CO (10 μM) also had no effect on K_{Ca} channels in these diabetic cells (n = 4), similar to the lack of effect of CO on freshly isolated diabetic SMCs.

To examine whether hyperglycemia or hyperosmolality caused the diminished sensitivity of diabetic SMCs to CO, normal SMCs were cultured with 25 mM glucose or 25 mM 3-O-methylglucose (3-OMG). After 8 days in culture, the stimulatory effect of CO to K_{Ca} channels of normal SMCs was consistently diminished; at 10 μM, CO did not affect the mean NPo of single K_{Ca} channels. Since 3-OMG is a non-metabolizable glucose analogue, the diminished sensitivity of K_{Ca} channels in cells cultured with high concentrations of 3-OMG indicates that the glycation of K_{Ca} channels rather than the metabolism of glucose by cultured vascular SMCs may be the mechanism for the altered K_{Ca} channel functionality in diabetes.

Similarly, McGinty et al.[50] showed that in bovine retinal pericytes cultured with 25 mM glucose, calcium influx evoked by endothelin-1 or Bay K8644 was reduced compared with the cells cultured with 5 mM glucose. 3-OMG mimicked this effect of high concentration of glucose. Furthermore, chronically culturing normal SMCs for 8 days with 25 mM mannitol in the culture medium did not alter the effect of CO on single-channel behaviors of K_{Ca} channels in our experiments.[18] A $73 \pm 9\%$ increase in the mean NPo of K_{Ca} channels was observed in the presence of CO ($10 \, \mu M$). Thus, the role played by hyperosmolality in the diminished effect of CO on K_{Ca} channels in diabetes can be minimized.

Hyperglycemia-induced protein glycation and lipid peroxidation are enhanced in diabetic subjects.[64] Several mechanisms may account for the glycation-induced diminished sensitivity of K_{Ca} channels to CO:

1. Glycation of K_{Ca} channels may produce steric hindrance for the exposure of the CO-acting sites on the K_{Ca} channel proteins.[65] Although the major glycation sites on proteins are asparagine, glutamine, and lysine,[66,67] glycation will also affect the microenvironments of other amino acid residues in proteins, including histidine. Altered accessibility to the surface histidines has been shown in the glycated RNase A protein.[66] CO mainly interacts with histidine residues located on the extracellular domains of K_{Ca} channels.[59] This interaction may be impeded by the glycation of K_{Ca} channels.

2. Glycation of channel proteins may lead to protein thiol oxidation, protein aggregation, and cross-linking.[68] The glycation of the gap junction protein has been shown to alter the C terminus arm, thus decreasing channel permeability.[68] The glycation of K_{Ca} channels may also cause the channel gates to become inflexible as a consequence of the conformational changes, thus decreasing open probability that would be otherwise enhanced by CO.

3. Glycation of ion channel proteins may damage the structural integrity of channel proteins by targeting histidine and other side chains.[67]

E. DEGLYCATION OF K_{CA} CHANNEL PROTEINS RESTORES THE SENSITIVITY OF K_{CA} CHANNELS IN DIABETIC SMCs TO CO

If glycation of K_{Ca} channels is responsible for decreased sensitivity to CO, deglycation of K_{Ca} channels should restore channel sensitivity. To follow up this reasoning, we cultured tail artery SMCs from 1-mo diabetic rats with 5 mM glucose for different periods.[18] Culturing these diabetic SMCs for 8 days with 5 mM glucose did not restore their responsiveness to CO. This may simply represent the insufficient non-enzymatic deglycation associated with relatively short culture duration (8 days). Even in the presence of high concentrations of certain deglycosylating enzymes, the deglycation of proteins was hardly completed in 10 to 20 days.[69]

We used the deglycation enzyme, aminoguanidine (0.1 M), in the culture medium to facilitate deglycation, but the result was deteriorated cell viability (unpublished observation). Therefore, a prolonged culture period beyond 8 days in the absence of deglycation enzyme became the choice for the purpose of deglycating K_{Ca} channels.

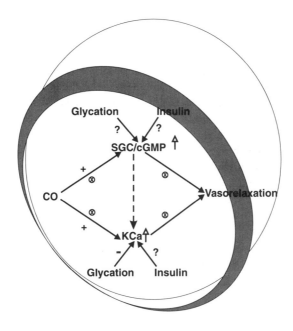

⊗ Indicates supressed reactions in diabetes

FIGURE 12.3 Altered vascular effects of CO in diabetes and underlying mechanisms.

The activities of K_{Ca} channels of diabetic SMCs cultured for about 5 weeks with 5 mM glucose in the culture medium were significantly increased by CO. CO (10 µM) increased the mean NPo levels of the single K_{Ca} channels in these cells by $62 \pm 8\%$ (n = 5, p <0.05). The regained sensitivity to CO was probably not related to the prolonged incubation period, as CO (10 µM) with 25 mM glucose still had no effect on NPo of K_{Ca} channels in diabetic SMCs cultured for 35 days. The control experiment showed that K_{Ca} channels in diabetic SMCs cultured for the same period (35 days) with 25 mM glucose still exhibited significantly lower sensitivity to CO.[18]

Our data demonstrated a decreased vasorelaxant function of CO in diabetes. The underlying mechanisms for this alteration are summarized in Figure 12.3. The CO-evoked generation of cGMP in diabetic vascular tissues was significantly lower as compared to normal tissues. This could partially explain the reduced vasorelaxant effect of CO in diabetes. More importantly, our tissue contraction study showed that the vasorelaxant effect of CO was completely eliminated by pretreating the diabetic tissues with ODQ which blocked the cGMP pathway. Considering the demonstrated low sensitivity of K_{Ca} channels of diabetic SMCs to CO, we can conclude that another leg of the CO reaction system, i.e., the K_{Ca} channel network, malfunctions in diabetes. Glycation of K_{Ca} channel proteins facing hyperglycemia is the potential mechanism for the reduced CO sensitivity of K_{Ca} channels in diabetic vascular SMCs. Further studies are essential to isolate K_{Ca} channel proteins from diabetic SMCs and directly determine the glycation/deglycation status of these channel proteins.

VI. CONCLUDING REMARKS

The HO/CO system is involved in the pathogenesis and maintenance of vascular complications of diabetes in three different ways. First, insulin secretion can be stimulated by CO and a lower CO level may decrease the stimulatory input for insulin secretion, thus constituting a pathogenic factor for the development of diabetes. This event may occur locally in pancreatic islets. Second, in established diabetes, the expression and activity of HO may be stimulated by hyperglycemia and increased oxidative stress. This happens ubiquitously and affects the cellular levels of heme, CO, and biliverdin, each responsible for different cellular functions. The increased CO production is reflected by the increased exhaled CO level, but the alteration of circulating level of HbA_{1C} is still uncertain. This compensatory increase in CO production could counteract a lower CO level in pancreatic islets to boost insulin secretion and the lower responses of CO targets. Third, vascular responses to CO, especially CO-induced vasorelaxation, are reduced in diabetes, likely reflecting the changes in the densities or the sensitivities of certain cellular components that are putative targets of CO. Although this clearly represents a local event on the vascular walls, different vascular beds have different responses to CO in diabetes. The altered HO expression and activity will no doubt lead to altered heme metabolism to modulate the cellular production of CO. However, in diabetes, the reduced vascular responses to CO play a predominant role. As a result, even increased endogenous CO production cannot help to restore normal vascular tone.

Hyperglycemia represents the major etiologic factor for the vascular complications of diabetes. The front line strategy in prevention and management of vascular complications of diabetes lies in the tight control of blood glucose level. Lowering the level will not only reduce the formation of AGEs, but also decrease the oxidative stress associated with the disease. More relative to the involvement of the HO/CO system in diabetes is that reduced formation of AGEs would restore the normal sensitivity of CO targets in vascular walls and normalize the vasorelaxant functions of CO.

The emphasis on the pathological importance of hyperglycemia does not minimize the impacts of insulin deficiency and insulin desensitization on the metabolism and vascular effects of CO. This is an area for intensive investigation. The application of human genome information to profile CO-modulated gene expression patterns in diabetes, and the over-expression of HO in pancreatic islets to restore normal insulin secretion are also expected. To conclude, the awareness of the important relationship of a functional HO/CO system and diabetes has accelerated momentum in this field. Every discovery will lead to new hypotheses, and our understanding of the mechanisms of diabetic vascular complications and the role of the HO/CO system will be greatly enhanced.

ACKNOWLEDGMENTS

This work is supported by research grants from the Canadian Institute of Health Research (CIHR), the Natural Science and Engineering Research Council of Canada, and the Heart and Stroke Foundation of Canada (HSF). L. Wu is supported by a post-doctoral fellowship award from HSF. R. Wang is supported by a scientist award from CIHR.

REFERENCES

1. Rodgers, P.A. et al., Sources of carbon monoxide (CO) in biological systems and applications of CO detection technologies, *Sem. Perinatol.*, 18, 2, 1994.
2. Bucalo, L.R. et al., Pulmonary excretion of carbon monoxide in the human infant as an index of bilirubin production. IIc. Evidence for the possible association of cord blood erythropoietin levels and postnatal bilirubin production in infants of mothers with abnormalities of gestational glucose metabolism, *Am. J. Perinatol.*, 1,177, 1984.
3. Stevenson, D.K. et al., Pulmonary excretion of carbon monoxide in the human infant as an index of bilirubin production. IIb. Evidence for the possible effect of maternal prenatal glucose metabolism on postnatal bilirubin production in a mixed population of infants, *Eur. J. Pediatr.*, 137, 255, 1981.
4. Nikberg, I.I., Murashko, V.A., and Leonenko, I.N., Carbon monoxide concentration in the air exhaled by the healthy and the ill, *Vrach. Delo.*, 12, 112, 1972.
5. Paredi, P. et al., Exhaled carbon monoxide levels elevated in diabetes and correlated with glucose concentration in blood: a new test for monitoring the disease? *Chest,* 116, 1007, 1999.
6. Miyahara, S., Biological CO evolution, *J. Biochem.,* 69, 231, 1971.
7. Ditzel, J., Changes in red cell oxygen release capacity in diabetes mellitus, *Fed. Proc.,* 38, 2484, 1979.
8. Bourdon, E., Loreau, N., and Blache, D., Glucose and free radicals impair the antioxidant properties of serum albumin, *FASEB J.,* 13, 233, 1999.
9. Horvath, I. et al., Raised levels of exhaled carbon monoxide are associated with an increased expression of heme oxygenase-1 in airway macrophages in asthma: a new marker of oxidative stress, *Thorax,* 53, 668, 1998.
10. Belli, R. and Givliani. V., Recerche sull'ossicarbonismo ossicarbone mia endogena e diagnosi di ossicarbonismo cronico, *Folia Med.*, 38, 127, 1955.
11. Crosetti, L., Pettinati, L., and Rubino, G.F., Alcune considerazional in tema di preuenzione tecnica e biologica dell' intossicatzione da ossido di carbonio, *Med. Lavoro.*, 56, 604, 1965.
12. Takano, T., Honma, K., and Maeda, H., Comparative study on endogenous carbon monoxide production in alloxanized rats and normal rats, *Jap. J. Hyg.*, 31, 237, 1976.
13. Desoille, H., Cremer, G., and Girard, C., On the subject of a supposed blood carbon monoxide of endogenous origin in diabetics, *Arch. Mal. Prof.*, 26,625, 1965.
14. Hodgkin, J.E. and Chan, D.M., Diabetic ketoacidosis appearing as carbon monoxide poisoning, *JAMA*, 231,1164, 1975.
15. Ljubic, S. et al., Reduction of diffusion capacity for carbon monoxide in diabetic patients, *Chest,* 114,1033, 1998.
16. Wang, R., Resurgence of carbon monoxide: an endogenous gaseous vasorelaxing factor, *Can. J. Physiol. Pharmacol.*, 76,1, 1998.
17. Nishio, Y. et al., Altered activities of transcription factors and their related gene expression in cardiac tissues of diabetic rats, *Diabetes*, 47, 1318, 1998.
18. Wang, R. et al., Reduced vasorelaxant effect of carbon monoxide in diabetes and the underlying mechanisms, *Diabetes,* 50, 166, 2001.
19. Hammes, H.P. et al., Antioxidant treatment of experimental diabetic retinopathy in rats with nicanartine, *Diabetologia,* 40, 629, 1997.
20. Schmidt, A.M. et al., Advanced glycation endproducts (AGEs) induce oxidant stress in the gingiva: a potential mechanism underlying accelerated periodontal disease associated with diabetes, *J. Periodontal Res.*, 31, 508, 1996.

21. da Silva, J.L. et al., Diminished heme oxygenase-1 mRNA expression in RPE cells from diabetic donors as quantitated by competitive RT/PCR, *Curr. Eye Res.*, 16, 380, 1997.
22. Bitar, M. and Weiner, M., Diabetes-induced metabolic alterations in heme synthesis and degradation and various heme-containing enzymes in female rats, *Diabetes*, 33, 37, 1984.
23. Bitar, M. and Weiner, M., Heme and hemoproteins in streptozotocin-diabetic female rats, *Biochem. Pharmacol.*, 32,1921, 1983.
24. Alm, P. et al., Morphological evidence for the existence of nitric oxide and carbon monoxide pathways in the rat islets of Langerhans: an immunocytochemical and confocal microscopical study, *Diabetologia,* 42,978, 1999.
25. Henningsson, R. et al., Chronic blockade of NO synthase paradoxically increases islet NO production and modulates islet hormone release, *Am. J. Physiol.*, 279, E95, 2000.
26. Henningsson, R. et al., Heme oxygenase and carbon monoxide: regulatory roles in islet hormone release: a biochemical, immunohistochemical, and confocal microscopic study, *Diabetes*, 48, 66, 1999.
27. Henningsson, R., Alm, P., and Lundquist, I., Occurrence and putative hormone regulatory function of a constitutive heme oxygenase in rat pancreatic islets, *Am. J. Physiol.*, 273, C703, 1997.
28. Helqvist, S. et al., Heat shock protein induction in rat pancreatic islets by recombinant human interleukin 1β, *Diabetologia,* 34, 150, 1991.
29. Strandell, E. et al., Interleukin-1β induces the expression of HSP70, heme oxygenase and Mn-SOD in FACS-purified rat islet β-cells, but not in α-cells, *Immunol. Lett.*, 48, 145, 1995.
30. Welsh, N. and Sandler, S., Protective action by hemin against interleukin-1β induced inhibition of rat pancreatic islet function, *Mol. Cell. Endocrinol.*, 103, 109, 1994.
31. Cellek, S., Kasakov, L., and Moncada, S., Inhibition of nitrergic relaxation by a selective inhibitor of the soluble guanylyl cyclase, *Br. J. Pharmacol.*, 118,137, 1996.
32. Moro, M.A. et al., cGMP mediates the vascular and platelet actions of nitric oxide: confirmation using an inhibitor of the soluble guanylyl cyclase, *Proc. Natl. Acad. Sci. U.S.A.,* 93,1480, 1996.
33. Ingi, T., Cheng, J., and Ronnett, G.V., Carbon monoxide: an endogenous modulator of the nitric oxide-cyclic GMP signaling system, *Neuron,* 16, 835, 1996.
34. Takano, T., Honma, K., and Maeda, H., Endogenous carbon monoxide production in alloxanized rats, *Bull. Tokyo Med. Dent. Univ.*, 24, 67, 1977.
35. Welsh, N. et al., Differences in the expression of heat-shock proteins and antioxidant enzymes between human and rodent pancreatic islets: implications for the pathogenesis of insulin-dependent diabetes mellitus, *Mol. Med.*, 1, 806, 1995.
36. Shinohara, M. et al., Overexpression of glyoxalase-I in bovine endothelial cells inhibits intracellular advanced glycation endproduct formation and prevents hyperglycemia-induced increases in macromolecular endocytosis, *J. Clin. Invest.*, 101, 1142, 1998.
37. Brownlee, M., Advanced protein glycosylation in diabetes and aging, *Rev. Med.*, 46, 223, 1995.
38. Yan, S.D. et al., Enhanced cellular oxidant stress by the interaction of advanced glycation end products with their receptors/binding proteins, *J. Biol. Chem.*, 269, 9889, 1993.
39. Baynes, J.W., Role of oxidative stress in the development of complications in diabetes, *Diabetes*, 40, 405, 1991.

40. Stocker, R., Induction of haem oxygenase as a defence against oxidative stress, *Free Radical Res. Commun.* 9, 101, 1990.
41. Stocker, R. et al., Bilirubin is an antioxidant of possible physiological importance, *Science*, 235, 1043, 1987.
42. Vogt, B.A. et al., Acquired resistance to acute oxidative stress. Possible role of heme oxygenase and ferritin, *Lab. Invest.*, 72, 474, 1995.
43. Morris, T. et al., Reactive oxygen species and iron: a dangerous partnership in inflammation, *Int. J. Biochem. Cell. Biol.*, 27, 109, 1995.
44. Stevens, M.J. et al., The linked roles of nitric oxide, aldose reductase and (Na^+, K^+)-ATPase in the slowing of nerve conduction in the streptozotocin diabetic rat, *J. Clin. Invest.*, 94, 853, 1994.
45. Lee, T.S. et al., Activation of protein kinase C by elevation of glucose concentration: proposal for a mechanism in the development of diabetic vascular complications, *Proc. Natl. Acad. Sci. U.S.A.*, 86,5141, 1989.
46. Sakthivel. R. et al., Regulation of the ligand binding activity of the human very low density lipoprotein receptor by protein kinase C-dependent phosphorylation, *J. Biol. Chem.*, 276, 555, 2001.
47. Carmines, P.K., Ohishi, K., and Ikenaga, H., Functional impairment of renal afferent arteriolar voltage-gated calcium channels in rats with diabetes mellitus, *J. Clin. Invest.*, 98, 2564, 1996.
48. Wang, R. et al., Altered L-type voltage-dependent calcium channels in diabetic vascular smooth muscle cells, *Am. J. Physiol.*, 278, H714, 2000.
49. Wang, R. et al., Diabetes-related abnormal calcium mobilization in smooth muscle cells is induced by hyperosmolality, *Mol. Cell. Biochem.*, 183, 79, 1998.
50. McGinty, A. et al., Effect of glucose on endothelin-1-induced calcium transients in cultured bovine retinal pericytes, *J. Biol. Chem.*, 274, 25250, 1999.
51. Rivera, A.A. et al., Hyperglycemia alters cytoplasmic Ca^{2+} responses to capacitative Ca^{2+} influx in rat aortic smooth muscle cells, *Am. J. Physiol.*, 269, C1482, 1995.
52. Christlieb, A.R., Diabetes and hypertensive vascular disease: mechanisms and treatment, *Am. J. Cardiol.*, 32, 592, 1973.
53. Epstein, M. and Soweres, J.R., Diabetes mellitus and hypertension, *Hypertension*, 19, 403, 1992.
54. Williams, R.H. and Porte, D., Jr., The pancreas: specific organ involvement, in *Textbook of Endocrinology*, Williams, R.H., Ed., W.B. Saunders, Philadelphia, 1974, 572.
55. Wang, Z., Wu, L., and Wang, R., Kinin B2 receptor-mediated contraction of tail artery from normal or streptozotocin-induced diabetic rats, *Br. J. Pharmacol.*, 125, 143, 1998.
56. Wang, R., Wang, Z.Z., and Wu, L., Carbon monoxide-induced vasorelaxation and the underlying mechanisms, *Br. J. Pharmacol.*, 121, 927, 1997.
57. Quast, U., Do the K^+ channel openers relax smooth muscle by opening K^+ channels? *Trends Pharmacol. Sci.*, 14, 332, 1993.
58. Wang, R., Wu, L., and Wang, Z.Z., The direct effect of carbon monoxide on K_{Ca} channels in vascular smooth muscle cells, *Pflügers Arch.*, 434, 285, 1997.
59. Wang, R. and Wu, L., The chemical modification of K_{Ca} channels by carbon monoxide in vascular smooth muscle cells, *J. Biol. Chem.*, 272, 8222, 1997.
60. Jourdon, P. and Feuvray, D., Calcium and potassium currents in ventricular myocytes isolated from diabetic rats, *J. Physiol. (Lond.)*, 470, 411, 1993.
61. Shimoni, Y. et al., Short-term diabetes alters K^+ currents in rat ventricular myocytes, *Circ. Res.*, 74, 620, 1994.

62. Magyar, J. et al., Action potentials and potassium currents in rat ventricular muscle during experimental diabetes, *J. Mol. Cell. Cardiol.*, 24, 841, 1992.
63. Stoffel, M. et al., Cloning of rat K_{ATP}-2 channel and decreased expression in pancreatic islets of male Zucker diabetic fatty rats, *Biochem. Biophys. Res. Commun.*, 26, 894, 1995.
64. Lyons, T.J., Lipoprotein glycation and its metabolic consequence, *Diabetes*, 41 (Suppl. 2), 67, 1992.
65. D'Andera, G. et al., Kinetic features of ascorbic acid oxidase after partial deglycation, *Biochem. J.*, 264, 601, 1989.
66. Baek, W.O. and Vijayalakshmi, M.A., Effect of chemical glycosylation of Rnase A on the protein stability and surface histidines accessibility in immobilized metal ion affinity electrophoresis (IMAGE) system, *Biochim. Biophys. Acta,* 1336, 394, 1997
67. Coussons, P.J. et al., Glucose modification of human serum albumin: a structural study, *Free Rad. Biol. Med.*, 22, 1217, 1997.
68. Swamy, M.S. and Abraham, E.C., Glycation of lens MIP26 affects the permeability in reconstituted liposomes, *Biochem. Biophys. Res. Commun.*, 186, 632, 1992.
69. Kobayashi, K. et al., Deglycation of glycated proteins with hydrazine analogues, *Life Sci.*, 53, 291, 1993.

13 Selective Increase in Human Heme Oxygenase-1 Gene Expression Attenuates Development of Hypertension and Increases Body Growth in Spontaneously Hypertensive Rats

Nader G. Abraham, Shuo Quan, Sylvia Shenouda, and Attallah Kappas

CONTENTS

I. ABSTRACT

Perturbations in heme metabolism are known to affect the levels and activities of hemoprotein-dependent processes, including cytochrome P450-mediated arachidonic acid (AA) metabolism. We studied the effects of heme arginate and of $SnCl_2$, inducers of heme oxygenase (HO) on cytochrome P450 levels and blood pressure in spontaneously hypertensive rats (SHRs). Administration of heme arginate or heme alone at doses of 9 to 30 mg/kg body weight/day for 4 days resulted in a marked decrease of blood pressure in SHRs compared to controls.

Administration of heme resulted in an accumulation of HO mRNA, accompanied by an increase in HO activity. The increase was prevented by Sn protoporhyrin (SnPP). The effect of $SnCl_2$ on the transcription of the HO gene in SHRs was examined during development of blood pressure over time. An increase in renal HO-1 mRNA levels was observed in response to $SnCl_2$ treatment. As a consequence of $SnCl_2$ activation of HO-1 gene transcription, renal enzyme activity increased eight-fold at 16 hours and reached 16-fold over controls (maximal activity) 32 hours after injection. Cytochrome P450-AA ω/ω-1 hydroxylase(s) activity and formation of 19- and 20-hydroxyeicosatetraenoic acid (19- and 20-HETE) products were significantly reduced 24 hours after administration of $SnCl_2$ and remained lower than control levels at 48 and 72 hours after treatment. In addition, blood pressure was reduced from 151 ± 2.5 mmHg to 133 ± 2.3 mmHg 48 hours after $SnCl_2$ treatment (p <0.05). The reduction preceded natriuresis.

A selective increase in HO-1 gene activity was achieved by retroviral-mediated human HO-1 (HHO-1) gene transfer to SHRs. A single intracardiac injection of the concentrated infectious viral particles (expressing HHO-1) to 5-day-old SHRs resulted in functional expression of the human HO-1 gene and development of hypertension. Rats expressing HHO-1 showed significant increases in total body growth, decreases in urinary excretion of a vasoconstrictor AA metabolite, and reductions in myogenic response to increased intraluminal pressure in isolated arterioles. These biochemical and physiological changes brought about a selective decrease in the synthesis of 19- and 20-HETE, arachidonate metabolites having prohypertensive properties and associated with blood pressure reduction to normal levels. It is suggested that pharmacologic or genetic manipulation leading to a selective increase in HO activity and a decrease in cytochrome P450-AA ω-hydroxylase expression may be of therapeutic importance in regulating blood pressure. The relation of HO to body growth rate is a newly defined aspect of this enzyme activity that has broad significance for this metabolic system.

II. INTRODUCTION

As the key enzyme in heme degradation, heme oxygenase (HO) governs cellular heme concentrations.[1,2] To date, three HO isoforms (HO-1, HO-2, and HO-3) — the products of three distinct genes — have been identified in mammals.[3,4] HO and its metabolic products have been implicated in the regulation of numerous biological processes.[4-11] Carbon monoxide (CO) derived from HO activity has been shown to

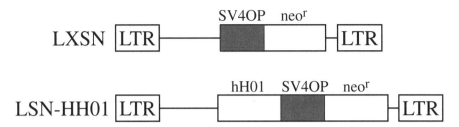

FIGURE 13.1 Schematic diagram of retroviral vectors LSN–HHO-1 and LXSN (SV40P = Simian virus 40 promoter; LTR = long terminal repeat).

function as a neurotransmitter,[12,13] a vasodilator,[14] and an endogenous modulator of the nitric oxide (NO)–cGMP signaling system in the brain.[4,13]

Recent studies indicate that administration of HO inhibitors increases arterial pressure in normotensive rats.[15] These observations suggest that endogenous HO-derived CO plays a role in the regulation of basal vascular tone and contributes to setting the level of arterial blood pressure. The development of gene transfer techniques provided the opportunity to deliver a functional HO-1 gene and to evaluate the direct effects of this gene on blood pressure.[16-18] We used a retroviral vector to deliver the human HO-1 (HHO-1) gene to spontaneously hypertensive rats (SHRs) to explore the role of this enzyme in the genesis of hypertension.

III. METHODS

A. CONSTRUCTION OF THE RETROVIRAL VECTOR LSN–HHO

The human HO-1 gene expressing replication-deficient retrovirus vector LSN–HHO-1 was constructed. A 987-bp HindIII–HindIII HHO-1 cDNA fragment was released from plasmid pRC–CMV–HHO-1 and inserted at the HindIII site of the pGEM-7zf(+) vector.[19] After digestion with ApaI, the transcription-orientational clones were selected and designated pGEM7–HHO. LSN–HHO-1 was constructed by cloning the HHO-1 cDNA fragment from pGEM7–HHO-1 at the EcoRI–BamHI sites of retroviral vector LXSN (Figure 13.1).

B. TRANSFECTION AND VIRUS PRODUCTION

PA317 retroviral packaging cells (3×10^5/ml) were seeded in 60-mm tissue culture dishes and incubated for 24 h. The attached cells were washed twice with serum-reduced Opti-MEM (GIBCO-BRL). The cells were added separately to 5 µg of retroviral vector (LSN–HHO-1 or LXSN) incubated in 20 µl of plasmid lipo-fectamine reagent (GIBCO-BRL) for 30 min at room temperature (22°C). After incubation at 37°C for 5 h, 3 ml of DMEM, containing 20% FBS were added to the culture dishes, which were further incubated for 18 h. The culture medium was replaced with fresh complete medium and incubated for another 24 h. The cells were passaged 1:10 into the G418-containing medium (600 μg/ml) (GIBCO-BRL). After a 14-day culture at 37°C in 5% CO_2, individual G418-resistant clones were selected.

C. ANIMALS

Male spontaneously hypertensive rats (SHRs) and normotensive Wistar–Kyoto (WKY) rats (5 to 6 weeks old) were purchased from Charles River Breeding Laboratories (Wilmington, MA). They were fed and housed under identical conditions, 4 to 5 days before the beginning of the study. SHRs and WKY rats were injected subcutaneously with $SnCl_2$ (15 mg/100 g body weight) or heme (3 mg/100g). The control SHRs and WKY rats were injected with empty virus. Blood pressure was measured from the tail, without anesthesia, using a plethysmograph prior to and 1 to 4 days after injection. Urine was collected in metabolic cages over 24-h periods, and urine volume, K^+ and Na^+ concentrations were measured.

Three control and four treated animals were sacrificed at different time points after $SnCl_2$ administration. One kidney from each rat was immediately frozen in liquid nitrogen for RNA extraction; the other was used for enzyme measurement of cytochrome P450 and HO activity.

D. ANIMALS TREATED WITH RETROVIRAL-MEDIATED HHO-1 GENE

Pregnant SHR mothers were purchased from Taconic Laboratories (Germantown, NY). Five-day-old rats from the same litters were divided into three treatment groups: vehicle (HBSS), LXSN (viral control), and LSN–HHO-1 (experimental). Treatments were administered by bolus injection of 10μL HBSS with or without LXSN or LSN–HHO-1 viral particles (1×10^{10} CFU/ml) directly into the left ventricle under methoxyflurane anesthesia. Survival was 96%. Animals were weaned at 21 days of age; males were separated and utilized for all experiments. Systolic blood pressure was measured by tail cuff sphygmomanometry twice weekly, starting at 4 weeks of age. Average daily food intake and total body weight were measured for all treatment groups. At 4 weeks of age, animals were subjected to radiography (n = 6). They were sacrificed at different times (4, 6, and 8 weeks), and tissues were isolated for determination of HHO-1 expression and HO activity. Analysis of HO-1/HO-2 proteins, HHO-1, HO activity, and blood pressure were performed.[20-22]

IV. RESULTS AND DISCUSSION

A. EFFECT OF HEME ARGINATE AND HEME ON BLOOD PRESSURE

We determined the dose–response relationships of heme arginate and heme with respect to blood pressure. Administration of heme arginate at all three doses significantly reduced blood pressure (Figure 13.2). Because the heme moiety of heme arginate plays an important role in the maintenance of cellular cytochrome P450 and because arginine is a substrate for nitric oxide (NO), we examined the effects of both on the blood pressure of SHRs. As shown in Figure 13.2, heme alone administration caused a decrease in blood pressure. This decrease was about

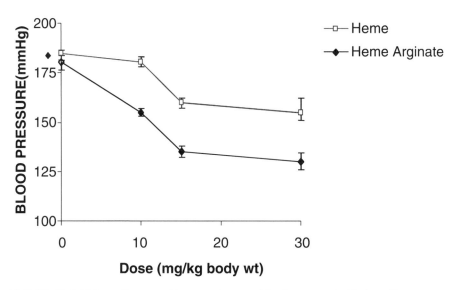

FIGURE 13.2 Effect of heme and heme arginate on blood pressure in 45-day-old spontaneously hypertensive rats injected with heme or heme arginate (0 to 30 mg/kg body weight) for 4 consecutive days. Control rats were injected with vehicle. Systolic blood pressure was measured as described in Section II. Results represent the mean ± SE; n = 4 per group. The results for heme- and heme-arginate-treated groups at all doses tested were significantly different from those of controls; p <0.01.

60% of that which occurred after heme arginate administration, suggesting that the effect of heme arginate may be the result of the additive effect of L-arginine and heme.

Pharmacological agents such as Sn mesoporphyrin (SnMP), an inhibitor of HO, can inhibit HO activity significantly and have been shown to be highly effective in single doses in controlling hyperbilirubinemia in newborns and other patients.[23-27] ZnPP, also an HO inhibitor, has been shown to inhibit bone marrow and macrophages growth. CrPP, which exerts similar activity, is also quite toxic to whole animals.[28] Therefore, SnMP was used in the experiments. As shown in Figure 13.3, inhibition of HO activity by SnPP completely abolished the lowering effect of hemin (30 mg/kg body weight) on blood pressure in SHRs, suggesting that the heme effect is mediated via activation of HO.

B. EFFECT OF HEME ON RENAL HEME OXYGENASE ACTIVITY

SHRs and WKY rats were treated with heme alone or in combination with SnPP. Renal and hepatic HO activities were assessed. When SHRs were treated with heme alone, a marked increase in renal HO activity (240%) was observed (Table 13.1). SnPP alone inhibited the basal levels of HO in untreated SHRs by 87%. When administered with heme, SnPP completely abolished the induced HO activity as well as the basal tone.

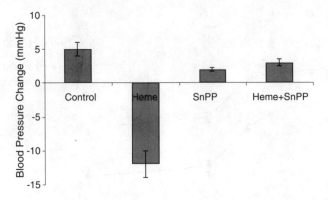

FIGURE 13.3 Effect of SnPP on heme-induced blood pressure changes. SnPP (3.75 mg/kg body weight) was given subcutaneously 30 min before heme administration (30 mg/kg body weight). Results represent the mean ± SE; n = 4.

TABLE 13.1
Effect of Heme and SnPP
on Renal HO Activities[a]

Treatment Group	Heme Oxygenase (nmol of bilirubin/mg/h)
Control	0.791 ± 0.102
Hemin (15 mg/kg)	1.891 ± 0.274[d]
Hemin (15 mg/kg) plus SnPP (3.75 mg/kg)	0.148 ± 0.086[c,d]
SnPP	0.101 ± 0.042[b]

[a] Results are mean ± SD; N = 3.
[b] p <0.001 vs. control.
[c] p <0.0001 vs. treatment without SnPP.
[d] p <0.01 vs. control.

C. EFFECT OF STANNOUS CHLORIDE ON HO-1 mRNA AND ENZYME ACTIVITIES

We postulated that the effect of $SnCl_2$ on systolic blood pressure is related to the induction of HO activity because inhibition of HO activity abolished the blood pressure-reducing effects of $SnCl_2$ and heme arginate as well.[21] We examined the time-dependent effect of $SnCl_2$ on HO-1 mRNA levels and on HO activity, and correlated the effect with the decrease in P450-AA metabolism and blood pressure in SHRs. As shown in Figure 13.4a, renal HO activity increased 2.3-fold over control levels within 4 h after $SnCl_2$ administration (i.e., from 0.90 ± 0.04 nmol bilirubin/mg/h to 2.10 ± 0.10 nmol bilirubin/mg/h), confirming our earlier findings.[29] Twenty-four and 32 h later, HO activity increased 12- and 16-fold, respectively, over control levels.

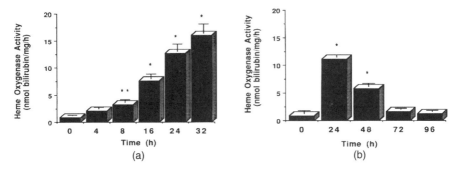

FIGURE 13.4 Effect of $SnCl_2$ treatment on renal (a) and hepatic HO activities (b). Rats were treated with a single dose of $SnCl_2$ (15mg/100g body weight). Kidneys and livers were removed at different times. Microsomal HO activity was measured as described in Section II. Each bar represents the mean ± SE of four experiments. *$p < 0.01$; **$p < 0.05$ when compared with control levels (time 0).

The effect of $SnCl_2$ was highly selective to renal HO. Hepatic HO activity also increased, but to a lesser extent, i.e., from 1.53 ± 0.04 nmol/mg/h to 3.08 ± 0.51 nmol/mg/h and 5.24 ± 0.96 nmol/mg/h at 4 and 32 h after $SnCl_2$ treatment, respectively (Figure 13.4b).

Determination of HO over a 4-day, post-injection period revealed that the maximal increase in hepatic HO activity occurred 24 h after $SnCl_2$ injection, gradually declined at 48 h, and returned to control level 72 h after injection (Figure 13.4b). Similarly, HO activity increased in WKY rats, i.e., 1.1 ± 0.1 nmol/mg/h and 13.4 ± 0.6 nmol/mg/h before and 24 h after $SnCl_2$ injection.

To evaluate whether the increased enzyme activity is a consequence of the activation of existing protein or represents *de novo* synthesis of protein, we determined the time-dependent effect of $SnCl_2$ on HO-1 mRNA. Northern blot hybridization of total RNA with a specific cDNA probe quantified by autoradiography (Figure 13.5, bottom) and densitometry scanning (Figure 13.5, top) demonstrated maximal induction of renal HO-1 mRNA (24-fold) 8 h after injection. The observed increase in HO-1 mRNA returned to control levels 32 h after injection (see Figure 13.2). A similar induction in HO-1 mRNA also was seen in WKY rats.

D. EFFECT OF STANNOUS CHLORIDE ON BLOOD PRESSURE AND RENAL FUNCTION

Concomitant with the increase in HO-1 mRNA levels and HO activity and the decrease in cytochrome P450 AA ω/ω-1 hydroxylation, $SnCl_2$ caused significant changes in blood pressure and urinary electrolyte excretion. Administration of a single dose to 6-week-old SHRs markedly decreased blood pressure in a time-dependent manner (Figure 13.6). A decrease in blood pressure was observed 24 h after injection, which, when compared with the untreated group, was significant ($p < 0.05$). The effect on blood pressure was followed by an increase in urine volume and urinary K^+ and Na^+ excretion.

HEME OXYGENASE EXPRESSION

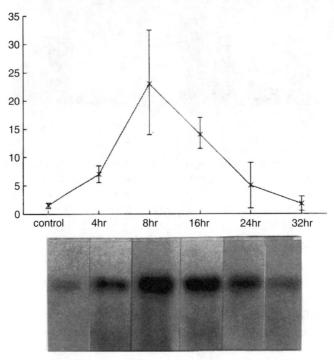

FIGURE 13.5 Time-dependent changes in HO-1 mRNA levels after $SnCl_2$ treatment. Top: Densitometry ratios of renal HO (RHO)/GAPDH. Each point represents the mean ± SE of four experiments. *p <0.05 when compared with control levels (time 0). Bottom: Northern Blot analysis. Total RNA (10 μg) isolated from the kidneys of control and treated rats were analyzed for HO-1 mRNA level.

Significant increases in urinary K^+ and Na^+ excretion and urine volume were achieved after 96 h after treatment. $SnCl_2$ treatment did not affect food intake or body weight. Administration of $SnCl_2$ to age-matched WKY rats had no effect on blood pressure, urine volume, or electrolyte excretion. Injection of the retroviral HHO-1 gene construct into 5-day-old SHRs resulted in expression of the gene in several tissues. HHO-1 mRNA was detected by reverse transcriptase/polymerase chain reaction (RT/PCR) in the kidneys, livers, lungs, and brains of 12-week-old SHRs treated with LSN–HHO-1 but not with LXSN viral particles (Figure 13.7).

Rat HO-1 mRNA expression was comparable in SHRs treated with LXSN and LSN–HHO-1 viruses. The average level of expression of HHO-1 mRNA in kidneys, estimated by competitive RT/PCR using an internal standard,[30] was 1.81×10^6 molecules of HHO-1 mRNA/ng total RNA. Immunoblot analysis, using specific antibodies that discriminate between human and rat HO-1, revealed expression of HHO-1 protein only in tissues of SHRs treated with LSN–HHO-1, but not with LXSN viral particles.

Rat HO-1 and HO-2 GAPDH were comparable in tissues of SHR treated with LSN–HHO-1 or LXSN viral particles (Figure 13.7). HO-1 protein expression was

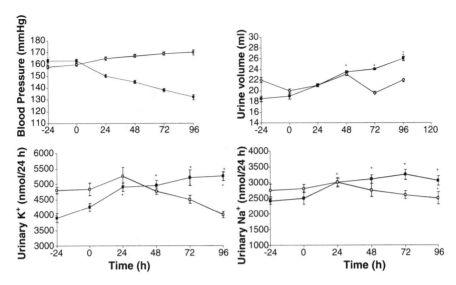

FIGURE 13.6 Effects of $SnCl_2$ on blood pressure, urine volume, and electrolytes in 6-week-old spontaneously hypertensive rats. $SnCl_2$ was injected subcutaneouly at day 0 (15 mg/100g body weight). Each point represents the mean ± SE of five experiments. Blood pressure; urine volume; urinary K^+ excretion; and urinary K^+ excretion were measured every 24 hours for 4 days. *p <0.05 when comparing treated and untreated rats at each time point.

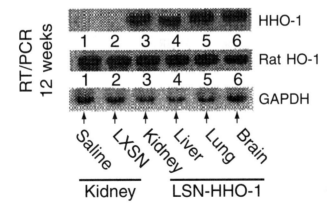

FIGURE 13.7 Expression of HHO-1 in cultured RLMV cells and tissues from spontaneously hypertensive rats. A representative RT/PCR autoradiogram of HHO-1 and rat HO-1 mRNA from kidney of control vehicle treated rat (Lane 1), kidney of LXSN-treated rat (Lane 2), and kidney, liver, lung and brain (Lanes 3 through 6, respectively) of LSN–HHO-1 treated rat. Five-day-old rats were given single 10 μl intracardiac injections of LXSN and HHO-1 viral particles (1×10^{10}CFU/ml).

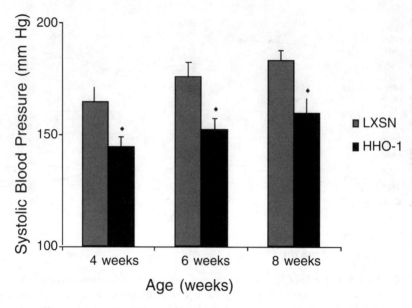

FIGURE 13.8 Effect of LSN–HHO-1 treatment on systolic blood pressure in spontaneously hypertensive rats. At 5 days of age, animals were injected with LXSN or LSN–HHO-1 (1×10^{10} CFU/ml). Blood pressure was determined twice weekly by the tail cuff method at 4, 6, and 8 weeks of age. Results are mean ± SE. Blood pressure of LSN–HHO-1 treated rats (n = 32) was significantly different (*p <0.001) from vehicle-treated spontaneously hypertensive rats (n = 10) or LXSN-treated rats (n = 23) by ANOVA and the Student's *t* test.

shown by immunohistochemical analysis to increase in SHR tissues. Expression of HHO-1 in rat tissues was associated with increased HO activity. Similarly, we observed an increase in HO activity in both liver and lung microsomes from SHRs treated with LSN–HHO-1 compared to SHRs treated with LXSN viral particles (data not shown). The levels of HO activity in LXSN-treated SHRs were comparable to those of vehicle-treated SHRs.

Blood pressure increased as a function of age in all treatment groups; however, up to 20 weeks of age, the blood pressure values of LSN–HHO-1-treated SHRs were significantly lower than those of vehicle-treated or LXSN-treated SHRs (Figure 13.8). The fact that hypertension is attenuated in SHRs expressing the HHO-1 gene implies that a mechanism dependent upon the function of this human gene lowers blood pressure in SHRs. Thus, the attenuating influence of LSN–HHO-1 treatment on the development of hypertension in SHRs is most likely the result of increased HO activity consequent to HHO-1 expression. This is in agreement with reports that other interventions that increase HO activity in SHRs also attenuate the development of hypertension.[31]

The association of increased HO activity and attenuation of hypertension in SHRs expressing the HHO-1 gene suggests that the heme–HO system in this type of rat either interferes with the expression of prohypertensive mechanisms or promotes the expression of antihypertensive mechanisms. The development of hypertension in SHRs has been linked to increased expression of a prohypertensive mechanism mediated by a metabolite of AA derived from the cytochrome P450 system, presumably, 20-hydroxyeicosatetraenoic acid (20-HETE).[32,33] HO has been implicated as a major regulator of cytochrome P450 hemoproteins, including those responsible for the formation of 20-HETE, by limiting the amounts of heme and/or by producing CO which strongly binds to the heme moiety of cytochrome P450, causing enzyme inhibition.

Beginning at 4 weeks of age, body weights of SHRs treated with LSN–HHO-1 viral particles surpassed those of SHRs treated with vehicle alone or with LXSN viral control.[34] The nose-to-tail lengths and fibula lengths of SHRs treated with LSN–HHO-1 also exceeded the corresponding values in rats treated with vehicle or LXSN. However, food intake was similar in all treatment groups. Rats expressing the HHO-1 gene grew faster than those lacking the HHO-1 gene, particularly during the first 12 weeks. The increase in somatic growth associated with HHO-1 expression was proportionate. This latter observation, striking and unexpected, implies that SHRs expressing the HHO-1 gene are, in metabolic terms, more efficient than their counterparts lacking the HHO-1 gene, and thus can develop faster somatically without consuming greater amounts of food.

Recent reports indicate that both humans[35] and mice[36] lacking the HO-1 gene display severe growth retardation. HO-1 gene expression has been shown to play a role in cell proliferation and cell death; indeed, previous studies demonstrated that elevation of HO-1 activity by gene transfer to rabbit coronary microvessel endothelial cells enhances cell proliferation[37] and increases angiogenesis.[38] In contrast, Lee et al.[39] demonstrated that overexpression of HO-1 in pulmonary epithelial human cell line results in cell growth arrest, highlighting the cell-specific effects of HO-1 on cellular proliferation.

A priori, a consequence of HO activity may directly impact somatic growth by influencing the production and/or cellular actions of hormones and other factors that stimulate or inhibit growth. Cheriathundam et al.[41] found a significant correlation between hepatic levels of HO-1 and growth hormone in transgenic mice. Moreover, consensus binding sites for NF-κβ, AP-1, AP-2, and IL-6 responsive elements and other transcription factors have been reported in the promoter region of the HO-1 gene.[40] Whether these transcription factors activate certain elements involved in promoting SHR growth remains to be investigated. The present study provides no information on the mechanisms responsible for the observed growth-promoting effect of HHO-1 expression in SHRs. However, the finding is highly important since it links, for the first time, the human HO system to the regulation of somatic growth.

ACKNOWLEDGMENTS

This work was supported by National Institutes of Health Grants RO1 HL54138 and PO1 HL34300. The authors thank Barbara Stern for editorial assistance.

REFERENCES

1. Yoshida, T. and Kikuchi, G., Purification and properties of heme oxygenase from pig spleen microsomes, *J. Biol. Chem.*, 253, 4224, 1978.
2. Abraham, N.G. et al., Biological significance and physiological role of heme oxygenase, *Cell Physiol. Biochem.*, 6, 129, 1996.
3. McCoubrey, W.K., Jr., Huang, T.J., and Maines, M.D., Isolation and characterization of a cDNA from the rat brain that encodes hemoprotein heme oxygenase-3, *Eur. J. Biochem.*, 247, 725, 1997.
4. Maines, M.D., The heme oxygenase system; a regulator of second messenger gases, *Annu. Rev. Pharmacol. Toxicol.*, 37, 517, 1997.
5. Zakhary, R. et al., Heme oxygenase 2: endothelial and neuronal localization and role in endothelium-dependent relaxation, *Proc. Natl. Acad. Sci. U.S.A.*, 93, 795, 1996.
6. Choi, A.M.K. and Alam, J., Heme oxygenase-1: function, regulation, and implication of a novel stress-inducible protein in oxidant-induced lung injury, *Am. J. Respir. Cell. Mol. Biol.*, 15, 9, 1996.
7. Lutton, J.D. et al., Differential induction of heme oxygenase in the hepatocarcinoma cell line (Hep3b) by environmental agents, *J. Cell. Biochem.*, 49, 259, 1992.
8. Neil, T.K. et al., Modulation of corneal heme oxygenase expression by oxidative stress agents, *J. Ocul. Pharmacol. Ther.*, 11, 455, 1995.
9. Dennery, P.A. et al., Heme oxygenase-mediated resistance to oxygen toxicity in hamster fibroblasts, *J. Biol. Chem.*, 272, 14937, 1997.
10. Lu, T.H. et al., Molecular cloning, characterization, and expression of the chicken heme oxygenase-1 gene in transfected primary cultures of chick embryo liver cells, *Gene*, 207, 177, 1998.
11. Mitani, K. et al., Heme oxygenase is a positive acute phase reactant in human Hep3B hepatoma cells, *Blood*, 79, 1255, 1992.
12. Verma, A. et al., Carbon monoxide: a putative neural messenger, *Science*, 259, 381, 1993.
13. McCoubrey, W.K., Jr., Ewing, J.F., and Maines, M.D., Human heme oxygenase-2: characterization and expression of a full-length cDNA and evidence suggesting that the two HO-2 transcripts may differ by choice of polyadenylation signal, *Arch. Biochem. Biophys.*, 295, 13, 1992.
14. Zhang, F. et al., Carbon monoxide produced by isolated arterioles attenuates pressure-induced vasoconstriction, *Am. J. Physiol.*, 14, 625, 2001.
15. Johnson, R.A. et al., Role of endogenous carbon monoxide in central regulation of arterial pressure, *Hypertension*, 30, 962, 1997.
16. Abraham, N.G., Jiang, S., Yang, L., Zand, B.A., Marji, J., Drummond, G.S., and Kappas, A., Adenoviral vector-mediated transfer of human heme oxygenase in rats virtually decreases renal heme-dependent arachidonic acid epoxygenase activity, *J. Exp. Pharm. Ther.*, 293, 494, 2000.
17. Sabaawy, H.E. et al., Transfer of the human heme oxygenase-1 gene decreases blood pressure and promotes growth in spontaneously hypertensive rats, 54th Annual Conference of the Council for High Blood Presure, Fall 2000, p. 52.
18. Gadano, A.C. et al., Endothelial calcium–calmodulin dependent nitric oxide synthase in the *in vitro* vascular hyporeactivity of portal hypertensive rats, *J. Hepatol.*, 26, 678, 1997.
19. Yang, L., Quan, S., and Abraham, N.G., Retrovirus-mediated HO gene transfer into endothelial cells protects against oxidant-induced injury, *Am. J. Physiol.*, 277, L127, 1999.
20. Martasek, P. et al., Hemin and L-arginine regulation of blood pressure in spontaneous hypertensive rats, *J. Am. Soc. Nephrol.*, 2, 1078, 1991.

21. Levere, R.D. et al., Effect of heme arginate administration on blood pressure in spontaneously hypertensive rats, *J. Clin. Invest.,* 86, 213, 1990.
22. da-Silva, J.L. et al., Tin-mediated heme oxygenase gene activation and cytochrome P450 arachidonate hydroxylase inhibition in spontaneously hypertensive rats [published erratum appears in *Am. J. Med. Sci.,* 308, 138. 1994], *Am. J. Med. Sci.,* 307, 173, 1994.
23. Kappas, A. and Drummond, G., Control of heme metabolism with synthetic metalloporphyrins, *J. Clin. Invest.,* 77, 335, 1986.
24. Kappas, A.., Simionatto, C.S., Drummond, G.S., Sassa, S., and Anderson, K.E., The liver excretes large amounts of heme into bile when heme oxygenase is inhibited competitively by Sn-protoporphyrin, *Proc. Natl. Acad. Sci. U.S.A.,* 82, 896, 1985.
25. Kappas, A., Drummond, G.S., Manola, T., Petmezaki, S., and Valaes, T., Sn-protoporphyrin use in the management of hyperbilirubinemia in term newborns with direct Coombs-positive ABO incompatibility, *Pediatrics,* 81, 485, 1988.
26. Kappas, A. et al., Direct comparison of Sn-mesoporphyrin, an inhibitor of bilirubin production, and phototherapy in controlling hyperbilirubinemia in term and near-term newborns, *Pediatrics,* 95, 468, 1995.
27. Kappas, A., Drummond, G.S., and Vallaes, J., A single dose of Sn-mesoporphyrin prevents development of significant hyperbilirubinemia in glucose-6 phosphate dehydrogenase deficient newborns, *Pediatrics,* 108, 25, 2001.
28. Lutton, J.D. et al., Zinc porphyrins: potent inhibitors of hematopoiesis in animal and human bone marrow, *Proc. Natl. Acad. Sci. U.S.A.,* 94,1432, 1997.
29. Kappas, A. and Maines, M.D., Tin: a potent inducer of heme oxygenase in kidney, *Science,* 192, 60, 1976.
30. Abraham, N.G., Quantitation of heme oxygenase (HO-1) copies in human tissues by competitive RT/PCR, *Methods Mol. Biol.,* 108,199, 1998.
31. Sacerdoti, D. et al., Treatment with tin prevents the development of hypertension in spontaneously hypertensive rats, *Science,* 243, 388, 1989.
32. Omata, K. et al., Age-related changes in renal cytochrome P-450 arachidonic acid metabolism in spontaneously hypertensive rats, *Am. J. Physiol.,* 262, F8, 1992.
33. Imig, J.D. et al., Elevated renovascular tone in young spontaneously hypertensive rats. Role of cytochrome P-450, *Hypertension,* 22, 357, 1993.
34. Sabaawy, H.E. et al., Human heme oxygenase-1 gene transfer lowers blood pressure and promotes growth in spontaneously hypertensive rats, *Hypertension,* 2001, in press.
35. Yachie, A. et al., Oxidative stress causes enhanced endothelial cell injury in human heme oxygenase-1 deficiency, *J. Clin. Invest.,* 103, 129, 1999.
36. Poss, K.D. and Tonegawa, S., Reduced stress defense in heme oxygenase-1 deficient cells, *Proc. Natl. Acad. Sci. U.S.A.,* 94, 10925, 1997.
37. Deramaudt, B.M. et al., Gene transfer of human heme oxygenase into coronary endothelial cells potentially promotes angiogenesis, *J. Cell. Biochem.,* 68, 121, 1998.
38. Deramaudt, B.J.M., Remy, P., and Abraham, N.G., Upregulation of human heme oxygenase gene expression by Ets-family proteins, *J. Cell. Biochem.,* 72, 311, 1999.
39. Lee, P.J. et al., Overexpression of heme oxygenase-1 in human pulmonary epithelial cells results in cell growth arrest and increased resistance to hyperoxia, *Proc. Natl. Acad. Sci. U.S.A.,* 93, 10393, 1996.
40. Lavrovsky, Y. et al., Activation of nuclear factor kappa B and oncogene expression by 12(R)-hydroxyeicosatrienoic acid, an angiogenic factor in microvessel endothelial cells, *J. Biol. Chem.,* 269, 24321, 1994.
41. Cheriathundam, E., Doi, S.Q., Knapp, J.R., Jasser, M.Z., Kopchick, J.J., and Alvares, A.P., Consequences of overexpression of growth hormone in transgenic mice on liver cytochrome P450 enzymes, *Biochem. Pharmacol.,* 55, 1481, 1998.

Section 3

Techniques Used in Carbon Monoxide Research

14 Studies on the Development of Carbon Monoxide-Releasing Molecules: Potential Applications for the Treatment of Cardiovascular Dysfunction

Roberto Motterlini, Roberta Foresti, and Colin J. Green

CONTENTS

I. INTRODUCTION

Carbon monoxide (CO) is, by common definition, a colorless, odorless, tasteless, non-corrosive gas of about the same density as that of air and is the most commonly encountered and pervasive poison in our environment. It is generally produced by the incomplete combustion of fossil fuels such as natural gas, propane, coal, gasoline, and wood. In the atmosphere, the average global levels are estimated to be 0.19 parts per million (ppm), 90% of which comes from natural sources including ocean microorganism production, and 10% of which is generated by human activity. Thus, inhalation of even small quantities of CO is inevitable for living organisms.

Depending on the extent and time of exposure, CO is capable of producing myriad of debilitating and harmful residual effects.[1] The most immediate effect, and perhaps the most notorious one, is the binding to hemoglobin in the blood stream, which rapidly decreases the oxygen transport capability of the cardiovascular system. Paradoxically, more than half a century ago it was found that CO is constantly formed in humans in small quantities,[2] and that under certain pathophysiological conditions, this endogenous production of CO may be considerably increased.[3-5] The discovery that hemoglobin, a heme-dependent protein, is required as substrate for the production of CO *in vivo*,[6,7] and the identification of the heme oxygenase enzyme as the crucial pathway for the generation of this gaseous molecule in mammals,[8] set the basis for the early investigation of an unexpected and still unrecognized role of CO in the vasculature.[9]

The subsequent cloning[10] and characterization of constitutive (HO-2) and inducible (HO-1) isoforms of heme oxygenase[11-13] and studies of the kinetics and tissue distribution of these enzymes[14] revealed a major importance of this pathway in the physiological degradation of heme. That is, the end products of heme degradation (CO, biliverdin, and bilirubin) might have crucial biological activities.[15-17]

The recognition that CO possesses vasodilatory properties when applied to blood vessels[18-20] is, perhaps, the most significant evidence in favor of a pharmacological function of CO. Although the molecular mechanisms and the chemical modifications required to transduce the signals mediated by CO into a specific biological effect need to be fully elucidated, convincing scientific reports recently highlighted the signaling properties of endogenously generated CO.[21-24]

It is remarkable how the physiological effect produced by CO in the vasculature is similar to that elicited by another renowned diatomic gas, nitric oxide (NO). NO, which like CO has been known for years as a noteworthy environmental pollutant, is a gaseous molecule once thought produced only by bacteria. In 1987, when researchers first demonstrated that metabolic pathways in mammalian arteries and veins could also produce NO,[25,26] the fields of cardiovascular pharmacology, immunology, neurobiology, and toxicology began to take a profound interest in this area. Since then, evidence has mounted in support of NO's crucial role in a variety of clinical conditions, including septic shock, stroke, hemorrhagic shock, inflammation, and injury caused by ischemia and reperfusion.[27]

With the advent of NO research, experimental studies were largely facilitated by the development of a wide variety of organic compounds that spontaneously release NO and can be easily acquired to reproduce a physiological or pathophysiological function of NO. Abundant literature now discusses the different types of NO donors and NO-releasing agents that, depending on their stability and half-lives, can be used in disparate *in vitro* and *in vivo* models to simulate the biological activity of this important signaling molecule.[28,29]

In clinical practice, compounds such as sodium nitroprusside and glyceryl trinitrate that deliver NO into the circulation are used to lower blood pressure and treat certain cardiovascular diseases.[30] Drugs containing a functional NO group that can selectively target an organ or tissue are currently under development or are in clinical trials for the treatment of specific pathophysiological states.[31,32] However, no compounds capable of carrying or delivering CO have been examined as potential effectors in cells or tissues. The synthesis of molecules containing carbonyl groups that possess distinct physiological effects will extend our understanding of the chemistry of CO, its interaction with intracellular targets, and its biological importance in physiology and disease. In the long term, studies in this area may promote the design of vasodilatory drugs as alternatives to organic nitrates, which are known to lead to tolerance when continuously used.

This chapter will summarize our knowledge of the functional role of CO in the cardiovascular system with a major emphasis on the active participation of the heme oxygenase pathway in the mitigation of myocardial ischemia–reperfusion injury. The discussion will lead to the description of novel experimental data concerning the effect of certain CO-releasing molecules (CO-RMs) that might be used as prototypes for the development of carriers of CO into biological systems; their potential application for the treatment of vascular dysfunction will also be discussed.

II. GENERATION OF CARBON MONOXIDE IN THE CARDIOVASCULAR SYSTEM

Heme oxygenase is the rate-limiting enzyme in the degradation of heme that catalyzes the opening of iron protoporphyrin IX at the α-methene bridge to form biliverdin IX, iron, and CO. This pathway is ubiquitous in nature and the enzyme is highly conserved throughout the animal and plant kingdoms.

Although the regulation of enzymatic activity and expression of the various isoforms of heme oxygenase (HO-1 and HO-2) have been extensively studied in a variety of mammalian organs for over 30 years, it was not until the early 1990s that scientists began to investigate the specific role of this enzyme and its products in the cardiovascular system. The putative signal transduction mechanism of vasorelaxation involving the activation of soluble guanylate cyclase by NO and CO[20,33] was proposed and circumstantial evidence for participation of the heme oxygenase pathway in the control of blood pressure was reported.[34]

Sacerdoti and colleagues observed that treatment of 7-week-old spontaneously hypertensive rats with stannous chloride, a potent inducer of heme oxygenase activity that is selective for the kidney, dramatically reduced the elevation of blood pressure typical in these young animals.[34] This striking effect was associated with a significant increase in renal heme oxygenase activity and reduction of both cytochrome P-450 (a heme-dependent protein) levels and arachidonic acid metabolite formation in the treated rats. Metabolites of arachidonic acid have the potential to alter blood pressure by affecting vascular tone and Na/K-ATPase. The data indicated that depletion of renal cytochrome P-450 by increased heme oxygenase in the kidney limited the production of these vasoconstrictor agents, thereby producing an anti-hypertensive effect. Retrospectively, this elegant study overlooked any direct contribution of heme oxygenase products in the observed effect, possibly because strong indications of the signaling properties of exogenous CO in vessels became apparent a few years later.[20]

Similar reports showed that heme oxygenase might be actively involved in the modulation of pressor responses. Administration of the heme oxygenase inhibitor, zinc deuteroporphyrin 2,4-bis glycol, into conscious rats produced significant increases in mean arterial pressure and total peripheral resistance, and decreased cardiac output without affecting heart rate.[35] Since infusion of biliverdin had no effect on arterial blood pressure in these animals, the data indicate that intracellular CO may affect pressor mechanisms mediated by the autonomic nervous system. Similarly, in spontaneously hypertensive rats, treatment with heme derivatives that stimulate the formation of heme oxygenase products elicited an antihypertensive effect[36]; the involvement of free iron was excluded in this model by showing that pre-treatment with deferoxamine did not influence the vasodepressive action mediated by heme.

The circumstantial evidence indicating a role for CO in the vasculature was supported by direct detection of this gas in biological systems[37]; this was reinforced by measurements of heme oxygenase activity in endothelial and smooth muscle cells and by localization of heme oxygenase isoforms in these types of tissues. Heme oxygenase activity, determined as CO production, has been reported in rat and rabbit aortas as well as in the human inferior mesenteric arteries.[38-40] Immunohistochemistry analysis revealed the presence of HO-2 and HO-1 proteins in bovine pulmonary arteries and veins, which correlated with heme oxygenase activity.[41] Enzymatic activity was found in the adventitia and medial layers of arteries, and protein isoforms were localized in the vasa vasorum of the adventitia and throughout the smooth muscle cells in the medial layer. Increased heme oxygenase activity has been detected in aortic endothelial cells in culture after exposure to heme or various forms of hemoglobins.[42-44]

Heme oxygenase activity and CO production were also found in smooth muscle cells after exposure to low oxygen tension.[21] This effect was associated with a significant increase in intracellular cGMP, which was abolished by a specific heme oxygenase inhibitor but remained unaltered by blockade of the NO synthase pathway. These data demonstrate that vascular cells generate CO in normal conditions and have the ability to markedly increase the production of CO when the inducible heme oxygenase system (HO-1) is appropriately stimulated.

The first evidence reporting the contribution of endogenously generated CO in the regulation of vascular function can be attributed to Suematsu and collaborators, who designed experiments to elucidate whether heme oxygenase-derived CO can serve as an active vasorelaxant in the hepatic microcirculation.[45,46] Using a model of isolated liver perfusion, they found that CO flux, directly measured in the venous effluent by trapping the gas with myoglobin, is in the order of 0.7 nmol/min/gr of tissue. Administration of low concentrations of zinc protoporphyrin IX (a heme oxygenase inhibitor) completely abrogated baseline CO production and caused significant vascular resistance associated with sinusoidal constriction and reduction of sinusoidal perfusion velocity. These effects were considerably attenuated by infusion of CO gas (1 μM) into the perfusate or by addition of a cGMP analogue, suggesting the involvement of the guanylate cyclase pathway in the signaling process. Interestingly, NO synthase inhibitors applied to this model did not have any effect on vascular resistance or sinusoidal hemodynamics. As these data were obtained in livers in a steady-state condition, it appears that the effect elicited by endogenously generated CO originates from constitutively expressed heme oxygenase (HO-2) or from HO-1 that is not maximally up-regulated. This is sustained by subsequent findings showing that distribution of the two enzymatic isoforms in rat liver has a distinct topographic pattern, with HO-1 present only in Kupffer cells and HO-2 localized in parenchymal cells but absent in hepatic stellate cells and sinusoidal endothelial cells.[47]

A contribution of constitutive HO-2 in regulating the diameters of resistance vessels has also been investigated by examining the effects of inhibitors of heme oxygenase in large and small arteries as well as in arterioles.[48] The important finding is that both descending aorta and gracilis muscle arterioles express HO-2 but not HO-1 protein. Furthermore, two different heme oxygenase inhibitors were shown to decrease the diameters of pressurized gracilis muscle arterioles. Although this might indicate a role for CO in the regulation of basal tone in resistance vessels, interpretation of the data is limited by the fact that a possible contribution of the NO pathway in this system has not been explored.

Zakhary and colleagues[49] detected prominent staining for HO-2 in the endothelium of blood vessels and evaluated a role for this constitutive enzyme in the control of vascular reactivity. In porcine distal pulmonary arteries, acetylcholine caused endothelium-dependent relaxation via both NO-dependent and -independent mechanisms. Specifically, concentrations of tin protoporphyrin IX that do not affect NOS activity inhibit the NO-independent component of relaxation with potency resembling the inhibition of heme oxygenase. Although the authors did not actually measure CO production in these vessels, they suggested that a heme oxygenase product, presumably CO, could function as an endothelium-derived relaxing factor. The authors also proposed that CO might act as an endogenous vasodilator when its concentration is sufficiently high or, alternatively, when endogenous production of NO is low.

In view of the known affinity of guanylate cyclase for NO, which is much higher compared to that for CO, these findings suggest that under normal physiological conditions it is unlikely that CO generated from constitutive HO-2 plays a major role in the regulation of vessel tone. This should not be emphasized too strongly as it cannot be excluded *a priori* that CO acts as a more prominent vasodilator in vessels with smaller diameters, in which relaxation following muscarinic cholinergic stimulation is resistant to reversal by NOS inhibitors. Nevertheless, as described in detail below, the effect of CO on vascular reactivity can become more prominent when the endogenous production of CO and, consequently, heme oxygenase activity are highly intensified.[23]

In contrast to HO-2 that generates only limited amounts of CO, up-regulation of HO-1 can result in substantial production of CO, provided that substrate heme is promptly available. Wang and colleagues demonstrated that relaxation of pre-contracted isolated rat tail artery with exogenous CO involves the activation of both cyclic GMP pathways and big conductance K_{Ca} channels.[50] Interestingly, phenylephrine-mediated contraction of tail arteries was suppressed in a concentration- and time-dependent manner by pre-incubation with hemin. The effect on vascular contractility mediated by hemin was abolished by incubation of arteries with either oxyhemoglobin or zinc protoporphyrin IX. This was the first report indicating that heme, substrate and potent inducer of HO-1 expression, can be utilized by vascular tissue to attenuate vessel contractility presumably via a product that is dependent on activation/induction of the heme oxygenase pathway.

In 1998, our laboratory reported that pre-treatment of isolated aortas *in vitro* with the NO-releasing agent, S-nitroso-N-acetyl penicillamine (SNAP), results in a rapid and marked induction of HO-1 mRNA and protein expression.[23] HO-1 protein, which was maximally expressed 5 h after SNAP treatment, was localized primarily in the endothelial layer and to a lesser extent in the smooth muscle cells. When vessels displaying high HO-1 expression were placed in an organ bath, phenylephrine failed to elicit vasoconstriction, an effect that was completely restored by pre-incubation with tin protoporphyrin IX but not with NO synthase inhibitors. Most importantly, SNAP-treated vessels were shown to generate significantly higher amounts of CO compared to untreated aortas as assessed by quantification of ^{14}CO released after loading tissues with [2-^{14}C]-L-glycine, a heme precursor. Predictably, the increased generation of CO was accompanied by a marked elevation in cGMP levels. These data revealed that, once HO-1 is highly up-regulated, vascular CO production is significantly augmented and contributes more than NO to the regulation of vessel contractility. These findings also highlight the importance of NO and NO derivatives as potent activators of the heme oxygenase system in the vasculature[23,51-57] and emphasize the pivotal role of heme oxygenase products in the modulation of NO synthase activity and function.[58-61]

As several lines of evidence point to the crucial role of inducible nitric oxide synthase (iNOS)-derived NO in diseases such as septic and hemorrhagic shock,[62-65] myocardial ischemia–reperfusion,[66] and inflammation,[67] it is clear that HO-1 induction as a consequence of increased NO production in the cardiovascular system may have important clinical and pharmacological implications.[68-73] Studies in our and others' laboratories are ongoing to unravel the biological significance of the interaction between NO and the heme oxygenase pathway[61] (see also Chapter 6).

The direct involvement of CO in governing vascular activities depends upon the concentration of CO locally generated by the activity of heme oxygenases and consequently by the expression of the two major isozymes. It is interesting that the action of CO may also be facilitated by migration of the heme oxygenase complex. In the lamb ductus arteriosus, HO-1 and HO-2 proteins were localized in endothelial and muscle cells, whereas HO-2 was confined to the muscle.[74] Within the muscle cells, HO-1 and HO-2 immunoreactivities appear to be limited to the perinuclear region and the Golgi apparatus. Upon exposure to endotoxin, HO-1 becomes more abundant and both isoforms are translocated to outer regions where the product CO can more easily diffuse to extracellular targets.

Of major importance is the observation that CO formation does not reach a threshold for a vasodilatory effect in the ductus arteriosus either at normal or reduced pO_2, unless the vessel is exposed to substances (endotoxins or bradykinins) that promote induction/activation of both HO isoforms. These data point to a major participation of CO in intracellular signaling mechanisms under conditions whereby the heme oxygenase pathway is maximally activated, and they reveal the dynamic features of these isozymes as well as their versatility in controlling vascular contractility. This is an important concept that finds its best example in conditions where stimulation of heme oxygenase is required to mediate a distinct physiological phenomenon or reverse a pathophysiological state. For instance, increased heme oxygenase activity and CO production are found in human pregnant myometrium and treatment with hemin completely inhibits spontaneous myometrial contraction. The fact that tin protoporphyrin IX inhibits CO production in this system suggests that this gas may limit uterine contractility and that heme oxygenase may play a role in maintenance of the quiescent state of the uterus during pregnancy.[75]

Induction of HO-1 and the consequent increase in the rate of CO production in vascular tissues have been shown to affect vessel contractility and blood pressure *in vitro*. In an attempt to study the mechanisms underlying the well known vasoconstrictor properties of cell-free hemoglobin solutions, it was found that failure to promote acute hypertension in rats transfused with αα-cross-linked hemoglobin coincided with transient HO-1 expression and increased heme oxygenase activity in aortic tissue, liver, and heart due to surgical stress.[76,77]

Interestingly, in rats displaying elevated tissue HO-1, mean arterial pressure remained unchanged even following infusion of an NOS inhibitor L-nitro-arginine methyl ester (L-NAME). Pre-treatment of these animals with zinc protoporphyrin IX restored the ability of either hemoglobin or L-NAME to increase blood pressure at the time HO-1 was maximally up-regulated in the vasculature. The results of this study are consistent with the hypothesis that HO-1, once stimulated, can actively utilize heme as substrate for CO production, resulting in the control of pressor responses. This hypothesis is sustained by the findings that stress-mediated induction of tissue heme oxygenase was associated with: (1) increased CO and cGMP production in aortic tissue; (2) accelerated metabolism of heme, as measured by an increased rate of plasma hemoglobin disappearance; and (3) increased excretion of urinary bilirubin, the end product of heme catabolism. The increase in aortic CO and the augmented catabolism of heme were both significantly attenuated by pre-treatment of animals with zinc protoporphyrin IX. In addition, CO release, aortic cGMP, and urinary bilirubin returned to basal levels when heme oxygenase activity returned to normal values.

These data strongly suggest that, in conditions of maximal expression of the HO-1 gene, the signaling properties of CO may prevail over the action mediated by NO. Their chemical differences (NO is a free radical; CO is not) and the recent evidence supporting a direct regulatory role of heme oxygenase products on NO function[61] may partly explain this intriguing observation.

Consistent with the hypothesis that the HO-1/CO pathway regulates pressor responses *in vivo* are the findings that HO-1 mRNA and protein expression are highly up-regulated in rat aortas following hypertension induced by angiotensin II[78] and in genetically hypertensive rats.[79] Increased HO-1 protein in both large and small blood vessels by endotoxin has also been found to contribute to the reduction of vascular tone associated with septic shock.[80]

Recent studies confirmed a direct involvement of overproduced CO and its predominance in the regulation of vascular function compared to NO. In perfused rat livers, overexpression of hepatic HO-1 resulted in a marked increase in venous CO flux and a reduction of basal resistance.[81] The reduction in resistance was abolished by administration of oxyhemoglobin, which scavenges both CO and NO, but not by methemoglobin, which captures only NO. In addition, livers overexpressing HO-1 became less sensitive to endothelin-1-mediated vasoconstriction than control livers through mechanisms involving CO. Hepatic arterial and portal venous vascular resistance appears instead to be differentially regulated by NO and CO.

In the normal rat liver *in vivo*, NO serves as a potent vasodilator in the hepatic arterial circulation, but exerts only a minor vasodilatory effect in the portal venous vascular bed.[82] In contrast, while there is no intrinsic CO-mediated vasodilatation in the hepatic artery, CO acts to maintain portal venous vascular tone in a relaxed state. It is conceivable that the precise biological activities of CO and/or NO may be dictated in defined tissues by local oxygen concentration, which is known to dramatically affect the bioavailability and signal transduction properties of NO in the form of S-NO-hemoglobin.[83]

Although the effect of tissue pO_2 on the vasodilatory action of endogenous CO awaits investigation, it is intriguing that the HO-1 gene is highly up-regulated in vascular cells exposed to reduced oxygen tension[21,57,84] and that both NO and S-nitrosothiols are regulators of this induction.[57] Most recently, a role for HO-1-derived CO in attenuating aortic and renal vasoreactivity following chronic hypoxia has been postulated.[85,86] It is expected that more refined measurements of CO generated within the vasculature[87] under physiological or pathophysiological conditions, and the possible identification of new intracellular targets, will improve our understanding of the exact vascular function of this biologically active molecule.

III. CARBON MONOXIDE IN THE HEART: ROLE OF HEME OXYGENASE IN THE MITIGATION OF MYOCARDIAL ISCHEMIA/REPERFUSION INJURY

A 1975 report by Scharf and colleagues[9] examined the myocardial function of isolated dog hearts following exposure of the animals to hypoxic hypoxia (5 to 10% O_2) or CO hypoxia (200 to 250 ppm CO). Not surprisingly, the responses to these stimuli consisted of an increase in coronary flow and a decrease in coronary vascular resistance. More specifically, coronary blood flow increased far less with hypoxic hypoxia than with CO and the increase in oxygen consumption was slightly greater with hypoxic than with CO hypoxia. Interestingly, when cardiac muscle cells in culture are grown in the presence of a mixture of CO (10 to 20%) and O_2 (10 to

20%) for prolonged periods, the growth rate of these cells is comparable to that of control cells.[88] Moreover, cardiomyocytes maintained their contractile activities when exposed to 20% CO and the structures of both myofibrils and mitochondria were well preserved.

These *ex vivo* data appear to indicate that: (1) the effect of CO on cardiac muscle performance relies on mechanisms controlling vascular contractility similar to those described earlier for other types of blood vessels; and (2) myocardial tissue can tolerate the exposure to relatively high concentrations of CO without affecting the growth of cardiomyocytes. Despite the fact that muscle tissue is metabolically active and contains a substantial number of mitochondria and abundant myoglobin that could be preferential targets for an undesired action of CO, the possibility that heme oxygenase-derived CO has a significant role in regulating important biological processes within cardiac cells deserves consideration. An analysis of the available data will allow us to touch on various aspects of the physiological role of heme oxygenases in the myocardium.

The induction of rat hepatic heme oxygenase by trace metals such as cobalt has been known for more than 25 years.[89] In 1976, this effect was seen to extend to other organs including the heart, which displayed reduced microsomal and mito-chondrial content of hemoproteins.[90] Regulation of cardiac heme oxygenase by cobalt was also examined in the rabbit heart and enzymatic activity was found in both ventricular and atrial microsomal fractions.[91] Similarly, expression of heme oxygenase mRNA was elevated in both ventricles after exposing rats to hypoxia for 3 days.[92] HO-1 and HO-2 mRNA induction and other heat shock proteins (HSPs) were studied in rats exposed to hyperthermia.[93] Unlike HSP70 and HSP27 which showed discordant patterns of tissue expression, HO-1 mRNA (but not HO-2) was expressed in a coordinated manner in the heart and all other organs examined. In another report, over-expression of cardiac HO-1 mRNA induced by heat shock correlated with a rapid increase in HO-1 protein and heme oxygenase activity.[94] Interestingly, the elevation in heme oxygenase activity caused by hyperthermia was accompanied by an increase in cardiac cGMP, which occurred in the absence of altered NOS activity. These early data indicate that heme oxygenase activity is present in the myocardium and suggest that, under stress conditions, HO-1 and its products may contribute to increased demand for messenger production in the cardiovascular system.

Studies conducted by Sharma and colleagues[95-98] revealed that the HO-1 gene is up-regulated by subjecting hearts to ischemia/reperfusion events. In a porcine model, in which the left anterior descending coronary artery was repeatedly occluded and reperfused, HO-1 mRNA expression was highly increased[95] and similar results were found in reperfused isolated rat hearts following a brief period of ischemia.[97] Immunohistochemical analysis of rat hearts after 1-h reperfusion demonstrated a moderate staining for HO-1 protein in cardiomyocytes and intense immunoreactivity in the perivascular regions of blood vessels.

In a subsequent study by the same group,[98] inhibitors of heme oxygenase and NOS activities were used to examine a role for cGMP in protection against myo-cardial ischemia/reperfusion injury. It was found that both the heme oxygenase and

NOS pathways contribute to the maintenance of hemodynamic parameters at reperfusion, and that CO and NO are likely to play an interactive role in this modulatory effect. Although circumstantial, the evidence that CO may be directly involved in the preservation of myocardial function started to attract investigators, and more work has been done to ascertain the contribution of the heme oxygenase pathway in protection of cardiac tissue against oxidative stress.

In primary cultures of rat neonatal cardiomyocytes, HO-1 protein expression was detected 12 h after isolation and this effect coincided with a major change in the glutathione redox state.[99] Exposure of myocyte-enriched cultures of rat heart cells to hypoxia or anoxia resulted in increased HO-1 mRNA expression,[100,101] whereas HO-2 protein levels remained unaltered. Interestingly, the hypoxia-mediated HO-1 stimulation was significantly attenuated by the glutathione precursor, N-acetyl-L-cysteine, suggesting that oxidative stress reactions involving glutathione are responsible for the induction of cardiac HO-1 gene.[101]

Raju and Maines reported an unprecedented finding on the intimate link between kidney and heart function in relation to expression of the HO-1 gene.[102] They showed that ischemia/reperfusion in rat kidney caused by occlusion of the renal artery *in vivo* is translated into a response in the cardiovascular system; this was reflected by increased cardiac HO-1 transcription, protein, and enzymatic activity, all of which remained elevated for more than 24 h after the ischemic event. Once again, this effect was accompanied by augmented intracellular cGMP concentrations in the heart with no increase in NOS activity. That study implied that the increased availability of hemoglobin-heme which results from ischemic insults to the kidneys could lead to a cGMP-mediated vasodilatory action in the myocardium. The observation that HO-1 over-expression was confined to the perivascular region is consistent with this hypothesis.

Sharma and colleagues found that, in the stunned porcine myocardium, HO-1 transcript and immunoreactivity are highly pronounced in the cytoplasm of cardiomyocytes as well as in the perivascular region.[103] Thus, it is possible that the ensuing increased CO production capacity in the heart may activate sensory components in control of vascular tone and, therefore, regulate the myocardial adaptive response to ischemia. The fact that HO-1 mRNA is highly expressed in the cardiac ventricles of spontaneously hypertensive rats[79] and in hearts in response to chronic administration of angiotensin II[104] supports the notion that the endogenous HO-1/CO system is an active component of the signal transduction mechanisms in this organ.

The induction of the HO-1 gene and consequent increased generation of its products, bilirubin and CO, are now regarded as a refined system to counteract oxidative and nitrosative stress in a diversity of tissues.[61] Activation of this pathway may represent an expedient to prevent or reverse myocardial dysfunction during the development of many pathological states that affect the cardiovascular system. If a biological role for HO-1 in protecting the heart against various forms of stress is postulated, then the effects of increased CO and bilirubin should be clearly established. Our group has attempted to address this important point by examining a direct link between cardiac HO-1 induction and endogenous bilirubin production in the ischemic rat heart.[105] Bilirubin is a naturally occurring potent antioxidant and is produced intracellularly in a 1:1 ratio with CO. Our studies revealed that up-regulation of the HO-1 gene by treatment of animals with hemin 24 h prior to ischemia ameliorates myocardial dysfunction and reduces infarct size upon reperfusion of isolated hearts. Increased cardiac HO-1 expression and heme oxygenase activity were associated with enhanced tissue bilirubin content and increased rate of bilirubin release into the perfusion buffer. Tin protoporphyrin IX completely abolished the improved postischemic myocardial performance and exacerbated cardiac tissue injury after heminmediated HO-1 induction. Interestingly, the addition of bilirubin (100 nM final concentration) to the perfusion buffer prior to ischemia significantly restored myocardial function and minimized both infarct size and mitochondrial damage upon reperfusion.

These data provide strong evidence for a primary role of HO-1-derived bilirubin in cardioprotection against reperfusion injury. In addition, as the rise in coronary perfusion pressure was significantly less pronounced in post-ischemic cardiac tissue expressing high levels of HO-1, these results also indicate that increased endogenous CO plays a role in the maintenance of vascular tone during the reperfusion of ischemic hearts.

Recent evidence supports the cardioprotective effect of HO-1 gene activation prior to ischemia-reperfusion *in vivo*.[106] In line with the concept that stimulation of the HO-1 system may be a necessary step to mitigate vascular dysfunction in humans, a few intriguing reports show an inverse correlation between plasma bilirubin levels and the risk of coronary artery disease.[107,108] In addition, the severe and persistent vascular damage that characterized the first human case of HO-1 deficiency is the best direct example of the essential function of the HO-1 gene in the vessel wall.[109]

The role of HO-1 in counteracting the pathophysiological consequence of myocardial dysfunction is not confined to ischemia/reperfusion injury and can be extended to other vascular complications. In a canine model of right-sided congestive heart failure, HO-1 transcript and protein significantly increased in the right, but not the left, ventricle and, as previously reported for other organ models, no changes in NOS activity and HO-2 expression were observed.[110] The increase in HO-1 in the failing ventricle was accompanied by an increase in cGMP levels and was simulated by norepinephrine infusion, which is known to be elevated in the failing myocardium. This differential regulation of HO-1 induction might be a defensive mechanism to protect cardiac tissue from stress caused by congestive heart failure.

In the diabetic myocardium, abnormalities in gene expression involve changes in the mRNA content for HO-1, which is markedly increased 4 weeks after induction of diabetes in rats by treatment with streptozotocin; this effect is consistently prevented by insulin treatment.[111] Up-regulation of HO-1 and increased heme oxygenase activity in isolated hearts from both non-diabetic and diabetic rats was found following ischemia/reperfusion. This induction was related to the occurrence of ventricular fibrillation with down-regulation of both HO-1 and enzymatic activity associated with post-ischemic ventricular fibrillation.[112]

These data indicate that HO-1 can be selectively and differentially regulated, depending on the type of biochemical and hemodynamic consequence originating from a defined stressful stimulus. In a model of mouse cardiac xenograft transplantation into rats, the expression of the HO-1 gene is functionally associated with preservation of myocardial activities and long-term (>60 days) graft survival.[113]

Mouse hearts lacking the HO-1 gene and transplanted into rats were rejected 3 to 4 days after transplantation, primarily due to: (1) vascular thrombosis associated with platelet aggregates expressing P-selectin; (2) infiltration by activated host leukocytes; and (3) widespread apoptosis of endothelial cells and cardiomyocytes. Similarly, in a model of cardiac allograft transplantation, long-term survival and prevention of atherosclerosis appeared to coincide with the expression of vascular antioxidant and anti-apoptotic genes, including HO-1.[114]

Although the mechanism by which HO-1 protects cardiac muscle from being rejected remains to be fully established, the possibility that the antiinflammatory properties of heme oxygenase-derived CO contribute to this effect has been postulated.[115] The antiinflammatory action of HO-1 may also rely on the increased production of both biliverdin and bilirubin as these bile pigments have been shown to suppress venular leukocyte adhesion, inhibit the expression of P- and E-selectin in the vasculature by oxidative stress,[116,117] and prevent monocyte transmigration induced by mildly oxidized LDL in human aortic endothelial cells.[118]

Thus, the concerted and/or synergistic actions of CO and bilirubin in the cardiovascular system appear to reflect the versatile biological role of HO-1 as both intracellular defensive weapon and modulator of physiological processes during the progression of various vascular dysfunctions.[119] Consequently, therapeutic strategies to exploit the beneficial properties of heme oxygenase should be rigorously designed and optimized. At least two approaches can be envisioned: (1) targeted and selective up-regulation of the HO-1 protein either by genetic or pharmacological means[120-123]; and (2) delivery of heme degradation products to organs and tissues that require bilirubin and/or CO to timely counteract stressful stimuli. In the past few years, our laboratory has been working on a group of substances that have the potential to release CO in biological systems; the next paragraphs will describe in detail the findings related to these compounds.

IV. USE OF TRANSITION METAL CARBONYLS AS CARBON MONOXIDE-RELEASING MOLECULES

A. Chemistry of Transition Metal Carbonyls

Carbon monoxide is the most common π-acceptor ligand in organometallic chemistry. This feature of CO is best exemplified in transition metal carbonyl complexes, compounds that contain a heavy metal such as nickel, cobalt, or iron surrounded by carbonyl (CO) groups as coordinated ligands.[124] These chemicals are useful as precursors to many other organometallic complexes as the bonding of the carbonyl to the metal center activates in such a way that it can undergo organic chemistry which otherwise would be difficult. Consequently, they are used in the preparation of metals of exceptionally high purity and as catalysts in organic syntheses. Some common metal carbonyls include tetracarbonylnickel [$Ni(CO)_4$], octacarbonyldicobalt [$Co_2(CO)_8$], iron pentacarbonyl [$Fe(CO)_5$] and dimanganese decacarbonyl [$Mn_2(CO)_{10}$].

The electronic structures of most metal carbonyls containing one metal atom per molecule (mononuclear carbonyls) bear striking resemblance to the structures of noble gas elements; they are typically saturated 18-electron species and thus relatively inert. However, certain spectator ligands in a metal complex can promote dissociation of CO sterically or electronically. Several papers have demonstrated that following introduction of a π-donor ligand into the metal complex, the CO group tends to be labilized.[125-127] Interestingly, formation of metal-centered radicals from dinuclear metal carbonyl complexes upon exposure to light has been reported[128] and dissociation of CO from these compounds has long been recognized as an alternative primary photoprocess.[129,130]

Photodissociation and consequent elimination of CO groups from metal carbonyls is a function of the intensity and wavelength of the irradiating light, and the general equation for this reaction can be written as follows:

$$M_x(CO)_n \underset{k'}{\overset{hv}{\rightleftharpoons}} M_x(CO)_{n-1} + CO$$

where M is the transition metal, hv is the irradiating light and k' is the rate constant for recombination of the metal with CO. For each CO group that dissociates or is released from these molecules, a defined energy is required to cleave the bond with the metal center. Several studies have been conducted to determine the strength of this CO-metal interaction in a variety of compounds.[131] The CO loss process has been observed in a flash photolysis study of ethanol solutions of $Mn_2(CO)_{10}$ which results in a relatively long-lived transient absorption product ($\lambda_{max} = 480$ nm) characterized as $Mn_2(CO)_9$ or an ethanol adduct of $Mn_2(CO)_9$.[132] Further studies using time-resolved infrared spectroscopy confirmed that, following irradiation of $Mn_2(CO)_{10}$, a thermally unstable species is formed and designated $Mn_2(CO)_9$.[133] These results constitute considerable evidence that dissociation of CO occurs as an alternative process to metal–metal bond homolysis upon irradiation of $Mn_2(CO)_{10}$.

Although all the studies on the chemistry of carbonyl complexes have been conducted in organic solvents, we decided to examine the abilities of certain metal carbonyls to release CO in aqueous solutions and investigate whether these substances promote physiological responses *in vitro*. The development of carriers of CO with physiological bioactivities that resemble those elicited by NO-releasing agents would facilitate the research in the heme oxygenase/CO field and enable scientists to address important questions related to the chemistry of CO and its intracellular interaction with important structural and functional targets. Moreover, the synthesis of compounds that specifically release known concentrations of CO to targeted organs or tissues should provide an elegant tool to simulate the action of heme oxygenase-derived CO. Thus, can transition metal carbonyls act as CO-releasing molecules (CO-RMs) in biological systems?

B. DETECTION OF CO FROM CO-RMS

Iron pentacarbonyl ($Fe(CO)_5$, 99.9%) and dimanganese decacarbonyl ($Mn_2(CO)_{10}$, 13 mM in DMSO) were first selected as transition metal carbonyls to act as CO-RMs. This choice was based on the fact that both iron and manganese are vital constituents of plant and animal life; they are commonly found in enzymes and proteins. The release of CO from metal carbonyl complexes was assessed spectro-photometrically by measuring the conversion of deoxymyoglobin (deoxy-Mb) to carbonmonoxymyoglobin (MbCO). Since CO loss from $Fe(CO)_5$ and $Mn_2(CO)_{10}$ occurs only by photodissociation, the release of CO was induced by continuously exposing CO-RMs to a cold light source and allowing the gas to diffuse through a membrane before reacting with myoglobin, using a modification of a device previously described.[23,77]

A CO-RM (500 μl) was placed in a plastic tube and a cell culture insert was sealed at the top to create two separate chambers; 1.5 ml of deoxy-Mb solution (66 μM final concentration in 0.04 M phosphate buffer, pH 6.8) was placed in the insert, which was then covered with parafilm. Aliquots of the myoglobin solution were taken from the insert at different times for assessment of the spectrum.

As shown in Figure 14.1A, MbCO (trace a) is rapidly formed with a distinctive absorption spectrum between 500 and 600 nm when deoxy-Mb (trace b) is reacted with CO gas. Interestingly, a very similar pattern is observed when a CO-RM is irradiated for 1 h with light, thus confirming the release of CO from these compounds (Figure 14.1B and C). In addition, changes at 540 nm (maximal absorbance for MbCO) were used to quantify the amount of CO liberated by $[Mn(CO)_{10}]$ over time (Figure 14.1C).

These novel data reveal that transition metal carbonyls release CO in aqueous solutions when appropriately stimulated and, therefore, could be tested as CO-RMs in biological systems. As no studies have been conducted in this respect, it must be emphasized that these experiments were initially performed to evaluate the potential of exploiting these molecules as CO carriers, with full awareness of their likely cytotoxic effect if used at relatively high concentrations. Since we noticed that exposure of $Fe(CO)_5$ to light rapidly resulted in deposition of a green–brown precipitate, possibly iron metal, we decided to abandon the studies on this metal carbonyl.

In the case of $Mn_2(CO)_{10}$, no visible precipitate was observed, and preliminary studies on the use of this compound revealed no major cytotoxicity on endothelial cells after exposure for 24 h to low concentrations (0 to 100 μM). Therefore, our subsequent experiments were conducted using $Mn_2(CO)_{10}$ to explore a possible biological activity of this specific CO-RM.

C. Biological Activity of CO-RMs

Isolated rat heart preparation was used as an experimental model to examine the vasodilatory properties of $Mn_2(CO)_{10}$. Hearts from male Lewis rats were perfused according to the Langendorff method.[105] The hearts were excised, the aortas cannulated, and retrograde perfusion was established at a constant flow of 15 ml/min using Krebs–Henseleit buffer bubbled with 95% O_2 and 5% CO_2 at 37°C (pH 7.4). Coronary perfusion pressure (CPP), a parameter of coronary vessel contractility, was continuously measured by a pressure transducer connected to the aortic cannula and data analyzed with AcqKnowledge software. Hearts were initially equilibrated for 20 min on the Langendorff apparatus and then perfused with the NOS inhibitor, L-nitro-arginine methyl ester (L-NAME, 25 μM), to elicit vasoconstriction. The extent

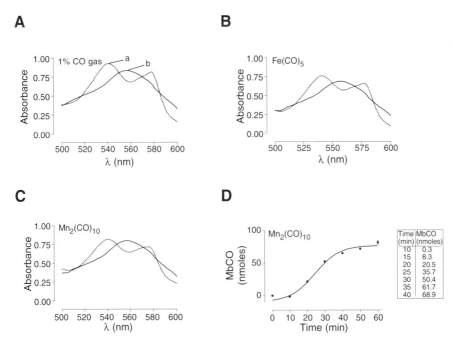

FIGURE 14.1 Detection of CO released from CO-releasing molecules (CO-RMs). The conversion of deoxy-myoglobin (deoxy-Mb, 66 µM in phosphate buffer, pH 7.4) to carbon monoxide–myoglobin (MbCO) measured spectrophotometrically was used as an index of CO release. (A) Spectra showing the formation of MbCO (trace a) from deoxy-Mb (trace b) after bubbling the myoglobin solution with 1% CO gas for 45 s. (B) Release of CO from iron pentacarbonyl [Fe(CO)₅] after exposing the transition metal carbonyl complex for 1 h to light. (C) Release of CO from dimanganese decacarbonyl [Mn₂(CO)₁₀] after exposing the transition metal carbonyl complex to light. (D) Quantification of the amount of CO released from Mn₂(CO)₁₀ over time measured as MbCO.

of CPP increase by L-NAME was monitored over time and the data are reported in Figure 14.2 (control).

In a second group, hearts were perfused with buffer supplemented with Mn₂(CO)₁₀ (13 µM final concentration) prior to L-NAME infusion and changes in CPP monitored over time. Since [Mn₂(CO)₁₀] releases CO only by photodissociation, Krebs buffer containing Mn₂(CO)₁₀ was exposed to a cold light source immediately before passing through the aortic cannula. As shown, treatment with Mn₂(CO)₁₀ significantly delayed the increase in CPP caused by L-NAME and maintained CPP at much lower levels compared to controls at the end of the experiment (Figure 14.2).

When the buffer containing Mn₂(CO)₁₀ was not subjected to light exposure, thus omitting the light-induced CO release, the increase in CPP mediated by L-NAME was found to be similar to controls; in addition, manganese chloride (negative control) had no effect on CPP (data not shown). These results demonstrate that Mn₂(CO)₁₀ attenuates vasoconstriction in the heart via delivery of CO from this specific CO-RM. Notably, the effect mediated by CO-RM was simulated by

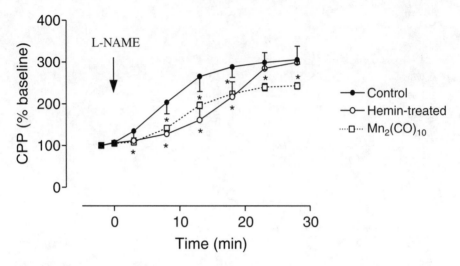

FIGURE 14.2 Effect of CO-RMs on coronary perfusion pressure in isolated rat heart. The vasoconstrictor L-nitro-arginine methyl ester (L-NAME) was added to the perfusion buffer (25 µ*M* final concentration) and changes in coronary perfusion pressure (CPP) were monitored over time in untreated hearts (control), hearts displaying high levels of heme oxygenase-1 (hemin-treated), and hearts perfused with a CO-RM [$Mn_2(CO)_{10}$, 13 µ*M* final concentration]. Each line represents the mean ± SEM of five experiments; *$p < 0.05$ vs. control.

increased production of endogenous CO. In fact, the increase in CPP mediated by L-NAME was markedly attenuated in hearts from hemin-treated animals (see Figure 14.2, hemin-treated group) characterized by elevated cardiac HO-1 expression and increased heme oxygenase activity.[105] These unprecedented findings concerning the vasodilatory action of $Mn_2(CO)_{10}$ in relation to its inherent property to carry and release CO in cardiac tissues should be viewed as the basis for the development of other CO-RMs with specific biological activities.

V. CONCLUSIONS

Substantial experimental evidence sustaining a role for the heme oxygenase/CO pathway in the control of cardiovascular functions has been collected. However, more work is necessary to unequivocally establish whether the heme oxygenase system is an important factor in the amelioration and prevention of vascular dysfunction. Further investigation is required to unravel the mechanisms of HO-1 regulation in cardiac and vascular tissue during the progression of pathophysiological states. How heme oxygenase can be finely modulated prior to or after a specific challenge to tissues and to what extent the products of this pathway can participate in the control of cellular homeostasis and restoration of functional activities remain to be assessed.

As both bilirubin and CO appear to be equally important to fully justify an active biological role for heme oxygenases, a major effort should be made to engineer molecules that will enable scientists to determine the exact role of heme oxygenase products and define their specific targets within the cells. To this end, the use of molecules that carry and timely deliver CO in a very selective fashion (CO-RMs) would certainly facilitate this task. Developing CO-RMs with different chemical stabilities and controlled rates of CO release and making them more compatible with the cellular environment will aid in the design of drugs that can function as alternatives to or in combination with NO-releasing agents for the cure of vascular disease, amelioration of post-ischemic myocardial activities, and regression of other pathophysiological states.

ACKNOWLEDGMENTS

We are grateful to Dr. James Clark for expert technical assistance. This work was supported by grants from the British Heart Foundation (PG/99005 to R.M. and PG/2000047 to R.F.), the National Heart Research Fund (to R.M.), the National Kidney Research Fund (R30/1/99 to R.M.), the Dunhill Medical Trust, and the Northwick Park Institute for Medical Research.

REFERENCES

1. Piantadosi, C.A., Toxicity of carbon monoxide: hemoglobins vs. histotoxic mechanisms, in *Carbon Monoxide,* Penney, D.G., Ed., CRC Press, Boca Raton, FL, 1996, Chap. 8.
2. Sjostrand, T., Endogenous formation of carbon monoxide in man under normal and pathological conditions, *Scand. J. Clin. Lab. Invest.,* 1, 201, 1949.
3. Coburn, R.F., Blakemore, W.S., and Forster, R.E., Endogenous carbon monoxide production in man, *J. Clin. Invest.,* 42, 1172, 1963.
4. Coburn, R.F., Williams, W.J., and Forster, R.E., Effect of erythrocyte destruction on carbon monxide production in man, *J. Clin. Invest.,* 43, 1098, 1964.
5. Coburn, R.F., Williams, W.J., and Kahn, S.B., Endogenous carbon monoxide production in patients with hemolytic anemia, *J. Clin. Invest.,* 45, 460, 1966.
6. Sjostrand, T., The formation of carbon monoxide by *in vitro* decomposition of haemoglobin in bile pigments, *Acta Physiol. Scand.,* 26, 328, 1952.
7. Coburn, R.F. et al., The production of carbon monoxide from hemoglobin *in vivo*, *J. Clin. Invest.,* 46, 346, 1967.
8. Tenhunen, R., Marver, H.S., and Schmid, R., Microsomal heme oxygenase. Characterization of the enzyme, *J. Biol. Chem.,* 244, 6388, 1969.
9. Scharf, S.M., Permutt, S., and Bromberger–Barnea, B., Effects of hypoxic and CO hypoxia on isolated hearts, *J. Appl. Physiol.,* 39, 752, 1975.
10. Shibahara, S. et al., Cloning and expression of cDNA for rat heme oxygenase, *Proc. Natl. Acad. Sci. U.S.A.,* 82, 7865, 1985.
11. Maines, M.D., Trakshel, G.M., and Kutty, R.K., Characterization of two constitutive forms of rat liver microsomal heme oxygenase: only one molecular species of the enzyme is inducible, *J. Biol. Chem.,* 261, 411, 1986.
12. Cruse, I. and Maines, M.D., Evidence suggesting that the two forms of heme oxygenase are products of different genes, *J. Biol. Chem.,* 263, 3348, 1988.
13. Trakshel, G.M. and Maines, M.D., Multiplicity of heme oxygenase isozymes: HO-1 and HO-2 are different molecular species in rat and rabbit, *J. Biol. Chem.,* 264, 1323, 1989.

14. Maines, M.D., Heme oxygenase: function, multiplicity, regulatory mechanisms, and clinical applications, *FASEB J.*, 2, 2557, 1988.
15. Marks, G.S. et al., Does carbon monoxide have a physiological function? *Trends Pharmacol. Sci.*, 12, 185, 1991.
16. Stocker, R. et al., Bilirubin is an antioxidant of possible physiological importance, *Science*, 235, 1043, 1987.
17. McDonagh, A.F., Is bilirubin good for you? *Clin. Perinatol.*, 17, 359, 1990.
18. Coceani, F. et al., Cytochrome P 450-linked monooxygenase: involvement in the lamb ductus arteriosus, *Am. J. Physiol.*, 246, H640, 1984.
19. Vedernikov, Y.P., Graser, T., and Vanin, A.F., Similar endothelium-independent arterial relaxation by carbon monoxide and nitric oxide, *Biomed. Biochim. Acta*, 8, 601, 1989.
20. Furchgott, R.F. and Jothianandan, D., Endothelium-dependent and -independent vasodilation involving cGMP: relaxation induced by nitric oxide, carbon monoxide and light, *Blood Vessels*, 28, 52, 1991.
21. Morita, T. et al., Smooth muscle cell-derived carbon monoxide is a regulator of vascular cGMP, *Proc. Natl. Acad. Sci. U.S.A.*, 92, 1475, 1995.
22. Christodoulides, N. et al., Vascular smooth muscle cell heme oxygenases generate guanylyl cyclase-stimulatory carbon monoxide, *Circulation*, 91, 2306, 1995.
23. Sammut, I.A. et al., Carbon monoxide is a major contributor to the regulation of vascular tone in aortas expressing high levels of haeme oxygenase-1, *Br. J. Pharmacol.*, 125, 1437, 1998.
24. Coceani, F., Carbon monoxide in vasoregulation: the promise and the challenge, *Circ. Res.*, 86, 1184, 2000.
25. Palmer, R.M.J., Ferrige, A.G., and Moncada, S., Nitric oxide release accounts for the biological activity of endothelium-derived relaxing factor, *Nature*, 327, 524, 1987.
26. Ignarro, L.J., Buga, G.M., and Wood, K.S., Endothelium-derived relaxing factor produced and released from artery and vein is nitric oxide, *Proc. Natl. Acad. Sci. U.S.A.*, 84, 9265, 1987.
27. Gross, S.S. and Wolin, M.S., Nitric oxide: pathophysiological mechanisms, *Annu. Rev. Physiol.*, 57, 737, 1995.
28. Feelisch, M., The biochemical pathways of nitric-oxide formation from nitrovasodilators: appropriate choice of exogenous NO donors and aspects of preparation and handling of aqueous NO solutions, *J. Cardiovasc. Pharmacol.*, 17, S25, 1991.
29. Feelisch, M., The use of nitric oxide donors in pharmacological studies, *Naunyn–Schmiedeberg's Arch. Pharmacol.*, 358, 113, 1998.
30. Luscher, T.F., Endogenous and exogenous nitrates and their role in myocardial ischaemia, *Br. J. Clin. Pharmacol.*, 34, Suppl. 1, 29S, 1992.
31. Saavedra, J.E. et al., Targeting nitric oxide (NO) delivery *in vivo*. Design of a liver-selective NO donor prodrug that blocks tumor necrosis factor-alpha-induced apoptosis and toxicity in the liver, *J. Med. Chem.*, 40, 1947, 1997.
32. Saavedra, J.E. et al., Localizing antithrombotic and vasodilatory activity with a novel, ultrafast nitric oxide donor, *J. Med. Chem.*, 39, 4361, 1996.
33. Schmidt, H.H., NO, CO and OH. Endogenous soluble guanyl cyclase-activating factors, *FEBS Lett.*, 307, 102, 1992.
34. Sacerdoti, D. et al., Treatment with tin prevents the development of hypertension in spontaneously hypertensive rats, *Science*, 243, 388, 1989.
35. Johnson, R.A. et al., A heme oxygenase product, presumably carbon monoxide, mediates a vasodepressor function in rats, *Hypertension*, 25, 166, 1995.
36. Johnson, R.A. et al., Heme oxygenase substrates acutely lower blood pressure in hypertensive rats, *Am. J. Physiol.*, 271, H1132, 1996.

37. Rodgers, P.A. et al., Sources of carbon monoxide (CO) in biological systems and applications of CO detection technologies, *Semin. Perinatol.*, 18, 2, 1994.

38. Grundemar, L. et al., Haem oxygenase activity in blood vessel homogenates as measured by carbon monoxide production, *Acta Physiol. Scand.*, 153, 203, 1995.

39. Cook, M.N. et al., Heme oxygenase activity in the adult rat aorta and liver as measured by carbon monoxide formation, *Can. J. Physiol. Pharmacol.*, 73, 515, 1995.

40. Grozdanovic, Z. and Gossrau, R., Expression of heme oxygenase-2 (HO-2)-like immunoreactivity in rat tissues, *Acta Histochemica*, 98, 203, 1996.

41. Marks, G.S. et al., Heme oxygenase activity and immunohistochemical localization in bovine pulmonary artery and vein, *J. Cardiovasc. Pharmacol.*, 30, 1, 1997.

42. Balla, G. et al., A cytoprotective antioxidant stratagem of endothelium, *J. Biol. Chem.*, 267, 18148, 1992.

43. Balla, J. et al., Endothelial-cell heme uptake from heme proteins: induction of sensitization and desensitization to oxidant damage, *Proc. Natl. Acad. Sci. U.S.A.*, 90, 9285, 1993.

44. Motterlini, R. et al., Oxidative-stress response in vascular endothelial cells exposed to acellular hemoglobin solutions, *Am. J. Physiol.*, 269, H648, 1995.

45. Suematsu, M. et al., Carbon monoxide as an endogenous modulator of hepatic vascular perfusion, *Biochem. Biophys. Res. Commun.*, 205, 1333, 1994.

46. Suematsu, M. et al., Carbon monoxide: an endogenous modulator of sinusoidal tone in the perfused rat liver, *J. Clin. Invest.*, 96, 2431, 1995.

47. Goda, N. et al., Distribution of heme oxygenase isoforms in rat liver. Topographic basis for carbon monoxide-mediated microvascular relaxation, *J. Clin. Invest.*, 101, 604, 1998.

48. Kozma, F. et al., Contribution of endogenous carbon monoxide to regulation of diameter in resistance vessels, *Am. J. Physiol.*, 276, R1087, 1999.

49. Zakhary, R. et al., Heme oxygenase 2: endothelial and neuronal localization and role in endothelium-dependent relaxation, *Proc. Natl. Acad. Sci. U.S.A.*, 93, 795, 1996.

50. Wang, R., Wang, Z.Z., and Wu, L.Y., Carbon monoxide-induced vasorelaxation and the underlying mechanisms, *Br. J. Pharmacol.*, 121, 927, 1997.

51. Motterlini, R. et al., NO-mediated activation of heme oxygenase: endogenous cytoprotection against oxidative stress to endothelium, *Am. J. Physiol.*, 270, H107, 1996.

52. Yee, E.L. et al., Effect of nitric oxide on heme metabolism in pulmonary artery endothelial cells, *Am. J. Physiol.*, 271, L512, 1996.

53. Foresti, R. et al., Thiol compounds interact with nitric oxide in regulating heme oxygenase-1 induction in endothelial cells. Involvement of superoxide and peroxynitrite anions, *J. Biol. Chem.*, 272, 18411, 1997.

54. Hartsfield, C.L. et al., Regulation of heme oxygenase-1 gene expression in vascular smooth muscle cells by nitric oxide, *Am. J. Physiol.*, 273, L980, 1997.

55. Durante, W. et al., Nitric oxide induces heme oxygenase-1 gene expression and carbon monoxide production in vascular smooth muscle cells, *Circ. Res.*, 80, 557, 1997.

56. Foresti, R. et al., Peroxynitrite induces haem oxygenase-1 in vascular endothelial cells: a link to apoptosis, *Biochem. J.*, 339, 729, 1999.

57. Motterlini, R. et al., Endothelial heme oxygenase-1 induction by hypoxia: modulation by inducible nitric oxide synthase (iNOS) and S-nitrosothiols, *J. Biol. Chem.*, 275, 13613, 2000.

58. Kim, Y.M. et al., Loss and degradation of enzyme-bound heme induced by cellular nitric oxide synthesis, *J. Biol. Chem.*, 270, 5710, 1995.

59. Albakri, Q.A. and Stuehr, D.J., Intracellular assembly of inducible NO synthase is limited by nitric oxide-mediated changes in heme insertion and availability, *J. Biol. Chem.*, 271, 5414, 1996.

60. Turcanu, V., Dhouib, M., and Poindron, P., Nitric oxide synthase inhibition by haem oxygenase decreases macrophage nitric-oxide-dependent cytotoxicity: a negative feedback mechanism for the regulation of nitric oxide production, *Res. Immunol.*, 149, 741, 1998.

61. Foresti, R. and Motterlini, R., The heme oxygenase pathway and its interaction with nitric oxide in the control of cellular homeostasis, *Free Rad. Res.*, 31, 459, 1999.

62. Thiemermann, C. et al., Vascular hyporeactivity to vasoconstrictor agents and hemo-dynamic decompensation in hemorrhagic shock is mediated by nitric oxide, *Proc. Natl. Acad. Sci. U.S.A.*, 90, 267, 1993.

63. Moncada, S., Palmer, R.M.J., and Higgs, E.A., Nitric oxide: physiology, pathophys-iology, and pharmacology, *Pharmacol. Rev.*, 43, 109, 1991.

64. Nava, E., Palmer, R.M.J., and Moncada, S., Inhibition of nitric oxide synthesis in septic shock: how much is beneficial? *Lancet*, 338, 1555, 1991.

65. Taille, C. et al., Protective role of heme oxygenases against endotoxin-induced dia-phragmatic dysfunction in rats, *Am. J. Resp. Crit. Care Med.*, 163, 753, 2001.

66. Dusting, G.J., Nitric oxide in coronary artery disease: roles in atherosclerosis, myo-cardial reperfusion and heart failure, *EXS*, 76, 33, 1996.

67. Tomlinson, A. et al., Cyclo-oxygenase and nitric oxide synthase isoforms in rat carrageenin-induced pleurisy, *Br. J. Pharmacol.*, 113, 693, 1994.

68. Willis, D. et al., Heme oxygenase: a novel target for the modulation of inflammatory response, *Nature Med.*, 2, 87, 1996.

69. Hauser, G.J. et al., HSP induction inhibits iNOS mRNA expression and attenuates hypotension in endotoxin challenged rats, *Am. J. Physiol.*, 271, H2529, 1996.

70. Tomlinson, A. et al., Temporal and spatial expression of the inducible isoforms of cyclooxygenase, nitric oxide synthase and heme oxygenase in tissues from rats infused with LPS in the conscious state, *Br. J. Pharmacol.*, 123, P178, 1998.

71. Katori, M. et al., Prior induction of heat shock proteins by a nitric oxide donor attenuates cardiac ischemia/reperfusion injury in the rat, *Transplantation*, 69, 2530, 2000.

72. Guo, Y. et al., The late phase of ischemic preconditioning is abrogated by targeted disruption of the inducible NO synthase gene, *Proc. Natl. Acad. Sci. U.S.A.*, 96, 11507, 1999.

73. Kanno, S. et al., Attenuation of myocardial ischemia/reperfusion injury by superin-duction of inducible nitric oxide synthase, *Circulation*, 101, 2742, 2000.

74. Coceani, F. et al., Carbon monoxide formation in the ductus arteriosus in the lamb: implications for the regulation of muscle tone, *Br. J. Pharmacol.*, 120, 599, 1997.

75. Acevedo, C.H. and Ahmed, A., Hemeoxygenase-1 inhibits human myometrial con-tractility via carbon monoxide and is up-regulated by progesterone during pregnancy, *J. Clin. Invest.*, 101, 949, 1998.

76. Motterlini, R., Interaction of hemoglobin with nitric oxide and carbon monoxide: physiological implications, in *Blood Substitutes: New Challenges,* Vandegriff, K., Intaglietta, M., and Winslow, R.M., Eds., Birkauser, Boston, 1996, Chap. 5.

77. Motterlini, R. et al., Heme oxygenase-1-derived carbon monoxide contributes to the suppression of acute hypertensive responses *in vivo*, *Circ. Res.*, 83, 568, 1998.

78. Ishizaka, N. et al., Angiotensin II-induced hypertension increases heme oxygenase-1 expression in rat aorta, *Circulation*, 96, 1923, 1997.

79. Seki, T. et al., Roles of heme oxygenase carbon monoxide system in genetically hypertensive rats, *Biochem. Biophys. Res. Commun.*, 241, 574, 1997.

80. Yet, S.F. et al., Induction of heme oxygenase-1 expression in vascular smooth muscle cells. A link to endotoxic shock, *J. Biol. Chem.*, 272, 4295, 1997.

81. Wakabayaski, Y. et al., Carbon monoxide overproduced by heme oxygenase-1 causes a reduction of vascular resistance in perfused rat liver, *Am. J. Physiol.*, 277, G1088, 1999.

82. Pannen, B.H. and Bauer, M., Differential regulation of hepatic arterial and portal venous vascular resistance by nitric oxide and carbon monoxide in rats, *Life Sci.*, 62, 2025, 1998.

83. McMahon, T.J. et al., Functional coupling of oxygen binding and vasoactivity in S-nitrosohemoglobin, *J. Biol. Chem.*, 275, 16738, 2000.

84. Lee, P.J. et al., Hypoxia-inducible factor-1 mediates transcriptional activation of the heme oxygenase-1 gene in response to hypoxia, *J. Biol. Chem.*, 272, 5375, 1997.

85. Caudill, T.K. et al., Role of endothelial carbon monoxide in attenuated vasoreactivity following chronic hypoxia, *Am. J. Physiol.*, 275, R1025, 1998.

86. O'Donaughy, T.L. and Walker, B.R., Renal vasodilatory influence of endogenous carbon monoxide in chronically hypoxic rats, *Am. J. Physiol. Heart Circ. Physiol.*, 279, H2908, 2000.

87. Morimoto, Y. et al., Real-time measurements of endogenous CO production from vascular cells using an ultrasensitive laser sensor, *Am. J. Physiol. Heart Circ. Physiol.*, 280, H483, 2001.

88. Nag, A.C., Chen, K.C., and Cheng, M., Effects of carbon monoxide on cardiac muscle cells in culture, *Am. J. Physiol.*, 255, C291, 1988.

89. Maines, M.D. and Kappas, A., Cobalt induction of hepatic heme oxygenase; with evidence that cytochrome P450 is not essential for this enzyme activity, *Proc. Natl. Acad. Sci. U.S.A.*, 71, 4293, 1974.

90. Maines, M.D. and Kappas, A., The induction of heme oxidation in various tissues by trace metals: evidence for the catabolism of endogenous heme by hepatic heme oxygenase, *Ann. Clin. Res.*, 8, 39, 1976.

91. Abraham, N.G. et al., Identification of heme oxygenase and cytochrome P-450 in the rabbit heart, *J. Mol. Cell. Cardiol.*, 19, 73, 1987.

92. Katayose, D. et al., Separate regulation of heme oxygenase and heat shock protein 70 mRNA expression in the rat heart by hemodynamic stress, *Biochem. Biophys. Res. Commun.*, 191, 587, 1993.

93. Raju, V.S. and Maines, M.D., Coordinated expression and mechanism of induction of HSP32 (heme oxygenase-1) mRNA by hyperthermia in rat organs, *Biochim. Biophys. Acta*, 1217, 273, 1994.

94. Ewing, J.F., Raju, V.S., and Maines, M.D., Induction of heart heme oxygenase-1 (HSP32) by hyperthermia: possible role in stress-mediated elevation of cyclic 3′:5′-guanosine monophosphate, *J. Pharmacol. Exp. Ther.*, 271, 408, 1994.

95. Sharma, H.S. et al., Coordinated expression of heme oxygenase-1 and ubiquitin in the porcine heart subjected to ischemia and reperfusion, *Mol. Cell. Biochem.*, 157, 111, 1996.

96. Maulik, N. et al., Nitric oxide: a retrograde messenger for carbon monoxide signaling in ischemic heart, *Mol. Cell. Biochem.*, 157, 75, 1996.

97. Maulik, N., Sharma, H.S., and Das, D.K., Induction of the heme oxygenase gene expression during the reperfusion of ischemic rat myocardium, *J. Mol. Cell. Cardiol.*, 28, 1261, 1996.

98. Maulik, N. et al., Nitric oxide/carbon monoxide: a molecular switch for myocardial preservation during ischemia, *Circulation*, 94 (Suppl. II), 398, 1996.

99. Hoshida, S. et al., Heme oxygenase-1 expression and its relation to oxidative stress during primary culture of cardiomyocytes, *J. Mol. Cell. Cardiol.*, 28, 1845, 1996.

100. Eyssenhernandez, R., Ladoux, A., and Frelin, C., Differential regulation of cardiac heme oxygenase-1 and vascular endothelial growth factor messenger RNA expressions by hemin, heavy metals, heat shock and anoxia, *FEBS Lett.*, 382, 229, 1996.

101. Borger, D.R. and Essig, D.A., Induction of HSP32 gene in hypoxic cardiomyocytes is attenuated by treatment with N-acetyl-L-cysteine, *Am. J. Physiol.*, 274, H965, 1998.

102. Raju, V.S. and Maines, M.D., Renal ischemia/reperfusion up-regulates heme oxygenase-1 (HSP32) expression and increases cGMP in rat heart, *J. Pharmacol. Exp. Ther.*, 277, 1814, 1996.

103. Sharma, H.S., Das, D.K., and Verdouw, P.D., Enhanced expression and localization of heme oxygenase-1 during recovery phase of porcine stunned myocardium, *Mol. Cell. Biochem.*, 196, 133, 1999.

104. Ishizaka, N. et al., Heme oxygenase-1 is up-regulated in the rat heart in response to chronic administration of angiotensin II, *Am. J. Physiol.*, 279, H672, 2000.

105. Clark, J.E. et al., Heme oxygenase-1-derived bilirubin ameliorates post-ischemic myocardial dysfunction, *Am. J. Physiol.*, 278, H643, 2000.

106. Hangaishi, M. et al., Induction of heme oxygenase-1 can act protectively against cardiac ischemia/reperfusion *in vivo*, *Biochem. Biophys. Res. Commun.*, 279, 582, 2000.

107. Breimer, L.H. et al., Serum bilirubin and risk of ischemic-heart-disease in middle-aged British men, *Clin. Chem.*, 41, 1504, 1995.

108. Hopkins, P.N. et al., Higher serum bilirubin is associated with decreased risk for early familial coronary artery disease, *Atherioscler. Thromb. Vasc. Biol.*, 16, 250, 1996.

109. Yachie, A. et al., Oxidative stress causes enhanced endothelial cell injury in human heme oxygenase-1 deficiency, *J. Clin. Invest.*, 103, 129, 1999.

110. Raju, V.S., Imai, N., and Liang, C.S., Chamber-specific regulation of heme oxygenase-1 (heat shock protein 32) in right-sided congestive heart failure, *J. Mol. Cell. Cardiol.*, 31, 1581, 1999.

111. Nishio, Y. et al., Altered activities of transcription factors and their related gene expression in cardiac tissues of diabetic rats, *Diabetes*, 47, 1318, 1998.

112. Csonka, C. et al., Heme oxygenase and cardiac function in ischemic/reperfused rat hearts, *Free Rad. Biol. Med.*, 27, 119, 1999.

113. Soares, M.P. et al., Expression of heme oxygenase-1 can determine cardiac xenograft survival, *Nature Med.*, 4, 1073, 1998.

114. Hancock, W.W. et al., Antibody-induced transplant arteriosclerosis is prevented by graft expression of antioxidant and anti-apoptotic genes, *Nature Med.*, 4, 1392, 1998.

115. Otterbein, L.E. et al., Carbon monoxide has antiinflammatory effects involving the mitogen-activated protein kinase pathway, *Nature Med.*, 6, 422, 2000.

116. Hayashi, S. et al., Induction of heme oxygenase-1 suppresses venular leukocyte adhesion elicited by oxidative stress. Role of bilirubin generated by the enzyme, *Circ. Res.*, 85, 663, 1999.

117. Vachharajani, T.J. et al., Heme oxygenase modulates selectin expression in different regional vascular beds, *Am. J. Physiol.*, 278, H1613, 2000.

118. Ishikawa, K. et al., Induction of heme oxygenase-1 inhibits the monocyte transmigration induced by mildly oxidized LDL, *J. Clin. Invest.*, 100, 1209, 1997.

119. Lane, N.J., Blood ties, *Sciences (New York)*, 38, 24, 1998.

120. Panahian, N., Yoshiura, M., and Maines, M.D., Overexpression of heme oxygenase-1 is neuroprotective in a model of permanent middle cerebral artery occlusion in transgenic mice, *J. Neurochem.*, 72, 1187, 1999.

121. Otterbein, L.E. et al., Exogenous administration of heme oxygenase-1 by gene transfer provides protection against hyperoxia-induced lung injury, *J. Clin. Invest.*, 103, 1047, 1999.

122. Motterlini, R. et al., A precursor of the nitric oxide donor SIN-1 modulates the stress protein heme oxygenase-1 in rat liver, *Biochem. Biophys. Res. Commun.*, 225, 167, 1996.

123. Motterlini, R. et al., Curcumin, an antioxidant and antiinflammatory agent, induces heme oxygenase-1 and protects endothelial cells against oxidative stress, *Free Rad. Biol. Med.*, 28, 1303, 2000.

124. Herrmann, W.A., 100 years of metal carbonyls. A serendipitous chemical discovery of major scientific and industrial impact, *J. Organomet. Chem.*, 383, 21, 1990.

125. Darensbourg, D.J., Klausmeyer, K.K., and Reibenspies, J.H., CO-labilizing ability of the fluoride ligand in tungsten (0) carbonyl fluorides. X-ray structure of $[Et_4N]_3[W_2(CO)_6F_3]$, *Inorg. Chem.*, 34, 4933, 1995.

126. Darensbourg, D.J., Klausmeyer, K.K., and Reibenspies, J.H., Coordinatively unsaturated derivatives of group 6 metal carbonyls containing the π-donating ligand 3,5-di-tert-butylcatecholate, *Inorg. Chem.*, 35, 1529, 1996.

127. Pearson, J. et al., Alkyne ligand enhancement of the substitution lability of mononuclear osmium, ruthenium, and iron carbonyls, *J. Am. Chem. Soc.*, 120, 1434, 1998.

128. Abrahamson, H.B. and Wrighton, M.S., Ordering the reactivity of photodegenerated, 17 valence electron, metal carbonyl radicals, *J. Am. Chem. Soc.*, 99, 5510, 1977.

129. Wrighton, M.S. and Ginley, D.S., Photochemistry of metal–metal bonded complexes. II. The photochemistry of rhenium and manganese carbonyl complexes containing a metal–metal bond, *J. Am. Chem. Soc.*, 97, 2065, 1975.

130. Hughey, J.L., Bock, C.R., and Meyer, T.J., Flash photolysis evidence for metal–metal bond cleavage and loss of CO in the photochemistry of $[n^5C_5H_5)Mo(CO)_3]_2$, *J. Am. Chem. Soc.*, 97, 4440, 1975.

131. Decker, S.A. and Klobukowski, M., The first carbonyl bond dissociation energies of $M(CO)_5$ and $M(CO)_4(C_2H_2)$ (m = Fe, Ru, and Os): the role of the acetylene ligand from a density functional perspective, *J. Am. Chem. Soc.*, 120, 9342, 1998.

132. Rothberg, L.J. et al., Picosecond dynamics of solution-phase photofragmentation of $[Mn_2(CO)_{10}]$, *J. Am. Chem. Soc.*, 104, 3536, 1982.

133. Hepp, A.F. and Wrighton, M.S., Relative importance of metal–metal bond scission and loss of carbon monoxide from photoexcited dimanganese decacarbonyl: spectroscopic detection of a coordinatively unsaturated, CO-bridged dinuclear species in low-temperature alkane matrices, *J. Am. Chem. Soc.*, 105, 5934, 1983.

15 Sources, Sinks, and Measurement of Carbon Monoxide

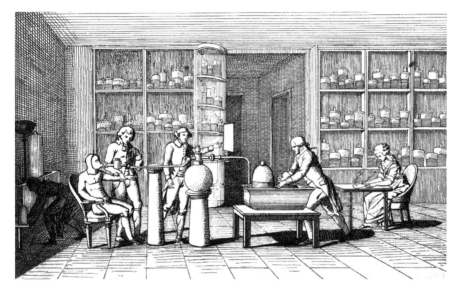

Early breath gas measurements by Lavoisier (1743–1794) and co-workers. Copyright 2000, Corbis.

Hendrik J. Vreman, Ronald J. Wong, and David K. Stevenson

CONTENTS

0-8493-1041-5/02/$0.00+$1.50

I. INTRODUCTION

Carbon monoxide (CO) has been long considered an exogenous toxic byproduct of combustion processes. Sjöstrand,[1] Tenhunen,[2] and many others have shown that CO is also produced endogenously, in equimolar amounts with biliverdin, from the degradation of heme during normal and pathologic erythrocyte turnover by the enzyme heme oxygenase (HO).[3] In humans, biliverdin is reduced immediately by biliverdin reductase to form bilirubin, a potent neurotoxin and antioxidant.[4-6] Evidence now indicates that endogenously produced CO has a physiologic role similar to that of nitric oxide (NO).[7-10]

In previous review articles, the authors focused on aspects of heme degradation related to the diagnosis and treatment of neonatal jaundice through measurements of CO.[11-13] This chapter will emphasize CO measurements pertaining to the study the role of CO as a physiologically active compound. Methods for CO quantitation available as research tools may need further refinement and sophistication to handle

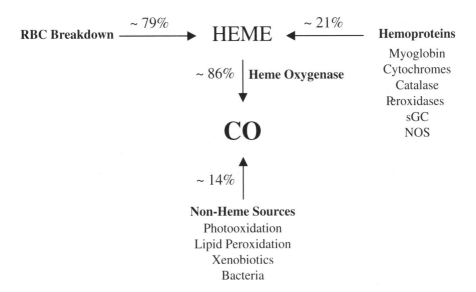

FIGURE 15.1 Heme degradation pathway.

the unique challenges presented by this new understanding. Various analytical techniques available for the quantitation of endogenously produced CO will be evaluated. Subsequently, the use of gas chromatography (GC) with specific and ultrasensitive reduction gas detection technology to measure CO generated *in vitro* and *in vivo* by heme degradation and other non-heme sources will be discussed.

II. QUANTITATION TECHNIQUES FOR CARBON MONOXIDE

The major challenge in the quantitation of CO generated for physiologic processes is to accurately determine these relatively small amounts against the large background concentrations of vascular and extravascular stores of CO. Under normal physiologic conditions, heme degradation catalyzed by HO is the predominant source of endogenous CO (Figure 15.1). Approximately 79% is derived from the heme of senescing red blood cells (RBCs).[14,15] The remaining heme-derived CO (21%) originates from the turnover of other hemoproteins such as myoglobins, cytochromes, catalase, and others.[2] Up to 14% of all CO produced in the body is estimated to arise from non-heme processes, such as photooxidation, lipid peroxidation, xenobiotic activity, bacterial activity in blood and intestines, and others.[15-18]

In vivo and *in vitro* investigations of the mechanisms of these processes require accurate, precise, sensitive, and relatively convenient measurements of CO in the gaseous, liquid, and non-liquid matrices found in biologic systems. Furthermore, because organisms ingest and subsequently produce a plethora of volatile organic compounds — each with differing biophysiological and biochemical properties — it is imperative that CO measuring methods are also tested for interfering compounds likely to be found in the matrices.[19,20] This section reviews some of the technologies and methods most commonly used for quantitation of CO.

A. TECHNIQUES FOR THE DIRECT MEASUREMENT OF BOUND CO

1. CO in Blood — CO-Oximetry

The most common method is the spectrophotometric determination of CO bound to hemoglobin (Hb) as carboxyhemoglobin (COHb) of circulating RBCs. This measurement made with CO-oximeters is primarily used for the clinical diagnosis of significant CO exposure and toxicity.[21] The determination of COHb is based upon the difference between the light absorption values of all hemoglobin derivatives and that of COHb in the blood. For each measurement, the spectral determinations are referenced to the absorption of a blank or zero solution. These measurements of absorbance are performed within a temperature-controlled 37°C cuvette.

Several instruments with different performance characteristics are produced by various manufacturers. However, the accuracy of most CO oximeters is often affected by the presence of clinically used dyes, bilirubin, and fetal hemoglobin.[22] Other disadvantages of these clinical instruments are their inaccuracy and irreproducibility in the normal ($\leq 2.5\%$ tHb) range and lack of sensitivity (COHb is measured only to 0.1% of the total hemoglobin concentration with an imprecision of 0.3%).[21]

For research purposes, especially in studies involving levels of CO $\leq 2.5\%$, the use of these instruments is not recommended. It is also unlikely that the sensitivity and accuracy of this methodology can be significantly improved to detect the small changes in COHb concentrations that occur due to physiologic processes, such as stimulation of vasodilation and neuronal functioning. A further complication is that these processes usually occur in only a portion (organ) of the total body mass, and thus the small amounts of CO produced may not be measurable against the large background pool of circulating COHb.

For the most accurate determination of COHb, gas chromatography (GC) is the method of choice (see Section III.B.1.b).

B. TECHNIQUES FOR THE MEASUREMENT OF FREE CO

A number of techniques are based on measuring unbound gaseous or bound and subsequently liberated CO, such as CO in inhaled air and/or exhaled breath or from a variety of biologic matrices (blood, tissues). Most promising for the study of physiologically active CO are methods utilizing isolated biologic systems, such as cell cultures or excised and perfused tissues (aortic rings and liver), which have been removed from the CO accumulated in the blood. However, due to the usually small sample sizes and relatively low CO concentrations generated in *in vitro* and *in vivo* biological experiments, few techniques are adequate.

1. Isotopes

These methods are based upon the use of radioisotope-labeled ^{14}C-heme precursors to measure the rate of [14]CO production. These precursors are incorporated into hemoproteins that have high turnover rates to produce early-labeled ^{14}CO, or into RBCs that then release the labeled ^{14}CO months later.[23]

Motterlini et al.[24] and Sammut et al.[25] in 1998 designed a device for trapping and measuring early-labeled ^{14}CO released from aortic tissues. 2-^{14}C-L-glycine was administered to the tissues, then incorporated into the heme of hemoproteins. As the labeled hemoproteins were metabolized, the produced ^{14}CO was trapped with deoxyhemoglobin or reduced Hb and then quantitated by scintillation counting.

Another method developed by Lincoln et al., used 5[5-^{14}C]aminolevulinate, another precursor, to label heme.[26] Upon heme degradation, ^{14}CO is produced in cultured hepatocytes and quantitated by scintillation counting.

In 1986, Salomon et al.,[27] using the method of Johnson et al.,[28] determined total and non-erythropoietic early-labeled bilirubin (and CO) formation by administering ^{14}C-ALA (a non-erythropoietic heme precursor) or ^{14}C-glycine (a total heme precursor) to bile duct-ligated adult rats. They found that short-term ligation increased RBC destruction.

These experiments demonstrated that the breakdown of heme occurred predominantly by the action of HO. However, this technique was successfully used only in experimental models, where newly synthesized and labeled heme is degraded rapidly.

2. Spectrophotometry

The majority of spectrophotometric methods are based upon the direct optical quantitation of CO trapped as COHb or carboxymyoglobin (COMb), utilizing laboratory based visible light spectrophotometers or CO-oximeters and the unique absorption spectra of the ferrous hemoglobin CO complexes.[21] Because the CO-trapping agents can be selected for purity and concentration, the method has the potential to be more sensitive and accurate than CO-oximetry of whole blood. Because of the high dissociation constants of COHb and COMb, only a small portion ($< 2\%$)[29] of the CO remains unbound and is thus not quantitated.

Suematsu[29] and Mori et al.[30] measured CO bound to myoglobin (Mb) in the effluent from perfused livers and spectrophotometrically quantitated the formed COMb. In an effort to discern the role of CO (and NO) in newborn infants with postasphyxial hypoxic–ischemic encephalopathy (HIE), Shi et al.[31] measured plasma CO levels by using a method described by Chalmers.[32] This method uses Hb to first trap unbound plasma CO, followed by a manual spectrophotometric measurement of COHb. In 1995, Nathanson et al. measured the rate of CO production in cerebellar slices by trapping the CO with Hb.[33] RBCs were separated from the slices, centrifuged, and analyzed for COHb with an automated, modified IL-482 CO-Oximeter (Instrumentation Laboratories, Lexington, MA).

3. Infrared Absorption Spectroscopy

Because CO production rates in living tissues are very low (< 10 nmol CO/h/mg protein), measurements of CO generated by small tissue masses have been limited to methods using GC and radioisotope counting.[34] These methods have the necessary sensitivity to measure small quantities of CO, but cannot readily measure CO production continuously in real time.

Infrared laser absorption spectroscopy may be potentially a superior method. Tunable infrared (4.61 µM) diode laser instruments are now being developed to measure CO in ambient air and in exhaled breath.[35,36] The instruments can measure CO in real time with sensitivity in the parts per billion (ppb) range and short response times (sec). In addition, no sample pre-treatment is needed. However, these instruments require relatively large sample volumes, are quite bulky and expensive, and are not commercially available.

In 1997, Topfer et al. successfully used an instrument with a sensitivity of 7 pmol,[37] to quantitate (every 20 sec) CO generated by smooth muscle cells in culture. They found that the rates of CO production for control, heme-, and tin mesoporphyrin-treated cells were 250, 490, and 20 pmol/h/mg protein, respectively.[38]

4. Electrochemistry

By far the least expensive and most frequently used CO detectors are the electrochemical (EC) sensors. A typical amperometric sensor contains two or three electrodes immersed in a liquid electrolyte. The key to the sensor's operation is the working electrode (WE) consisting of catalytic material, usually platinum or gold, on a porous hydrophobic polymer. The porous electrode allows the gas sample to reach the WE without allowing the electrolyte to leak out. The catalytic action either produces or consumes electrons, resulting in a flow of current through the WE terminal, which is converted to an analog signal.[39]

Electrochemical CO sensors have been incorporated into a number of CO detecting or quantitation devices used primarily for environmental exposure assessment,[40] smoking cessation programs,[41] jaundice diagnosis,[6] and treatment monitoring.[42] The use of EC sensors for physiologic studies, and in particular those measuring end tidal breath CO in relation to clinical conditions, needs to be carefully evaluated.[43] Considerations should include the sensor's selectivity toward CO, resolution [most often 1 part per million (ppm) or 0.5% of full scale], minimum detectable level (mostly 1 ppm), reproducibility (poor in the low, 0 to 5 ppm range), response time, sensitivity to interfering substances (of which there are large numbers with varying activities affecting the detector), and measurement drift. Furthermore, because this type of sensor is particularly sensitive to hydrogen, which is impossible to remove from gas mixtures, study protocols must be designed so that hydrogen production is minimized or averted.[44,45]

5. Gas Chromatography

Because few techniques at present are able to directly quantitate CO in mixtures of volatile organic compounds (VOCs), CO quantitation techniques require sample purification. Gas chromatography is such a technique capable of separating CO from other volatile compounds by passing a mixture through a heated column packed with a sorbant or a molecular sieve. A moving (carrier) inert gas phase elutes the CO and other compounds sequentially, based on their molecular sizes and/or absorption coefficients specific for each packing material. A detector located at the column exit quantitates the CO. A number of different types of GC detectors are available for the quantitation of CO and these are briefly discussed below.

6. Flame Ionization Detection

The flame ionization detector (FID) is the most commonly used detector in GC systems. For CO analysis, samples are dried, pre-concentrated, and separated from hydrocarbons on a pre-column. The CO and CH_4 (if present) are then separated on the analytical column. The emerging CO is reduced to CH_4 in a heated catalytic reduction tube (methanizer) and quantitated with the FID detector.[46-48] The technique has a sensitivity of 20 ppb and has no known interfering compounds. However, a trained operator is required for obtaining accurate results.

In 1968, Collison et al.[49] first described a classical method for the determination of CO in blood that is still in use, though modified, today (see Section III.B.1.b). The method is based on the principle that CO bound to Hb in RBCs is released by oxidation with $K_3Fe(CN)_6$ in a sealed reactor system. The CO liberated into the headspace of the reactor is then injected onto a molecular sieve column. After separation from other headspace gas components, CO is reduced to CH_4, followed by quantitation with an FID. The method had sufficient sensitivity to quantitate CO in 100 μl of normal blood (or approximately 100 nl CO) with a coefficient of variation of 1.8% and detection limit of 0.01% COHb. Since the introduction of this method, several improvements have increased the recovery of CO[50] and the sensitivity of the method.[51]

7. Mass Spectroscopy

Mass spectroscopy (MS), used in combination with GC, has emerged as the tool of choice for researchers who need to identify and quantitate individual compounds in complex volatile organic compound mixtures.[20] This type of GC detector is based on the bombardment of vapor phase molecules, like CO, emerging from the analytical GC column, with a stream of high-energy electrons, converting some of the molecules to ions, which are accelerated in an electric field. The accelerated ions are then separated according to their mass to charge (m/e) ratios in a magnetic or electric field. The ions, which have particular m/e ratios, are then counted by a detector. The instrument produces a graph with the number of detected particles for specific ratios. Because the molecular masses for CO and nitrogen are very similar, the quantitation of CO with this technique is not possible with a GC using nitrogen-containing carrier gas, unless a high resolution MS detector is used. The MS detector is especially useful for quantitating CO with stable isotopes other than $^{12}C^{16}O$ or ^{16}O.[52]

In order to study the role of HO-derived CO in vascular reactivity to vasopression, Kaide et al. quantitated CO released from incubated rat interlobal arteries via GC/MS.[53] They found that chromium mesoporphyrin (CrMP) treatment decreased the rate of CO formation from 95 ± 16 to 29 ± 5 pmol/h/mg protein.

In addition, a combination of GC, isotope measurements, and MS techniques was used by Balazy and Jiang to circumvent the lack of adequate standards for MS quantitation of CO.[54] This method appears to work successfully only with CO generated from cell cultures. It has not been demonstrated to be applicable in studies quantitating CO released from other systems.

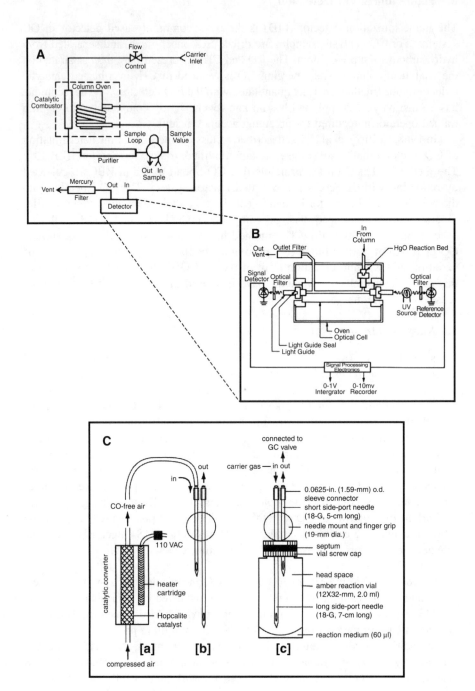

FIGURE 15.2

8. Reduction Gas Detection

The most sensitive method for quantitating CO is GC with a reduction gas detector (GC/RGD) or reduction gas analyzer (RGA, Trace Analytical, Inc., Menlo Park, CA). In the simplified diagram of the analyzer (Figure 15.2A), CO is separated from other potential reducing gases, such as hydrogen, with CO-free carrier gas at a flow rate of 30 ml/min on a stainless steel column (68×0.53 i.d.) packed with a 5A or 13X molecular sieve (Alltech Associates Inc., Deerfield, MI) and operated at 140°C. The CO then passes through an RGD, which contains a 5-mg solid mercuric oxide bed heated to 260°C. Upon oxidizing the CO to CO_2 and hydrogen to H_2O, gaseous mercury is released (Figure 15.2B). The concentration of the liberated mercury is measured spectrophotometrically in a 10-cm optical cell. The very high molar UV (254 nm) absorptivity of mercury is the basis of the very high sensitivity of the technique.[55]

This detector, initially designed for the continuous measurement of CO in ambient air, has also been used for the semi-continuous quantitation of CO (and hydrogen) generated via a variety of biological processes.[17,56,57] The GC/RGD presently in use has a sensitivity of 1 pmole of CO with a linearity of up to 120 pmoles. Much higher sensitivities can be achieved (10 fmole), but this generally offers no advantage in view of the biologic variations within tissues or animals studied.

In 1992, Nath et al.[58] measured HO activity through measurements of bilirubin in kidney microsomes as well as CO formation by kidney slices incubated overnight using a GC/RGD.

The same technique was used to measure the total body CO production (VCO) in adult male mice as well as CO generation from incubated feces and urine.[56] The reported VCO of fed and fasted mice was 1.0 ± 0.4 and 0.96 ± 0.07 nmol CO/h/g of body weight, respectively. Excreta exposed to oxygen generally produced significantly more CO than anaerobic excreta. These observations led to the conclusion that CO production by excreta may have affected measurements of heme turnover in previous animal studies, which used relatively long-term rebreathing techniques.

FIGURE 15.2 (opposite) Schematic representations of : (A) gas chromatograph; (B) reduction gas detector; and (C) catalytic converter [a]; double-needle assemblies for vial purging [b] and headspace sampling [c]. The assemblies are identical except for the direction of the gas flow through the needles. For the production of CO-free air, compressed air is passed through a heated (~120°C) catalytic converter [a] containing Hopcalite (CuO/MnO) catalyst (Trace Analytical, Inc.). The catalyst oxidizes any CO to CO_2. The resulting CO-free gas is used to purge the headspace of the reaction vial just prior to incubation. When the assembly [b] is removed from the vial after purging, the vial pressure will equilibrate to atmospheric pressure via the long needle after the shorter purging gas-inlet needle has been withdrawn. For headspace sampling [c], the long needle introduces carrier gas into the vial and the short needle serves as an outlet. Such an arrangement will prevent vial liquid from being forced into the injection valve by the flow of carrier gas. (A and B courtesy of Trace Analytical, Inc. Copyright 1996. C is reprinted from Vreman, H.J. et al., in *Current Protocols in Toxicology*, p. 9.2.1. John Wiley & Sons, Inc. Copyright 1999. With permission.)

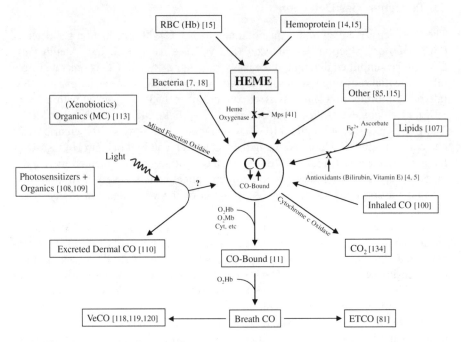

FIGURE 15.3 Sources and sinks of carbon monoxide.

Short-term flow-through studies were not expected to be significantly affected by this extraneous source of CO. Marks et al. used this technique for a number of inquiries into the physiologic role of CO.[59-62]

The authors selected GC/RGD technology for measurements of CO in any matrix because of the technique's selectivity, sensitivity, accuracy, and versatility. They applied this technology for *in vitro* measurements of HO activity and other processes, which represent the potential for CO production, the concentrations of CO in tissues, and total body CO excretion (VeCO) under normal, stimulated, and inhibited conditions (see Sections III.B and III.C).

III. METHODS OF CO QUANTITATION FOR EVALUATING SOURCES AND SINKS

The authors developed a number of *in vitro* and *in vivo* methods to evaluate the sources and sinks of CO (Figure 15.3) using GC/RGD. This section will first address pre-analytical considerations which may affect sample integrity and the accuracy of CO quantitation. Subsequently, specific methods for the quantitation of CO generated *in vitro* and *in vivo* will be outlined. Finally, some useful *in vitro* and *in vivo* accessory, non-CO producing methods will be discussed. The U.S. Environmental Protection Agency (EPA) publications of air quality criteria[63,64] provide especially helpful and comprehensive information regarding these topics.

A. PRE-ANALYTICAL CONSIDERATIONS

1. Inhaled CO

Studies investigating the sources, sinks, and physiologic role of CO in human subjects and animal models need to carefully assess or correct for inhaled CO. Ambient air normally contains approximately 0.5 ppm CO, but this concentration can vary dramatically and abruptly with time, depending on the subject's exposure to combustion processes from gas, charcoal, wood, and gasoline-fired devices, or from personal habits such as tobacco smoking.[64]

Cigarettes and cigars have been found to produce between 78 and 200 mg CO/g, respectively.[65] These sources expose the smoker[66] and, to a lesser extent, all others sharing an enclosed space to CO.[67] An important consideration is that approximately 10 to 40% of smokers fail to admit to the habit when interviewed.[68,69] The effect of prior CO exposure (dose, as well as time elapsed after each exposure) is an important consideration in view of the long half-life of CO in the circulation and extravascular (primarily as COMb) body stores.[70,71] The information on the dynamics of CO washout is incomplete, but the half-life values for CO in adult human blood have been found to range from 2 to 6 h.[72,73] For the smaller, more rapidly breathing human neonates, it is considerably lower (20 min to 3 h).[74] For small animal models, the half-life values are 30 to 60 min for adult mice and rats, respectively (authors' unpublished observations).

2. Materials (In)compatible with CO Measurements

In the course of collection, transfer, and storage, sample specimens can come in contact with a number of materials. Some of these are inert, such as glass, some types of stainless steel, aluminum, Teflon, Mylar, etc. Others may cause loss of CO through reversible (charcoal) and irreversible (soft steel) binding or loss through diffusion as observed with films of Teflon, polyethylene, etc. Other compounds such as natural rubber, silicone rubber, plastics, and a number of natural substances can generate CO, thereby changing the CO concentration in a sample.[51,75-77] The use of any materials except those proven inert must be carefully evaluated, particularly when elevated temperatures are involved.

3. Sample Collection

In studies quantitating CO generated *in vitro* or *in vivo*, samples must be collected, transported, and stored prior to analysis. These pre-analytical steps can present significant challenges with respect to obtaining representative samples of sufficient volumes free from CO contamination and loss.

For *in vitro* assays, CO is generally collected into glass reaction vials with silicone rubber septa allowing for access to the lumen. Although even the most carefully selected silicone septum material produces CO at low rates, this contamination can be corrected for with appropriate blank vials.[51] Also, cooling the vials, especially the septa, with wet or dry ice significantly reduces this interfering source of CO.

For *in vivo* studies, the sampling of breath can be accomplished most easily when the subject is placed in an air-supplied flow-through chamber and the CO is measured in the outlet air. However, for human subjects, the measurement of CO in alveolar or end tidal breath (ETCO) is a more convenient, reliable, and well studied index.[78] Breath can be sampled and analyzed continuously in real time using sensitive and rapidly responding near infrared (NIR)-based spectrophotometers. These instruments are, however, expensive and often not very portable. Intermittent sampling of end tidal breath can be accomplished after a 20-sec breath-hold with Priestley tube-type devices.[79] Alternatively, breath can be directly exhaled into an instrument with a quick response time for recording the peak (alveolar) CO concentration. For newborns, who cannot control their (fast and low volume) breathing, automatic sampling devices have been developed.[80-82] A commercially available instrument has now integrated the sampling and quantitation steps for ETCO, correcting for inhaled CO (ETCOc) measurements (see below).

4. Sample Cleanup

Because few detection techniques can directly quantitate CO in a complex gas mixture, most require some degree of sample cleanup. For NIR spectroscopy, only water vapor may need to be removed, but other detectors require more intensive removal of interfering substances. A wide variety of absorbents (for packing into gas filters) are available for more or less selective removal of interfering constituents such as CO_2, H_2O, VOCs, etc. in a physiologic sample.

However, care must be exercised so that the purifier does not remove CO as well. For example, when a breath sample is purified with some types of activated charcoal to remove VOCs, a significant amount of CO is absorbed as well[20] when the filter is of appropriate size.[45] Hydrogen is an interferent, especially for electrochemical-based devices, and is impossible to remove with current technology. However, if the CO quantitation technique is incapable of separating hydrogen from CO (like GC), steps can be taken to sample subjects during periods when hydrogen production is low[45] or suppressed through fasting.[79] Ethanol is another relatively common component of breath, which interacts with unprotected EC sensors leading to falsely elevated CO measurements.[39,83,84]

5. Standard Gas Supplies and Calibration

Accurate determination of CO requires appropriate instrument calibration procedures based on manufacturers' instructions. The necessary CO-containing gas mixtures, preferably certified, can be purchased[77] or carefully prepared using commercial gas mixers or even syringes.[51] Especially when using aqueous solutions of CO, solubility characteristics and gas/liquid phase physics must be carefully considered in order to obtain the most accurate experimental results.

B. *IN VITRO* METHODS USING GC/RGD

In vitro assays using organ preparations — from sonicates to perfused organs — have their limitations. At best, they can only provide an estimate of the potential for *in vivo* CO production. The removal of an organ eliminates its supply of substrates and prevents removal of products. Moreover, processing of tissue destroys cellular integrity and thereby alters the reaction environment for CO production. Also, the availabilities of substrates and co-reactants typically are fixed, at least initially. This is especially important, for instance in the HO reaction, where the concentration of 10 to 50 μM heme used in the *in vitro* assay is most likely greater than that found free in circulation, or possibly less than that available in spleen and liver. Furthermore, the selection of a heme concentration for the HO assay affects the measurable rate of CO generation,[85] and is also likely to affect the kinetics of metalloporphyrin inhibition of HO, which is competitive in nature[86] (see Section III.B.1.2).

For all *in vitro* CO quantitation assays, the authors use 2-ml septum-sealed glass reaction vials. Amber vials are used for all but photooxidation reactions, which are performed in clear, borosilicate vials. Sample and reagents for all *in vitro* assays are most rapidly, reproducibly, and accurately pipetted into the vials directly or through the septa, when appropriate, with fixed needle gas-tight syringes in repeating dispensers (Hamilton Co., Reno, NV). A double needle assembly (Figure 15.2C[b]) is used for purging the sealed vials of ambient CO with CO-free gas (Figure 15.2C[a]) before the reactions are started. A similar assembly is attached to the sample injection valve, allowing carrier gas to sweep through the attached vial in order to transfer the vial headspace gas onto the column for component separation and CO quantitation (Figure 15.2C[c]). The sample is injected for 15 sec and then analyzed for 90 sec as controlled by an interval timer (GraLab Model 451, Dimco–Gray, Dayton OH).

The detector response to the CO in the injected sample is displayed on an integrating recorder (Shimadzu Scientific Instruments Inc., Columbia, MD) and the sample's peak area (mV•S) is compared to a calibration curve prepared from injections of different volumes of standard gas containing 10.83 ppm CO (Scott Specialty Gases, Plumsteadville, PA). A mercury vapor filter is connected in line with the optical cell outlet for efficient removal of effluent mercury vapor. At a carrier gas flow rate of 30 ml/min, the retention time for CO is 0.7 min.

1. CO Generation from Heme

a. Heme Oxygenase Activity

In order to assess the relative potential for CO generation in tissues, the activity of HO is measured as follows.[85,87] Animal tissues are collected, rinsed, and immediately sonicated in four to nine volumes of ice cold 0.1 M KPO$_4$ buffer with a Microson™ ultrasonic cell disruptor (Misonix Inc., Farmingdale, NY) fitted with a microtip and operated at 50% maximum power. The HO activity in the 20-µl sonicate is determined in triplicate by measuring the amount of CO generated by the enzyme from 50 µM/11.2 µM metheme/albumin in the presence of 1.5 mM NADPH for 15 min at 37°C in the dark. Duplicate blank reactions contain no NADPH. Quantitation of the *in vitro* inhibition potential of, for instance, metalloporphyrins is determined by addition of small volumes (up to 3 µl) to the total 60 µl of reaction medium.

The ability of administered metalloporphyrins or HO activity up-regulating maneuvers to affect organ HO activity *in vivo* is determined in the same manner.

TABLE 15.1
In Vitro **CO Production (pmol CO/h/mg FW) via Different Processes by Adult Rat and Mouse Tissue Sonicates**

	Process			
	Heme Oxygenase		Lipid Peroxidation	
Tissue	Rat	Mouse	Rat	Mouse
Liver	193 ± 22	70 ± 7	4 ± 1	6 ± 1
Spleen	432 ± 152	167 ± 38	12 ± 3	126 ± 30
Kidney	60 ± 4	30 ± 12	161 ± 6	102 ± 9
Brain	99 ± 7	51 ± 6	258 ± 30	231 ± 10
Intestine	41 ± 12	21 ± 10	1 ± 2	4 ± 1
Heart	37 ± 8	25 ± 4	3 ± 1	86 ± 8
Lung	118 ± 10	109 ± 29	7 ± 1	75 ± 13
Testes	212 ± 27	143 ± 20	11 ± 3	147 ± 11
Blood	NM	NM	8 ± 5	NM
Muscle	NM	NM	NM	NM

Note: The data are based on the authors' unpublished preliminary results or reported in abstract form.[165] NM = not measured.

Tissues used for this purpose are usually harvested from the same animals used for the study of the effects of metalloporphyrin or HO activity up-regulating maneuvers on *in vivo* CO production rates (see Section III.C.1). HO activity, formerly expressed as nmol CO/h/mg protein,[85] is presently expressed in pmoles of CO produced/h/mg fresh weight.[86] This method is simple and rapid for the measurement of HO activity in the major organs of an animal (n = 10), usually taking 4 h from start to finish. Typical HO activity values for mouse and rat tissues are given in Table 15.1.

Metalloporphyrins and Inhibition of CO Production: A powerful and increasingly used tool for understanding the various aspects of a physiologic role for CO is the use of metalloporphyrins, competitive inhibitors of both HO-1 and HO-2.[62,88] However, each member of this category of natural and synthetic inhibitors has different physical and biochemical properties that may significantly impact the results of an *in vitro* or *in vivo* study.[89] Thus, metalloporphyrins are not magic bullets!

The authors have found that HO-1 and HO-2 activities are differentially sensitive to different metalloporphyrins,[90] although this difference is insufficient to allow for selective inhibition of HO-1 over HO-2. It is, however, large enough to affect the determination of I_{50} values for different tissues. Furthermore, some metalloporphyrins, after initially inhibiting HO activity, can increase HO-1 gene transcription and lead to subsequent HO activity up-regulation, with the potential for increased CO production.[3] Some metalloporphyrins are photoreactive; this can lead to unanticipated photogeneration of CO when significant light is not excluded during experimentation.

Some metalloporphyrins have been found to inhibit lipid peroxidation.[91,92] If this source of CO is functioning *in vivo,* the availability of CO from this source may decrease. The solubility of metalloporphyrins also needs to be considered for *in vivo* whole body (oral absorptivity) and intact cell studies because cellular uptake will differ for hydrophilic and hydrophobic compounds.[93-95]

Meffert et al. found that metalloporphyrins differentially inhibit nitric oxide synthase (NOS) and soluble guanylate cyclase (sGC) in hippocampal slices.[96] Appleton et al. found that a 5-μM concentration of CrMP was most selective for inhibiting HO in rat brain microsomes without affecting the activities of NOS and sGC.[62] All these and perhaps other undiscovered properties need to be considered when metalloporphyrins are used. However, of all the available metalloporphyrins, the natural zinc protoporphyrin (ZnPP), the synthetic, CrMP, and zinc bis glycol porphyrin (ZnBG) appear the most promising for physiologic studies.[13,97]

b. COHb in Blood

Carboxyhemoglobin concentrations in blood samples (120 to 140 µl) are determined within 1 month of storage at 4°C.[51,98] Briefly, 1 to 2 µl of blood is injected in triplicate into 2-ml septum sealed, CO-free, clear glass vials that contain 20 µl of 10% (w/v) $K_3Fe(CN)_6$ in 0.1 M potassium phosphate buffer, pH 6.0, containing 1% (w/v) saponin. The vials are incubated at 0°C (wet ice) for at least 30 min, but no longer than 1 h. The CO liberated into the vial headspace is then quantitated. The analyzer is standardized before and after each run of 16 sets of triplicate samples with volumes of standard gas containing 10.8 µl CO/l of air (Airco Air and Specialty Gases, Santa Clara, CA). The within-day and between-day coefficients of variation for reference blood samples using this method are 3% and 8%, respectively, with a minimum detectable concentration of 0.00005% COHb. COHb concentrations are traditionally expressed as a fraction of tHb saturation.[99] They are corrected for CO in inhaled air as follows[12,100]:

$$COHbc\ (\%\ tHb) = COHb\ (\%\ tHb) - 0.17\ \text{room air CO (ppm)}$$

The % tHb is used primarily because COHb measurements are made routinely for clinical evaluation of the effects of CO on oxygen transport and utilization. However, for the purpose of assessing the role of CO as a physiologically active agent, concentration units such as µmol or µl CO/ml blood or per mg Hb may be more appropriate.

Concentrations of tHb are measured with a manual cyanmethemoglobin method (Kit 525, Sigma Chemical Co., St. Louis, MO)[51] as follows. Triplicate samples of 4 µl of blood are reacted with 2.0 ml of Drabkin's reagent for a minimum of 2 h at room temperature. The absorbency of the resultant cyanmethemoglobin solution is determined at 540 nm with a spectrophotometer (Model UV-160, Shimadzu Scientific Instruments Inc., Columbia, MD). The within-day and between-day coefficients of variation for reference blood samples are 2.2% and 3.0%, respectively.[99] Typical COHb concentrations for human neonates and adults for different conditions are listed in Table 15.2. A preliminary COHb value for adult mice (n = 19) is 0.34 ± 0.11% tHb (authors' unpublished data).

Arterio–Venous COHb: The utilization or production of CO for physiologic processes can conceivably be quantitated via measurements of CO in arterial and venous blood. However, the potential for making such measurements is complicated

TABLE 15.2
Representative Values for Total Body Carbon Monoxide (CO) Measurements

Subject	COHb (% tHb)	Ref.	VeCO (µl/h/kg)	Ref.	ETCOc, µl/l (ppm)	Ref.
Fetus						
Normal	1.11 ± 0.14	99				
Hemolytic	1.59 ± 0.72	99				
Newborn						
Premature	0.86 ± 0.28[a]	98	17.2 ± 4.4	157	1.7 ± 0.5	98
Ventilated premature	1.06 ± 0.40	158	22.8 ± 5.5	158		
LGA-IDM	0.63 ± 0.13	157	19.9 ± 7.0	157		
Pulmonary dysfunction	0.49 ± 0.15	157	19.7 ± 6.8	157		
Term	0.45 ± 0.13	158	13.4 ± 3.2	158	1.6 ± 0.4	135
Hemolytic	2.13 ± 1.11	159				
Rh	2.13 ± 1.11	159	36.0 ± 22.2	159	5.7 ± 0.4	160
ABO	1.20 ± 0.42	159	17.4 ± 8.4	159	2.0 ± 0.7	160
Glucose-6-phosphate deficient	0.74 ± 0.14[a]	100			2.0 ± 0.5	161
Down's syndrome	0.92 ± 0.17[a]	162				
Child						
Normal					1.2 ± 0.5	82
Sickle cell					6.4 ± 2.9	82
Thalassemia					3.6 ± 1.5	82
Adults						
Normal	0.56 ± 0.11	44	6.6 ± 1.9	163	1.8 ± 0.7	82
Smoker	Up to 14	83			17.0 ± 8.2	
Asthmatic					5.6 ± 0.6	138
Sickle cell					4.9 ± 1.5	82
Thalassemia					6.3 ± 1.4	82
Bronchiectasis					6.0	164
Animals						
Rat			17.2 ± 4.7	*		
Mouse	0.34 ± 0.11	*	44.3 ± 10.7	*		

Note: The values listed were selected from a wide range reported in the literature or authors' unpublished results (*), and are for illustrative purposes only. The magnitude of each value depends on a number of factors, including the sensitivity and accuracy of methodology, the possibility of inhaled CO > 0.5 ppm, usually found in unpolluted air, sampling efficiency, etc. Most values were originally reported as mean ± SD; others were shown as mean ± SEM.

[a] Corrected for inhaled CO.

by the large pool of CO already bound to Hb. It is reasonable to assume that at most 0.1 µl/l (5%) of the 2.0 µl/l of CO excreted with breath at steady state conditions is derived from CO used for eliciting a physiologic response. This concentration represents 0.1 µl/l × 0.5 l breath = 0.05 µl CO produced during the 6 sec needed to equilibrate and excrete it with the breath (at 10 breaths per min). If this amount of CO were to be excreted into the blood flow, estimated at 1 ml/6 sec of an organ's arterial blood flow with a basal COHb concentration of 0.5% tHb (approximately 7 µl CO/ml blood) the method must be at least sensitive and accurate enough to detect an increase in venous baseline CO of 7 µl CO/ml blood with 0.05 µl CO/ml CO or 1%. This degree of sensitivity can be achieved with the most sensitive GC/RGD technique, but the measurement appears to be impossible due to the limited reproducibility of the method and other considerations. Special procedures need to be developed to detect such differences accurately and reproducibly.

c. CO in Plasma

The COHb method can also be applied to the measurement of free CO dissolved in the aqueous phase of blood plasma or CO possibly bound to circulating, non-hemolysis-derived hemoproteins. The authors made such measurements in human and mouse plasma, but found that when 40 µl of plasma samples were analyzed, no significant amounts (<1 pmol CO) of unbound or bound CO could be demonstrated (unpublished observations).

In contrast, Chalmers reported a simple, sensitive method for the measurement of CO in plasma, which should be applicable to estimations of CO in other aqueous body fluids, such as cerebrospinal fluid.[32] Fresh plasma from men (n = 17) and women (n = 8) was found to contain 0.14 to 0.60 mg CO/l with a mean of 0.36 mg/l or 13.0 µmol/l. This is an unlikely high CO concentration in water in the presence of a reported $1.0 \pm 0.8\%$ COHb and a large excess of oxyhemoglobin (O_2Hb). Also disturbing was the finding of no differences in plasma CO concentrations between smokers (mean COHb of $4.6 \pm 1.5\%$) and the control group.

In spite of these findings, Shi et al. used this method to identify a role for CO (and NO) in newborn infants with postasphyxial HIE.[31] Plasma CO levels in 28 neonates with HIE were significantly higher than those in five infants without HIE and in normal controls. The authors concluded that plasma CO levels (5.5 to 103 µmol/l) after perinatal asphyxia are related to the severity of neonatal HIE, brain damage, and neurological outcome. The detection limit of the plasma CO method was 3.5 µmol/l. The authors of this review question how so much free CO could be found in the presence of RBC O_2Hb. Others found that environmental exposure to CO resulted in interstitial CO concentrations in the nM range (11 nM at COHb of 3.8%).[101,102] It is clear that this issue needs to be examined in more detail, with appropriate methods.

d. CO in Tissues

To determine whether CO is indeed a biological messenger molecule, it is important to accurately measure the potential for CO production (activity of HO) in tissues[85] and also the concentration of CO in target tissues pre- and post- perturbations. Sokal et al. examined and measured CO concentrations in muscle and brain tissues and found that a combination of the greater affinity of Mb for CO and lower dissociation velocity constant for CO favored CO retention in muscular tissue. They also observed that certain, yet unidentified, mechanisms prevented equilibration between the vascular and extravascular components.[103] Other studies have shown that during exercise, CO has been found to diffuse from blood to skeletal muscle.[104] However, comprehensive studies on tissue concentrations have not yet been performed.

The authors developed the following sensitive method to quantitate the concentration of CO in rat and mouse tissue sonicates.[105] Tissues are harvested from experimental animals and immediately blanched with ice-cold 100 mM KPO$_4$ buffer. One part tissue is sonicated with three parts of ice-cold buffer. Forty µl of sonicate (10 mg tissue) is incubated in CO-free vials at 0°C with 10 µl of 50% (w/v) sulfosalicylic acid to dissociate CO bound to hemoproteins such as carboxyhemoglobin and carboxymyoglobin. After 30 min, the CO liberated into the vial headspace is quantitated.

The preliminary data on the native concentrations of CO in rat and mouse tissues indicate that only spleen and muscle tissue CO concentrations are significantly different in rats and mice. In addition, while blood has the highest CO concentration, tissues such as spleen, heart, kidney, muscle, and liver, which are rich in hemoproteins, also contain substantial amounts of CO. In contrast, the brain, lung, intestine, and testes, which have been reported to produce CO for physiologic processes, contained the lowest concentrations of CO. The method is being used to quantitate tissue CO concentrations after exogenous CO exposure and heme and methylene chloride (MC) administration, etc.

2.　CO Generation from Non-Heme Processes

a.　Lipid Peroxidation

A provocative, and possibly important, source of endogenous CO is through reactions not involving heme. Recently, the authors established that the *in vitro* iron-ascorbate-mediated peroxidation of cellular membranes can generate CO.[106] The CO generation correlated with the simultaneous production of thiobarbituric acid-reactive substances (TBARS), lipid peroxides, and conjugated dienes. Thus, it was concluded that CO is derived from the oxidation of membrane lipids. The following assay was developed for testing various tissues for susceptibility to lipid peroxidation or the absence of antioxidants.

Tissue sonicates, 20% w/v, in phosphate buffer are incubated for 30 min at 37°C in septum-sealed vials in the dark with Fe^{2+} (6 µM) and ascorbate (100 µM). Butylated hydroxytoluene (100 µM) is added for the blank reaction. CO produced into the headspace is quantitated. When sonicates of adult rat brain, kidney, and spinal cord are thus incubated, relatively large amounts of CO are produced. In contrast, other tissues appeared to be protected from oxidation by cytoplasmic antioxidants. Lipid peroxidation values for various tissues from rats and mice are shown in Table 15.2. When the *in vitro* rates of CO formation via lipid peroxidation and HO are compared for rat and mouse brain, lipid peroxidation produces 2.6- and 4.6-fold more CO, respectively. An intriguing question arises as to whether the production of CO via lipid peroxidation can be regulated by endogenously produced antioxidants (including biliverdin, bilirubin, and vitamin E) and iron chelators (including citrate).

b.　Photooxidation

A number of natural hydrocarbon-containing products have been found to generate CO upon exposure to fluorescent light, even in the absence of photosensitizers.[76,107]

Furthermore, riboflavin (vitamin B_6) has been studied as an endogenous photosensitizer.[108] Some metalloporphyrins have been reported to be photosensitizers — an undesirable side effect if these compounds are to be used clinically. The authors found that metalloporphyrins interact with light and oxygen to generate reactive oxygen species that in turn react with organic molecules, such as reduced nicotinamide adenine dinucleotide (NADH), to generate CO.[109] This reaction can be used for the identification of photoreactive compounds *in vitro* as follows.

Metalloporphyrins (or other potential photosensitizing compounds) are incubated at approximately 40 μM concentrations in 60 μl of 4.5 mM NADH or histidine (Sigma Chemical Co., St. Louis, MO) at 37°C in clear, CO-free septum-sealed 2-ml vials. The vials are then exposed to cool white fluorescent light (20 μW/cm^2/nm or 30 W/m^2) for 15 min. The generated CO diffused into the headspace is then quantitated. The results, corrected for dark control reactions determined simultaneously, are expressed in terms of pmoles of CO generated per vial per 15 min.

This method can also be used to determine the propensity of specific light sources to promote photooxidative reactions.[110,111] Irradiance is measured with a Joey Dosimeter (Healthdyne Technologies, Inc., Marietta, GA) over the range of 425 to 550 nm. For some light sources outside the latter range, light intensities are determined with a Model 2M thermopile detector with sapphire window and argon gas (Dexter Research Center, Dexter, MI). This detector has a flat spectral response from ultraviolet to far infrared and a linear signal output from 10^{-2} to 10^3 W/m^2.

c. Catabolism of Xenobiotics: Methylene Chloride

Methylene chloride (MC) is catabolized to CO in the liver via a microsomal mixed function oxidase (MFO)/cytochrome P-450 pathway and to carbon dioxide (CO_2) via a cytoplasmic glutathione-dependent pathway.[112] The CO pathway may have significance as an alternative source of endogenous CO which does not produce the biologically active byproducts (biliverdin, bilirubin, and Fe^{2+}) associated with heme catabolism.

The authors are studying the *in vitro* catabolism of MC to CO in mouse tissue sonicates in order to determine which tissues have this catabolic capability. The results should also produce further insight into the mechanism of MC toxicity. *In vitro* MC metabolism by tissue sonicates is determined via measurements of CO generated into the vial headspace of 2-ml septum-sealed reaction vials containing NADPH after 15 min incubation at 37°C. Blank reactions do not contain NADPH. The reactions are terminated by the addition of sulfosalicylic acid to 2% (w/v). Preliminary studies established that the rate of MC metabolism (pmol CO/h/mg fresh weight) by adult mouse organ sonicates was highest for the liver, blood, brain, and spleen. Lung, intestine, heart, kidney, and testes demonstrated significant but lower CO production rates.[113]

d. Other Sources of CO

A number of publications commented on the parallelism between the CO and NO pathways. The authors wish to point out that similarities exist, but fundamental differences that may be most important for understanding the physiologic effects of the two gases also exist. First, evidence indicates that the CO-generating enzymes,

HO-1 and HO-2, in contrast to the NOS enzymes, may have regulatory functions other than the catabolism of heme and, possibly, the production of CO. Second, in contrast to NO, a large pool of circulatory CO (as COHb) exists. Third, intracellular non-hemoglobin heme turnover is another significant source of CO. Finally, perhaps in parallel with NO, the authors speculate that a dedicated or at least a controlled pathway or process for the production and disposal of physiologically directed CO may exist. The CO may be derived from any of the processes mentioned above or other non-heme derived processes, such as lipid peroxidation, may deliver the intracellular CO.

The authors have evidence for the existence of other, still unidentified, sources. For example, the blank reaction (in the absence of NADPH or in the presence of all metalloporphyrin inhibitors of HO, except those with manganese as the central metal atom) for the *in vitro* HO assay (see Section III.B.1.a) produces significant amounts of CO, the rates of which appear to be dependent on the types of tissue.[114] Moreover, studies with manganese metalloporphyrin indicated that these compounds were metabolized. Upon closer examination, the blank CO production rate, in contrast to production in the presence of other metalloporphyrins, was depressed.[115] This observation may possibly provide a tool for the study of this "uninhibitable" source of CO.

Furthermore, the authors' inability to inhibit the VeCO of rodents with high doses of metalloporphyrins, even when HO activities in the major organs were completely inhibited, raises questions about the possible existence of other sources of CO (see Section III.C.1). These issues and others that may emerge need to be investigated. Finally, when investigating the role of CO as a physiologically active agent, an investigator should keep an open mind to allow for the discovery of possible minor sources of CO.

C. *In Vivo* CO Measurements Using GC/RGD

In vivo (or *ex vivo*) experimental models are needed to verify and extend the results of *in vitro* studies of CO production and oxidation via various pathways. The challenge for *in vivo* models is the difficult isolation and study of the organs responsible for CO production. More work in this area needs to be done. *Ex vivo* organ perfusion is one useful tool.[24] The presently available *in vivo* methods described below are variations of the VeCO method, in which an animal is studied in a flow-through chamber and the outlet air is analyzed for CO and other metabolic products such as CO_2, hydrogen, and water. Different inhibitory or stimulatory agents that affect the rate of CO production via the different CO generating processes, such as heme degradation (HO activity), lipid peroxidation, photooxidation, and xenobiotic metabolism can be administered to test subjects. These methods are only summarized; for more detail, the reader is directed to the referenced publications.

1. VeCO and Heme Degradation

The VeCO measurement represents the net result of the combined production rates of CO in all tissues by all CO producing processes and the oxidation of CO to CO_2 (Figure 15.3). However, the degradation of heme, mediated by the activities of HO-1, HO-2, and possibly HO-3 isozymes, is the primary source of CO.[3] VeCO measurements do not represent total body HO activity (such as measured *in vitro*), but rather the total body heme degradation rate or (possibly) the level of available heme in the organs, primarily in the spleen and liver. From *in vitro*[115] and *in vivo*[116,117] studies, the authors concluded that native HO activity appears to be in excess of heme availability in all organs except the spleen. A corollary to this concept is that, when HO activity in tissues is increased, it will not result in increased CO production. It has been suggested that up-regulation of HO activity (enzyme) may increase the potential for heme degradation and CO production, and may also mediate other processes, such as cytoprotection against oxidative injury (personal communication from P.A. Dennery).

To study processes not involving HO (see below), it is important that CO production via the heme pathway is kept at steady state or controlled for, so that perturbations of the minor processes can be measured with an appropriate degree of accuracy.

The measurement of VeCO with a flow-through apparatus is performed as follows. The GC/RGD is first calibrated with various concentrations (0 to 2 µl/l) of CO in zero CO air. This zero CO air (≤1 ppb) is produced by passing compressed air through a catalytic combustion filter (Trace Analytical, Inc.) with Hopcalite (an MnO and CuO mixture, Mine Safety Appliances Co., Pittsburgh, PA) operated at 110°C.[118] Animals are then placed head first into sealed plexiglass or polypropylene containers of suitable size (approximately 2 ml/g body weight), which are supplied with an airflow of (measured and low) CO concentration, approximately 0.5 ml/min/g body weight for rats[119] and mice.[120] After an equilibration period of ≥30 min, the chamber outlet gas is passed into a sample loop (0.1 to 2 ml volume), attached between the sample inlet and outlet ports of the injection valve, and the CO concentration is quantitated regularly for the duration of the experiment.

Animals can be studied for 7 to 12 h without signs of discomfort. The method can be used to study the *in vivo* efficacy of HO inhibitors[115] and heme preparations[117,120] as well as precursors.[27] For example, the inhibitory potential of metalloporphyrins was studied in an iatrogenic hemolytic model.[117] Under normal physiologic conditions, the native VeCO of rats can be inhibited by no more than 30% by high concentrations of various metalloporphyrins.[119,121] However, the HO activities in major CO-producing organs, the liver and spleen, were nearly abolished. This results in excretion of heme into the intestine, where it is metabolized to produce the CO that was not generated in the liver and spleen. Alternatively, the incompletely inhibited VeCO may involve unequal distribution of the inhibitors to tissues or the possibility that the proportion of the total body CO derived from heme degradation may be less for rodents than for humans.[15] This issue requires further investigation.

Adapting technology from earlier studies with humans,[118] the authors refined the VeCO method with small animals to allow quantitation of pulmonary — separately from total body — CO excretion rates in neonatal rats and hairless mice.[110] Typical VeCO (µl CO/h/kg body weight) values for various species and conditions are presented in Table 15.2.

2. Lipid Peroxidation

Lipid peroxidation is an autocatalytic free radical process that degrades polyunsaturated fatty acids in cell membranes to a number of short chain organic compounds, including CO. An *in vivo* model for lipid peroxidation-mediated CO production not involving the heme degradation pathway has not yet been developed. Divalent heavy metal (Cd^{2+}, Co^{2+}, Cu^{2+}, Ni^{2+}, Pb^{2+}, and Sn^{2+}) toxicity is most likely a lipid peroxidation-mediated process.[122] However, exposure to heavy metal ions also greatly increases HO mRNA, protein and activity in several tissues.[123] Thus, heavy metal administration may result in increased CO production via both processes. The authors are attempting to duplicate in an animal model an earlier clinical observation: a human premature neonate was found to have increased VeCO after administration of 1.5 mg/kg iron. This elevation was abolished upon intramuscular administration of 30 mg antioxidant vitamin E/kg body weight.[124]

3. Phototoxicity

The authors found a strong correlation between *in vitro* photooxidation of bilirubin and other organic compounds[109,125] and *in vivo* phototoxicity in newborn rats.[126] Because the following *in vivo* method for the testing of photosensitizers[115] is likely to involve suffering of the animals, it should only be used as a last resort, perhaps only to confirm negative or positive *in vitro* results.

Metalloporphyrins or other potential photosensitizers such as riboflavin are administered at doses of 40 µmol/kg body weight to 12- to 24-h old neonatal Wistar rats or hairless mice. Animals are placed in plexiglass (30 ml) chambers supplied with air at 10 ± 2 ml/min. The chambers are placed over, under, or between a bank of four 24-inch cool white fluorescent light tubes (20 W each, providing an irradiance of 20 µW/cm^2/nm or 30 W/m^2) and the animals' behavior is continuously monitored. The temperature is maintained at $30 \pm 1°C$ with circulating air. The survival rate after 12 h of light exposure is used as an index of phototoxicity. Animals treated with 30 µmol tin protoporphyrin (SnPP)/kg body weight are used as positive controls. Animals treated with the test compound and kept in the dark and untreated animals exposed to the light should be used as controls. Additional useful parameters that can be measured simultaneously are hydrogen, CO_2, and H_2O excretion.[126]

This method can also be used to compare the relative photosafety levels of different light sources for phototherapy in conjunction with drug (metalloporphyrin or other photosensitizer) administration.[110,111]

Intriguing is an observation by Furchgott and Jothianandan who found that rat aorta relaxed when exposed to light.[9] They hypothesized that a photo-induced relaxing factor stimulated sGC and could be inactivated by superoxide and hemoglobin. CO seems to be a reasonable candidate.

a. Evaluation of Light Photosafety

The authors have shown that CO is generated *in vitro* during photooxidation of organic compounds in the presence of natural and synthetic photosensitizers.[109] During studies comparing the efficacy of 360° exposure to light-emitting diodes (LEDs) and fluorescent and fiberoptic lights to decrease plasma bilirubin levels in newborn Gunn rats, light exposure caused significant elevations of VeCO.[127] To elucidate the source of this CO generation, total body, head, and trunk VeCO levels were monitored in 1- to 7-day-old Wistar rat pups kept in the dark and during subsequent 30-min exposure to light sources emitting 100 μW/cm^2/nm irradiance.[110] The pups were enclosed in specially constructed dual-section plexiglass chambers supplied with 20 ml air/min. CO concentrations in chamber section exit air were quantitated. The total body VeCO was measured for each group exposed to each light source and increases from baseline levels were found to be the greatest in those exposed to fluorescent light, followed by fiberoptic, blue LED, and green LED light.

Subsequent separate CO measurements of the head and trunk demonstrated that only the head (representing pulmonary CO excretion) excreted CO in the dark. However, upon exposure to light, CO excretion of the head (~15% body surface area) and the trunk increased quickly (within 2 to 30 min) significantly, and returned to dark VeCO levels within 30 min of light exposure cessation. It was concluded that the wavelength-dependent photogeneration of CO is most likely the result of interactions of light with endogenous photosensitizers in the skin and that CO is subsequently excreted primarily through neonatal skin. Furthermore, the rate of CO excretion was found to be wavelength (light source)-dependent.

A follow-up study with intraperitoneally administered riboflavin (10 μM per rat pup) demonstrated that this vitamin, which is known to be destroyed upon photo-therapy,[128,129] may be one of the CO-generating endogenous photosensitizers.[111] No studies have yet been performed to determine whether vascular bed blood flow is affected by the superficial photogeneration of CO.

4. Catabolism of Xenobiotics: Methylene Chloride

CO is implicated in the regulation of cell function and communication. While CO derived from the degradation of heme is important, CO derived from potential non-heme sources, such as the peroxidation of cell membrane lipids[106] and the degradation of xenobiotics such as MC[112,130] is also important. Furthermore, because heme degradation yields other physiologically active compounds (biliverdin, bilirubin, Fe^{2+}), it is important to develop a less complex source of local CO. Hayashi et al. found that induction of HO-1 activity could serve as a potential strategy to prevent oxidant-induced microvascular leukocyte adhesion through the action of bilirubin rather than CO.[131]

The authors studied the *in vivo* metabolism of MC to CO in the mouse and developed a model for iatrogenic, non-heme-derived CO production as follows[113]: After intraperitoneal administration of 39 and 78 nmol MC (in mineral oil)/g body weight, VeCO rose immediately, peaked within 25 min, and returned to baseline by 3 h. The relatively high metabolic rate in blood observed in *in vitro* studies (see Section III.E.1) may account for the very rapid rise of exhaled CO. These preliminary studies demonstrate that administration of MC results in an immediate increase in endogenous CO production rates. Furthermore, although the liver appears to be the major site of CO production, all other organs studied are capable of producing CO locally from this substrate (see Section III.E.1). These findings may lead eventually to finding a means to deliver physiologically active CO to organs to study the physiologic role of CO. Planned measurements of tissue CO concentrations are expected to demonstrate which organs metabolize administered MC with the consequence of increased tissue CO concentrations. The findings may also offer a method for real-time non-invasive monitoring of the physiologic consequences of MC toxicity.

5.　Oxidation of CO to CO_2

We have known about oxidation of CO to CO_2 since 1932; the process is believed to play a minor role relative to the major CO-producing process of heme degradation.[132] Several studies reported on different aspects of CO oxidation mediated by cytochrome oxidase.[70,132-134] However, it seems prudent to re-examine the CO oxidation process, particularly with regard to the possiblility that it acts as a sink for "spent" physiologic CO and may function as a local destruction mechanism. No recent studies have been reported on this topic. However, using the more sensitive analytical CO quantitation methods presently available, the authors are engaged in re-examining the earlier work. It is hoped that a sensitive method can be developed to determine the rates of CO oxidation in the major tissues.

D.　CO MEASUREMENTS USING THE CO-STAT™ END TIDAL BREATH ANALYZER

Because of high breathing rates, small tidal volumes, and inability to hold their breaths, a sensitive and specific device needed to be developed for estimating the rate of bilirubin production in neonates.[45] The CO-Stat™ End Tidal Breath Analyzer using a single-patient disposable nasal sampler (Natus Medical Inc., San Carlos, CA), was developed for measuring end tidal CO in breath, corrected for inhaled CO (ETCOc).[81,82] Other measurements provided by the device include breath CO concentration uncorrected for ambient CO concentration (ETCO), ambient CO concentration (reflecting inhaled air), end tidal CO_2, and respiratory rate. The device utilizes side-stream sampling to continuously sample breath by drawing small volumes of air through a sampling catheter composed of a soft, clear polymer with an outside diameter of 2.0 mm. Adhesive "wings" allow a maximum insertion depth of 6 mm before the device comes into contact with the lower edge of the nostril. The ETCOc measurement is made when the subject is sleeping or quiet: movement should be minimal. The instrument has a range of 0 to 25 ppm with a resolution of 0.1 ppm CO. Its accuracy is 0.3 ppm or 10% of the reading (whichever is greater) at 0 to 60 breaths/min. It is insensitive to H_2 concentrations <50 ppm. Several studies on neonates, children, and adults have been conducted.[45,81,82,135]

　　A series of reports on the correlation of ETCO measurements with EC sensors and pulmonary inflammatory diseases have been published.[136,137] Initially, ETCOc values as high as 14 ppm with 5.6 ± 0.6 ppm (mean ± SEM) were reported.[138] ETCOc values of 2.5 vs. 1.8 ppm for untreated patients and normal individuals, respectively, were reported recently for similar clinical profiles.[137] It seems inconceivable that HO- or lipid peroxidation-mediated CO generation in the airways can be many-fold greater than the normal turnover of total body heme (approximately 2 ppm). The possibility exists that some of the early CO measurements were inaccurate due to the presence of interferents, leading to falsely elevated ETCOc readings.[43] One means to resolve the question of whether ETCOc measurement is an accurate marker for pulmonary insufficiency is to measure ETCOc with an analyzer, such as the CO-Stat, which is not affected by breath contaminants. It would also be instructive to obtain measurements of COHb with a sensitive and accurate method to determine whether the increase in ETCOc is due to systemic or pulmonary processes. Alternatively, pre- and post-treatment patient breath may be analyzed with GC/MS in order to identify breath components other than CO that could change in concentration after treatment.

E. Accessory Non-CO-Producing Methods

1. *In Vitro* Methods

Although accessory methods do not directly measure produced CO, they nevertheless are valuable tools that provide important pieces to the puzzle of the potential for CO production and utilization. However, it is not appropriate to directly equate the presence or induction of HO mRNA and protein with *in vivo* CO production. There are simply too many possible regulatory processes between transcription and product formation.

a. HO Activity via Bilirubin Measurements

The measurement of bilirubin as an index of HO activity was originally developed by Tenhunen et al.[2] and the method has provided much basic information regarding the biology of HO.[3] A major limitation of this method is that it is based on the spectrophotometric quantitation of bilirubin produced in the reaction mixture.[139] Bilirubin spectrophotometry requires particle-free homogeneous solutions with negligible light absorption by non-bilirubin components of the reaction mixture near the peak absorption of bilirubin (470 nm). However, because HO is a membrane-bound enzyme, it is difficult to eliminate its light-scattering properties even in purified microsomal membranes. Furthermore, the substrate (methemalbumin) and the metalloporphyrin inhibitors of HO also absorb light at 470 nm, so that only relatively low concentrations of these compounds can be used, with the result that only low rates of bilirubin are measured. In addition, bilirubin binds to proteins and this alters its molecular absorption coefficient in not totally predictable ways, introducing yet another complication and generally immeasurable error.[87] Efforts have been made to circumvent these problems by extraction of bilirubin followed by direct photometric determination or by high-pressure liquid chromatography purification followed by spectrophotometric quantitation. However, the labor-intensive extraction steps preclude the design of comprehensive experiments with small tissue samples.

b. HO Isozyme mRNA

HO-1 and HO-2 isozyme mRNA levels are quantitated by Northern blot hybridizations.[140] Total RNA is extracted from tissue sonicates using commercially available kits (Qiagen Inc., Valencia, CA) and usually 10 µg is analyzed on glyoxal gels. RNA is then transferred from the gels to a positively charged membrane (Hybond, Amersham Pharmacia Biotech, Piscataway, NJ) by passive absorbance of buffer (6× SSC) overnight. Hybridization with HO-1 cDNA probes[140] is conducted at 65°C in 5× SSC for 6 h followed by successive washes. Detection of probes by autoradiographs is visualized and quantitated by densitometry and normalized to β-actin.

c.   HO Isozyme Protein

Quantitation of HO isozyme protein levels is quantitated by Western blot hybridizations. Polyclonal rabbit anti-rat HO-1 antibodies are raised against 30-kD HO-1- and 36-kD HO-2 proteins expressed in *E. coli* from rat liver cDNA. Between 50 and 100 μg of tissue sonicates are subjected to 12% SDS/PAGE[141,142] and transferred to polyvinylidene difluoride membranes using a Bio-Rad electroblot device. HO-1- and HO-2 proteins are detected using primary rabbit polyclonal human HO-1 and/or HO-2 antibody (Stressgen, Toronto, Canada), secondary goat anti-rabbit IgG (H + L) (Bio-Rad, Hercules, CA). Bands are visualized by chemiluminescence according to manufacturer protocol (Bio-Rad) and then are quantitated by densitometry.

2. *In Vivo* Methods

Like methods for *in vitro* assays, *in vivo* methods are not based on direct CO measurements, but on quantitation of elements essential to the CO-producing pathways at the molecular or biochemical level to non-invasively determine how CO-producing processes are regulated.

a.   Plasma Bilirubin

Even though heme degradation yields equimolar amounts of CO and bilirubin, measurements of plasma and serum bilirubin are almost exclusively used clinically to assess the risk for developing excessive unconjugated jaundice, which may lead to life-threatening kernicterus in neonates.[143,144] The quantitation of bilirubin with clinical analyzers is subject to considerable variability due to a number of factors.[145] Measurements of plasma bilirubin are unlikely to be useful as indices for total body CO production because of the rapid distribution of bilirubin into tissues or excretion with bile. However, these measurements have been useful for understanding photooxidative processes which yield CO (Section III.C.3), particularly as studied in Gunn rats.[127] Furthermore, because bilirubin has been identified as a potent antioxidant,[4,5] it is expected to be a factor in the production of CO via lipid peroxidative processes.

b.   Transcutaneous Bilirubinometry

Like plasma bilirubin measurements, the measurement of bilirubin in the skin (jaundice) with transcutaneous (TcB) jaundice meters is not useful for quantitatively assessing rates of CO production or accumulation.[146,147] Jaundice in humans is most often due to unconjugated bilirubin accumulation in circulation, which is quantitated as plasma or serum bilirubin, due to increased bilirubin (and CO) production and a usually temporary diminished capacity of the liver to excrete bilirubin. Gunn rats[148,149] and mice,[150] like humans with the Crigler–Najjar Syndrome,[151] lack the glucuronosyl-transferase enzyme in the liver, which conjugates bilirubin with glucuronic acid. They therefore lack the mechanism to excrete bilirubin with the bile. The authors are using TcB measurements for studies involving photooxidative processes as well.

c. HO-1 Transcription

A novel method[152] has been developed for minimally invasive real-time monitoring of *in vivo* HO-1 transcription in a variety of organs. Whole body bioluminescence imaging using sensitive light imaging systems has been applied to quantitate expression of reporter genes that encode for the light-producing enzyme, luciferase (*luc*).[153,154] These *in vivo* measurements are approximately as sensitive as those obtained using *ex vivo luc* activity measurements. The detection limit in the liver is 35 pg of *luc* enzyme/g liver, and one cell in a million transduced liver cells.[155]

HO-1 transcription can be measured in transgenic mice, in which the transgene (HO-*luc* Tg) consists of the full-length HO-1 promoter directing expression of the *luc* reporter gene. Anesthetized HO-*luc* Tg mice are administered 150 mg luciferin kg of body weight intraperitoneally. Luciferin is then rapidly converted to oxyluciferin by luciferase in the presence of oxygen and ATP and results in the emission of a photon of light. Photon emission is detected and displayed using a cooled charge-coupled camera device. The light intensity of the collected image is then quantitated. Any changes in HO-1 promoter activity, and therefore transcription, are monitored through a change in reporter gene expression, which is proportional to the amount of light emitted.

Previous studies using this Tg mouse line have shown a correlation between *in vivo* light production and *in vitro luc* activity and protein levels. Therefore, to study the effects of inducers (such as heme) and inhibitors (such as metalloporphyrins) on HO-1 gene regulation, changes in transcription can be assessed via *luc* reporter gene expression in a transgenic mouse line (HO-*luc* Tg).[156] By integrating these *in vivo* findings with traditional *in vitro* assays of enzyme activity and protein levels, the mechanisms by which HO is regulated, i.e., at the level of transcription or somewhere downstream, may finally be fully elucidated.

IV. CONCLUSIONS

We now have available sensitive and accurate methods for measuring CO concentration in tissues as well as CO production rates *in vitro* and *in vivo*. We have also identified other sources of CO that should be considered in studies investigating a physiologic role for CO.

ACKNOWLEDGMENTS

We thank Jay G. Bryson, Ph.D., for his critical review of this manuscript. This work was supported by National Institutes of Health Grants HD14426, RR00070, and HL58013, and unrestricted gifts from the H. M. Lui Research Fund, the Hess Research Fund, and the Mary L. Johnson Research Fund.

Abbreviations

CO	carbon monoxide	MFO	mixed function oxidase
CO_2	carbon dioxide	NIR	near infrared
COHb	carboxyhemoglobin	NO	nitric oxide
COMb	carboxymyoglobin	NOS	nitric oxide synthase
CrMP	chromium mesoporphyrin	O_2Hb	oxyhemoglobin
EC	electrochemical	ppb	parts per billion
EPA	Environmental Protection Agency	ppm	parts per million
ETCO	end tidal carbon monoxide	RBCs	red blood cells
ETCOc	end tidal carbon monoxide, corrected	RGD	reduction gas detector
	for inhaled carbon monoxide	sGC	soluble guanylate cyclase
FID	flame ionization detection	SnPP	tin protoporphyrin
GC	gas chromatography	TBARs	thiobarbituric acid reactive substances
Hb	hemoglobin	TcB	transcutaneous bilirubinometer
HIE	hypoxic ischemic encephalopathy	tHb	total hemoglobin
HO	heme oxygenase	VCO	total body carbon monoxide production rate
LED	light emitting diode	VeCO	total body carbon monoxide excretion rate
MC	methylene chloride	VOCs	volatile organic compounds
MS	mass spectroscopy	ZnBG	zinc bis glycol porphyrin
Mb	myoglobin	ZnPP	zinc protoporphyrin

REFERENCES

1. Sjöstrand, T., Endogenous formation of carbon monoxide in man under normal and pathological conditions, *Scand. J. Clin. Lab. Invest.*, 1, 201, 1949.
2. Tenhunen, R., Marver, H.S., and Schmid, R., The enzymatic conversion of heme to bilirubin by microsomal heme oxygenase, *Proc. Natl. Acad. Sci. U.S.A.*, 61, 748, 1968.
3. Maines, M.D., *Heme Oxygenase: Clinical Applications and Functions*, CRC Press, Boca Raton, FL, 1992.
4. Stocker, R. et al., Bilirubin is an antioxidant of possible physiological importance, *Science*, 235, 1043, 1987.
5. Dennery, P.A. et al., Hyperbilirubinemia results in reduced oxidative injury in neonatal Gunn rats exposed to hyperoxia, *Free Radic. Biol. Med.*, 19, 395, 1995.
6. Yao, T.C. and Stevenson, D.K., Advances in the diagnosis and treatment of neonatal hyperbilirubinemia, *Clin. Perinatol.*, 22, 741, 1995.
7. Vedernikov, Y.P., Gräser, T., and Vanin, A.F., Similar endothelium-independent arterial relaxation by carbon monoxide and nitric oxide, *Biomed. Biochim. Acta*, 48, 601, 1989.
8. Marks, G.S. et al., Does carbon monoxide have a physiological function? *Trends Pharmacol. Sci.*, 12, 185, 1991.
9. Furchgott, R.F. and Jothianandan, D., Endothelium-dependent and -independent vasodilation involving cyclic GMP: relaxation induced by nitric oxide, carbon monoxide and light, *Blood Vessels*, 28, 52, 1991.
10. Wang, R., Resurgence of carbon monoxide: an endogenous gaseous vasorelaxing factor, *Can. J. Physiol. Pharmacol.*, 76, 1, 1998.
11. Vreman, H.J., Mahoney, J.J., and Stevenson, D.K., Carbon monoxide and carboxyhemoglobin, *Adv. Pediatr.*, 42, 303, 1995.
12. Vreman, H.J., Wong, R.J., and Stevenson, D.K., Carbon monoxide in breath, blood, and other tissues, in *Carbon Monoxide Toxicity*, Penney, D.G., Ed., CRC Press, Boca Raton, FL, 2000, 19.

13. Stevenson, D.K. et al., Carbon monoxide detection and biological investigations, *Trans. Am. Clin. Climatol. Assoc.*, 111, 61, 2000.
14. Coburn, R.F., Williams, W.J., and Forster, R.E., Effect of erythrocyte destruction on carbon monoxide production in man, *J. Clin. Invest.*, 43, 1098, 1964.
15. Berk, P.D. et al., Comparison of plasma bilirubin turnover and carbon monoxide production in man, *J. Lab. Clin. Med.*, 83, 29, 1974.
16. Tenhunen, R., Marver, H.S., and Schmid, R., Microsomal heme oxygenase. Characterization of the enzyme, *J. Biol. Chem.*, 244, 6388, 1969.
17. Engel, R.R. et al., Carbon monoxide production from heme compounds by bacteria, *J. Bacteriol.*, 112, 1310, 1972.
18. Levine, A.S. et al., Metabolism of carbon monoxide by the colonic flora of humans, *Gastroenterology*, 83, 633, 1982.
19. Matsumoto, K.E. et al., The identification of volatile compounds in human urine, *J. Chromatogr.*, 85, 31, 1973.
20. Phillips, M., Breath tests in medicine, *Sci. Am.*, July 1992, p. 74.
21. Mahoney, J.J. et al., Measurement of carboxyhemoglobin and total hemoglobin by five specialized spectrophotometers (CO-oximeters) in comparison with reference methods, *Clin. Chem.*, 39, 1693, 1993.
22. Mahoney, J.J. et al., Fetal hemoglobin of transfused neonates and spectrophotometric measurements of oxyhemoglobin and carboxyhemoglobin, *J. Clin. Monit.*, 7, 154, 1991.
23. Israels, L.G. et al., The early bilirubin, *Medicine*, 45, 517, 1966.
24. Motterlini, R. et al., Heme oxygenase-1-derived carbon monoxide contributes to the suppression of acute hypertensive responses, *Circ. Res.*, 83, 568, 1998.
25. Sammut, I.A. et al., Carbon monoxide is a major contributor to the regulation of vascular tone in aortas expressing high levels of haeme oxygenase-1, *Br. J. Pharmacol.*, 125, 1437, 1998.
26. Lincoln, B.C., Aw, T.Y., and Bonkovsky, H.L., Heme catabolism in cultured hepatocytes: evidence that heme oxygenase is the predominant pathway and that a proportion of synthesized heme is converted rapidly to biliverdin, *Biochim. Biophys. Acta*, 992, 49, 1989.
27. Salomon, W.L. et al., Red cell destruction and bilirubin production in adult rats with short-term biliary obstruction, *J. Pediatr. Gastroenterol. Nutr.*, 5, 806, 1986.
28. Johnson, J.D. et al., Developmental changes in bilirubin production in the rat, *J. Pediatr. Gastroenterol. Nutr.*, 2, 142, 1983.
29. Suematsu, M. et al., Carbon monoxide: an endogenous modulator of sinusoidal tone in the perfused rat liver, *J. Clin. Invest.*, 96, 2431, 1995.
30. Mori, M. et al., Carbon monoxide-mediated alterations in paracellular permeability and vesicular transport in acetaminophen-treated perfused rat liver, *Hepatology*, 30, 160, 1999.
31. Shi, Y. et al., Role of carbon monoxide and nitric oxide in newborn infants with postasphyxial hypoxic-ischemic encephalopathy, *Pediatrics*, 106, 1447, 2000.
32. Chalmers, A.H., Simple, sensitive measurement of carbon monoxide in plasma, *Clin. Chem.*, 37, 1442, 1991.
33. Nathanson, J.A. et al., The cellular Na^+ pump as a site of action for carbon monoxide and glutamate: a mechanism for long-term modulation of cellular activity, *Neuron*, 14, 781, 1995.
34. Esler, M.B. et al., Precision trace gas analysis by FT-IR spectroscopy. 1. Simultaneous analysis of CO_2, CH_4, N_2O, and CO in air, *Anal. Chem.*, 72, 206, 2000.
35. Stepanov, E.V., Zyrianov, P.V., and Khusnutdinov, A.N., Multicomponent gas analyzers based on tunable diode lasers, *SPIE*, 2834, 1996.

36. Stepanov, E.V. and Kouznetsov, A.I., Endogenous CO dynamics monitoring in breath by tunable laser, *SPIE,* 2682, 247, 1996.
37. Topfer, T. et al., Room-temperature mid-infrared laser sensor for trace gas detection, *Appl. Opt.,* 36, 8042, 1997.
38. Morimoto, Y. et al., Real-time measurements of endogenous CO production from vascular cells using an ultrasensitive laser sensor, *Am. J. Physiol. Heart Circ. Physiol.,* 280, H483, 2001.
39. Cao, Z., Buttner, W.J., and Stetter, J.R., The properties and applications of amperometric gas sensors, *Electroanalysis,* 4, 253, 1992.
40. Kwor, R., Carbon monoxide detectors, in *Carbon Monoxide Toxicity,* Penney, D.G., Ed., CRC Press, Boca Raton, FL, 2000, 61.
41. Jarvis, M.J. et al., Low cost carbon monoxide monitors in smoking assessment, *Thorax,* 41, 886, 1986.
42. Stevenson, D.K., Rodgers, P.A., and Vreman, H.J., The use of metalloporphyrins for the chemoprevention of neonatal jaundice, *Am. J. Dis. Child.,* 143, 353, 1989.
43. Vreman, H.J., Wong, R.J., and Stevenson, D.K., Exhaled carbon monoxide in asthma, *J. Pediatr.,* 137, 889, 2000.
44. Vreman, H., Mahoney, J., and Stevenson, D., Electrochemical measurement of carbon monoxide in breath: interference by hydrogen, *Atmos. Environ.,* 27A, 2193, 1993.
45. Vreman, H.J. et al., Semiportable electrochemical instrument for determining carbon monoxide in breath, *Clin. Chem.,* 40, 1927, 1994.
46. Porter, K. and Vollman, D.H., Flame ionization detection of carbon monoxide for gas chromatographic analyses, *Anal. Chem.,* 34, 748, 1962.
47. Sunderman, F.W., Jr. et al., Gas-chromatographic assay for heme oxygenase activity, *Clin. Chem.,* 28, 2026, 1982.
48. Hoell, J.M. et al., Airborne intercomparison of carbon-monoxide measurement techniques, *J. Geophys. Res. [Atmos.],* 92, 2009, 1987.
49. Collison, H.A., Rodkey, F.L., and O'Neal, J.D., Determination of carbon monoxide in blood by gas chromatography, *Clin. Chem.,* 14, 162, 1968.
50. Rodkey, F.L. and Collison, H.A., An artifact in the analysis of oxygenated blood for its low carbon monoxide content, *Clin. Chem.,* 16, 896, 1970.
51. Vreman, H.J., Kwong, L.K., and Stevenson, D.K., Carbon monoxide in blood: an improved microliter blood-sample collection system, with rapid analysis by gas chromatography, *Clin. Chem.,* 30, 1382, 1984.
52. Tsunogai, U. et al., Stable carbon and oxygen isotopic analysis of carbon monoxide in natural waters, *Rapid Commun. Mass Spectrom.,* 14, 1507, 2000.
53. Kaide, J.I. et al., Role of heme oxygenase-derived carbon monoxide on vascular reactivity to vasopressin, *Acta Haematol.,* 103, 68, 2000.
54. Balazy, M. and Jiang, H., Analysis of carbon monoxide in biological fluids by isotopic dilution GC/MS, *Acta Haematol.,* 103, 78, 2000.
55. Seiler, W. and Junge, C., Carbon monoxide in the atmosphere, *J. Geophys. Res.,* 75, 2217, 1970.
56. Levitt, M.D., Ellis, C.J., and Engel, R.R., CO production by feces and urine, *J. Lab. Clin. Med.,* 113, 241, 1989.
57. Coceani, F. et al., Carbon monoxide formation in the ductus arteriosus in the lamb: implications for the regulation of muscle tone, *Br. J. Pharmacol.,* 120, 599, 1997.
58. Nath, K.A. et al., Induction of heme oxygenase is a rapid, protective response in rhabdomyolysis in the rat, *J. Clin. Invest.,* 90, 267, 1992.
59. Cook, M.N. et al., Heme oxygenase activity in the adult rat aorta and liver as measured by carbon monoxide formation, *Can. J. Physiol. Pharmacol.,* 73, 515, 1995.

60. Cook, M.N. et al., Ontogeny of heme oxygenase activity in the hippocampus, frontal cerebral cortex, and cerebellum of the guinea pig, *Brain Res. Dev. Brain Res.,* 92, 18, 1996.

61. Odrcich, M.J. et al., Heme oxygenase and nitric-oxide synthase in the placenta of the guinea-pig during gestation, *Placenta,* 19, 509, 1998.

62. Appleton, S.D. et al., Selective inhibition of heme oxygenase, without inhibition of nitric oxide synthase or soluble guanylyl cyclase, by metalloporphyrins at low concentrations, *Drug Metab. Dispos.,* 27, 1214, 1999.

63. *Air Quality Criteria for Carbon Monoxide*, U.S. Environmental Protection Agency, Research Triangle Park, NC, 1991.

64. *Air Quality Criteria for Carbon Monoxide*, U.S. Environmental Protection Agency, Research Triangle Park, NC, 1999.

65. Klepeis, N.E., Ott, W.R., and Switzer, P., A multiple-smoker model for predicting indoor air quality in public lounges, *Environ. Sci. Technol.,* 30, 2813, 1996.

66. Lando, H.A. et al., Use of carbon monoxide breath validation in assessing exposure to cigarette smoke in a worksite population, *Health Psychol.,* 10, 296, 1991.

67. Seufert, K.T. and Kiser, W.R., End-expiratory carbon monoxide levels as an estimate of passive smoking exposure aboard a nuclear-powered submarine, *South. Med. J.,* 89, 1181, 1996.

68. Jamrozik, K. et al., Controlled trial of three different antismoking interventions in general practice, *Br. Med. J.,* 288, 1499, 1984.

69. Jarvis, M.J. et al., Comparison of tests used to distinguish smokers from nonsmokers, *Am. J. Public Health,* 77, 1435, 1987.

70. Luomanmäki, K. and Coburn, R.F., Effects of metabolism and distribution of carbon monoxide on blood and body stores, *Am. J. Physiol.,* 217, 354, 1969.

71. Shimazu, T. et al., Half-life of blood carboxyhemoglobin after short-term and long-term exposure to carbon monoxide, *J. Trauma,* 49, 126, 2000.

72. Landaw, S.A., The effects of cigarette smoking on total body burden and excretion rates of carbon monoxide, *J. Occup. Med.,* 15, 231, 1973.

73. Peterson, J.E. and Stewart, R.D., Absorption and elimination of carbon monoxide by inactive young men, *Arch. Environ. Health,* 21, 165, 1970.

74. Stevenson, D.K., Estimation of bilirubin production, in *Report of the Eighty-Fifth Ross Conference on Pediatric Research*, Levine, R.L. and Maisels, M.J., Eds., Ross Laboratories, Columbus, OH, 1983, 64.

75. Rodkey, F.L., Collison, H.A., and Engel, R.R., Release of carbon monoxide from acrylic and polycarbonate plastics, *J. Appl. Physiol.,* 27, 554, 1969.

76. Levitt, M.D. et al., Carbon monoxide generation from hydrocarbons at ambient and physiological temperature: a sensitive indicator of oxidant damage? *J. Chromatogr. A,* 695, 324, 1995.

77. *Air Quality Criteria for Carbon Monoxide*, U.S. Environmental Protection Agency, Research Triangle Park, NC, 1999, Chap. 2.

78. *Air Quality Criteria for Carbon Monoxide*, U.S. Environmental Protection Agency, Research Triangle Park, NC, 1991, Chap. 8.

79. Metz, G. et al., A simple method of measuring breath hydrogen in carbohydrate malabsorption by end-expiratory sampling, *Clin. Sci. Mol. Med.,* 50, 237, 1976.

80. Yeung, C.Y. et al., Automatic end-expiratory air sampling device for breath hydrogen test in infants, *Lancet,* 337, 90, 1991.

81. Vreman, H.J. et al., Evaluation of a fully automated end-tidal carbon monoxide instrument for breath analysis, *Clin. Chem.,* 42, 50, 1996.

82. Vreman, H.J. et al., Validation of the Natus CO-Stat™ End Tidal Breath Analyzer in children and adults, *J. Clin. Monit. Comput.,* 15, 421, 1999.

83. Wald, N.J. et al., Carbon monoxide in breath in relation to smoking and carboxyhaemoglobin levels, *Thorax,* 36, 366, 1981.

84. Wallace, L. et al., Comparison of breath CO, CO exposure, and Coburn Model prediction in the U.S. E.P.A. Washington-Denver Study, *Atmos. Environ.,* 22, 2183, 1988.

85. Vreman, H.J. and Stevenson, D.K., Heme oxygenase activity as measured by carbon monoxide production, *Anal. Biochem.,* 168, 31, 1988.

86. Vreman, H.J. et al., Haem oxygenase activity in human umbilical cord and rat vascular tissues, *Placenta,* 21, 337, 1999.

87. Vreman, H.J. and Stevenson, D.K., Detection of heme oxygenase activity by measurement of CO, in *Current Protocols in Toxicology,* Maines, M.D. et al., Eds., John Wiley & Sons, New York, 1999, 9.2.1.

88. Zakhary, R. et al., Heme oxygenase 2: endothelial and neuronal localization and role in endothelium-dependent relaxation, *Proc. Natl. Acad. Sci. U.S.A.,* 93, 795, 1996.

89. Grundemar, L. and Ny, L., Pitfalls using metalloporphyrins in carbon monoxide research, *Trends Pharmacol. Sci.,* 18, 193, 1997.

90. Vreman, H.J. et al., *In vitro* heme oxygenase isozyme activity inhibition by metalloporphyrins, *Pediatr. Res.,* 43, 202A, 1998.

91. Imai, K. et al., Antioxidative effect of several porphyrins on lipid peroxidation in rat liver homogenates, *Chem. Pharm. Bull. (Tokyo),* 38, 258, 1990.

92. Wong, R.J., Vreman, H.J., and Stevenson, D.K., (Metallo)porphyrin inhibitors of heme oxygenase also inhibit lipid peroxidation (LP), *Pediatr. Res.,* 47, 465, 2000.

93. Vallier, H.A., Rodgers, P.A., and Stevenson, D.K., Oral administration of zinc deuteroporphyrin IX 2,4 bis glycol inhibits heme oxygenase in neonatal rats, *Dev. Pharmacol. Ther.,* 17, 220, 1991.

94. Vallier, H.A. et al., Absorption of zinc deuteroporphyrin IX 2,4-bis-glycol by the neonatal rat small intestine *in vivo, Dev. Pharmacol. Ther.,* 17, 109, 1991.

95. Vallier, H.A., Rodgers, P.A., and Stevenson, D.K., Inhibition of heme oxygenase after oral vs. intraperitoneal administration of chromium porphyrins, *Life Sci.,* 52, L79, 1993.

96. Meffert, M.K. et al., Inhibition of hippocampal heme oxygenase, nitric oxide synthase, and long-term potentiation by metalloporphyrins, *Neuron,* 13, 1225, 1994.

97. Labbé, R.F., Vreman, H.J., and Stevenson, D.K., Zinc protoporphyrin: a metabolite with a mission, *Clin. Chem.,* 45, 2060, 1999.

98. Fischer, A.F. et al., Carboxyhemoglobin concentration as an index of bilirubin production in neonates with birth weights less than 1,500 grams: a randomized double-blind comparison of supplemental oral vitamin E and placebo, *J. Pediatr. Gastroenterol. Nutr.,* 6, 748, 1987.

99. Widness, J.A. et al., Direct relationship of fetal carboxyhemoglobin with hemolysis in alloimmunized pregnancies, *Pediatr. Res.,* 35, 713, 1994.

100. Kaplan, M. et al., Neonatal hyperbilirubinemia in glucose-6-phosphate dehydrogenase-deficient heterozygotes, *Pediatrics,* 104, 68, 1999.

101. Coburn, R.F., Endogenous carbon monoxide production, *New Engl. J. Med.,* 282, 207, 1970.

102. Göthert, M., Lutz, F., and Malorny, G., Carbon monoxide partial pressure in tissue of different animals, *Environ. Res.,* 3, 303, 1970.

103. Sokal, J.A., Majka, J., and Palus, J., The content of carbon monoxide in the tissues of rats intoxicated with carbon monoxide in various conditions of acute exposure, *Arch. Toxicol.,* 56, 106, 1984.

104. Werner, B. and Lindahl, J., Endogenous carbon monoxide production after bicycle exercise in healthy subjects and in patients with hereditary spherocytosis, *Scand. J. Clin. Lab. Invest.*, 40, 319, 1980.

105. Wong, R.J. et al., Concentration of carbon monoxide (CO) in tissue, *J. Invest. Med.*, 48, 123A, 2000.

106. Vreman, H.J. et al., Simultaneous production of carbon monoxide and thiobarbituric acid reactive substances in rat tissue preparations by an iron-ascorbate system, *Can. J. Physiol. Pharmacol.*, 76, 1057, 1998.

107. Wilson, D.F., Swinnerton, J.W., and Lamontagne, R.A., Production of carbon monoxide and gaseous hydrocarbons in seawater: relation to dissolved organic carbon, *Science*, 168, 1577, 1970.

108. Sanvordeker, D.R. and Kostenbauder, H.B., Mechanism for riboflavin enhancement of bilirubin photodecomposition *in vitro*, *J. Pharm. Sci.*, 63, 404, 1974.

109. Vreman, H.J. et al., *In vitro* generation of carbon monoxide from organic molecules and synthetic metalloporphyrins mediated by light, *Dev. Pharmacol. Ther.*, 15, 112, 1990.

110. Vreman, H.J. et al., Dermal carbon monoxide (CO) production and excretion in neonatal rats during light exposure, *Pediatr. Res.*, 47, 463, 2000.

111. Vreman, H.J. et al., Effect of fluorescent- and light emitting diode (LED) blue light exposure on riboflavin-treated Gunn rat pups, *Pediatr. Res.*, 49, 325A, 2001.

112. Andersen, M.E. et al., Physiologically based pharmacokinetics and the risk assessment process for methylene chloride, *Toxicol. Appl. Pharmacol.*, 87, 185, 1987.

113. Vreman, H.J. et al., Methylene chloride metabolism: an *in vivo* and *in vitro* model for carbon monoxide (CO) generation, *Pediatr. Res.*, 49, 453A, 2001.

114. Vreman, H.J. et al., Correlation of carbon monoxide and bilirubin production by tissue homogenates, *J. Chromatogr.*, 427, 315, 1988.

115. Vreman, H.J., Ekstrand, B.C., and Stevenson, D.K., Selection of metalloporphyrin heme oxygenase inhibitors based on potency and photoreactivity, *Pediatr. Res.*, 33, 195, 1993.

116. Cowan, B.E. et al., The effect of tin protoporphyrin on the bilirubin production rate in newborn rats, *Pediatr. Pharmacol.*, 3, 95, 1983.

117. Posselt, A.M. et al., Suppression of carbon monoxide excretion rate by tin protoporphyrin, *Am. J. Dis. Child.*, 140, 147, 1986.

118. Ostrander, C.R., Johnson, J.D., and Bartoletti, A.L., Determining the pulmonary excretion rate of carbon monoxide in newborn infants, *J. Appl. Physiol.*, 40, 844, 1976.

119. Hamori, C.J., Vreman, H.J., and Stevenson, D.K., Suppression of carbon monoxide excretion by zinc mesoporphyrin in adult Wistar rats: evidence for potent *in vivo* inhibition of bilirubin production, *Res. Commun. Chem. Pathol. Pharmacol.*, 62, 41, 1988.

120. Vreman, H.J. et al., Carbon monoxide production and up-regulation of heme oxygenase activity in mice after heme administration, *J. Invest. Med.*, 47, A27, 1999.

121. Vreman, H.J., Lee, O.K., and Stevenson, D.K., *In vitro* and *in vivo* characteristics of a heme oxygenase inhibitor: ZnBG, *Am .J. Med. Sci.*, 302, 335, 1991.

122. Sunderman, F.W., Jr. et al., Increased lipid peroxidation in tissues of nickel chloride-treated rats, *Ann. Clin. Lab. Sci.*, 15, 229, 1985.

123. Sunderman, F.W., Jr., Metal induction of heme oxygenase, *Ann. N.Y. Acad. Sci.*, 514, 65, 1987.

124. Stevenson, D.K. et al., Pulmonary excretion of carbon monoxide in the human newborn infant as an index of bilirubin production: III. Measurement of pulmonary excretion of carbon monoxide after the first postnatal week in premature infants, *Pediatrics*, 64, 598, 1979.

125. Vreman, H.J. and Stevenson, D.K., Metalloporphyrin-enhanced photodegradation of bilirubin *in vitro*, *Am. J. Dis. Child.*, 144, 590, 1990.
126. Hintz, S.R., Vreman, H.J., and Stevenson, D.K., Mortality of metalloporphyrin-treated neonatal rats after light exposure, *Dev. Pharmacol. Ther.*, 14, 187, 1990.
127. Chan, M.L. et al., *In vivo* efficacy of light-emitting diodes (LEDs) as a light source for phototherapy in neonatal jaundiced rats, *Pediatr. Res.*, 45, 1104, 1999.
128. Rudolph, N. et al., Postnatal decline in pyridoxal phosphate and riboflavin. Accentuation by phototherapy, *Am. J. Dis. Child.*, 139, 812, 1985.
129. Sisson, T.R., Photodegradation of riboflavin in neonates, *Fed. Proc.*, 46, 1883, 1987.
130. DiVincenzo, G.D. and Kaplan, C.J., Uptake, metabolism, and elimination of methylene chloride vapor by humans, *Toxicol. Appl. Pharmacol.*, 59, 130, 1981.
131. Hayashi, S. et al., Induction of heme oxygenase-1 suppresses venular leukocyte adhesion elicited by oxidative stress: role of bilirubin generated by the enzyme, *Circ. Res.*, 85, 663, 1999.
132. Fenn, W.O., The burning of CO in tissues, *Ann. N.Y. Acad. Sci.*, 174, 64, 1970.
133. Clark, R.T., Stannard, J.N., and Fenn, W.O., The burning of CO to CO_2 by isolated tissues as shown by the use of radioactive carbon, *Am. J. Physiol.*, 161, 40, 1950.
134. Young, L.J. and Caughey, W.S., Mitochondrial oxygenation of carbon monoxide, *Biochem. J.*, 239, 225, 1986.
135. Balaraman, V. et al., End-tidal carbon monoxide in newborn infants: observations during the 1st week of life, *Biol. Neonate*, 67, 182, 1995.
136. Paredi, P. et al., Changes in exhaled carbon monoxide and nitric oxide levels following allergen challenge in patients with asthma, *Eur. Respir. J.*, 13, 48, 1999.
137. Uasuf, C.G. et al., Exhaled carbon monoxide in childhood asthma, *J. Pediatr.*, 135, 569, 1999.
138. Zayasu, K. et al., Increased carbon monoxide in exhaled air of asthmatic patients, *Am. J. Respir. Crit. Care Med.*, 156, 1140, 1997.
139. McCoubrey, W.K., Detection of heme oxygenase 1 and 2 proteins and bilirubin formation, in *Current Protocols in Toxicology*, Maines, M.D. et al., Eds., John Wiley & Sons, New York, 1999, 9.3.1.
140. Dennery, P.A. et al., Hyperoxic regulation of lung heme oxygenase in neonatal rats, *Pediatr. Res.*, 40, 815, 1996.
141. Laemmli, U.K., Cleavage of structural proteins during the assembly of the head of bacteriophage T4, *Nature*, 227, 680, 1970.
142. Towbin, H., Staehelin, T., and Gordon, J., Electrophoretic transfer of proteins from polyacrylamide gels to nitrocellulose sheets: procedure and some applications, *Proc. Natl. Acad. Sci. U.S.A.*, 76, 4350, 1979.
143. Slusher, T.M. et al., Glucose-6-phosphate dehydrogenase deficiency and carboxyhemoglobin concentrations associated with bilirubin-related morbidity and death in Nigerian infants, *J. Pediatr.*, 126, 102, 1995.
144. Dennery, P.A., Seidman, D.S., and Stevenson, D.K., Neonatal hyperbilirubinemia, *New Engl. J. Med.*, 344, 581, 2001.
145. Vreman, H.J. et al., Interlaboratory variability of bilirubin measurements, *Clin. Chem.*, 42, 869, 1996.
146. Dai, J., Parry, D.M., and Krahn, J., Transcutaneous bilirubinometry: its role in the assessment of neonatal jaundice, *Clin. Biochem.*, 30, 1, 1997.
147. Wong, R.J. et al., Transcutaneous bilirubinometry: a new tool for studying neonatal jaundiced rats, *Pediatr. Res.*, 45, 1373, 1999.
148. Gunn, C.H., Hereditary acholuric jaundice in new mutant strain of rats, *J. Hered.*, 29, 137, 1938.

149. Swarm, R.L., *Congenital Hyperbilirubinemia in the Rat: An Animal Model for the Study of Hyperbilirubinemia*, National Academy of Science, Washington, 1971, 149.

150. Saxton, A.M. et al., New mutation causing jaundice in mice, *J. Hered.*, 76, 441, 1985.

151. Jansen, F.H. et al., Congenital non-hemolytic jaundice: Crigler–Najjar syndrome, *Biol. Neonat.*, 14, 53, 1969.

152. Contag, C.H. et al., Visualizing gene expression in living mammals using a bioluminescent reporter, *Photochem. Photobiol.*, 66, 523, 1997.

153. Zhang, W.S. et al., Selection of potential therapeutics based on *in vivo* spatiotemporal transcription patterns of heme oxygenase, *J. Mol. Med.*, 45, in press, 2001.

154. Zhang, W.S. et al., Rapid *in vivo* functional analysis of transgenes in mice using whole body imaging of luciferase expression, *Transgenic Res.*, in press, 2001.

155. Lipshutz, G.S. et al., *In utero* delivery of adeno-associated viral vectors: intraperitoneal gene transfer produces long-term expression, *Mol. Ther.*, 3, 284, 2001.

156. Wong, R.J. et al., Heme oxygenase gene transcription and enzyme activity after heme administration, *Pediatr. Res.*, 49, 323A, 2001.

157. Ostrander, C.R. et al., Paired determinations of blood carboxyhemoglobin concentration and carbon monoxide excretion rate in term and preterm infants, *J. Lab. Clin. Med.*, 100, 745, 1982.

158. Fischer, A.F. et al., Carbon monoxide production in ventilated premature infants weighing less than 1500 g, *Arch. Dis. Child.*, 62, 1070, 1987.

159. Fällström, S.P., Endogenous formation of carbon monoxide in newborn infants. IV. On the relation between the blood carboxyhaemoglobin concentration and the pulmonary elimination of carbon monoxide, *Acta Paediatr. Scand.*, 57, 321, 1968.

160. Smith, D.W. et al., Bilirubin production after supplemental oral vitamin E therapy in preterm infants, *J. Pediatr. Gastroenterol. Nutr.*, 4, 38, 1985.

161. Seidman, D.S. et al., Role of hemolysis in neonatal jaundice associated with glucose-6 phosphate dehydrogenase deficiency, *J. Pediatr.*, 127, 804, 1995.

162. Kaplan, M. et al., Neonatal bilirubin production, reflected by carboxyhaemoglobin concentrations, in Down's syndrome, *Arch. Dis. Child. Fetal Neonatal. Ed.*, 81, F56, 1999.

163. Lynch, S.R. and Moede, A.L., Variation in the rate of endogenous carbon monoxide production in normal human beings, *J. Lab. Clin. Med.*, 79, 85, 1972.

164. Horváth, I. et al., Raised levels of exhaled carbon monoxide are associated with an increased expression of heme oxygenase-1 in airway macrophages in asthma: a new marker of oxidative stress, *Thorax*, 53, 668, 1998.

165. Vreman, H.J., Wong, R.J., and Stevenson, D.K., Heme oxygenase activity in the developing mouse, *Acta Haematol.*, 103, 60 (A237), 2000.

Index

A

Acetylcholine, 27–28, 39, 253
  salt-sensitive hypertension and, 158
N-Acetyl-L-cysteine, 47
Activated charcoal, 284
Activator protein-1 (AP-1), 47
Acute respiratory disease, 15
Adrenal glands, HO-1 deficiency pathology, 189
Advanced glycation end products (AGEs), 214–215, 221, 228
Aldosterone system, 159–160
Aminoguanidine, 226
4-Aminopyridine, 85, 100
Amyloidosis, 16, 189, 191, 204
Anaphylaxis, *See* Cardiac anaphylaxis
Anesthetic agents, 70
Angeli's salt, 117
Angiogenesis, 187, 243
Angiotensin II, 47, 86, 159, 183, 256
AP-1, 167, 243
AP-2, 243
Apamin, 34, 74, 85, 86, 96, 97–98
Apoptosis, 15, 29, 53–55
Arachidonate, 168
Arachidonic acid metabolites, and hypertension in spontaneously hypertensive rats, 234, 243, 251–252
L-Arginine, 157, 219
Arrhythmias, 167, 169, 172
Arsenite, 72
Asplenia, and human HO-1 deficiency, 185, 187, 192
Asthma, 215
Atherosclerosis, 167–168, 183
  HO-1 deficiency case, 192
ATP-sensitive K^+ channels, 84, 86–88, 93–95, 100–101

B

Baroreceptors, 126, 152
Basophil activation, 169–170, 175
Bay K8644, 226
Bcl-2 proteins, 53–55
Bile canaliculi contraction, 72
Bilirubin, 5, 58, 154, 167, 175, 221–222, 274
  accumulation in heme- and NO-treated cells, 118

cardiac HO-1 induction in ischemic heart, 258
^{14}C labeling, 277
hemin-treated heart production, 173
measurement methods, 297–299
NO interaction, 119
Biliverdin, 5, 58, 119, 154, 175, 182, 221, 274, *See also* Bilirubin
Bioluminescence imaging, 299
Blood pressure regulation, carbon monoxide effects, 138, 149–161, 183, 255
  HO inducer effects, 31
  HO inhibitors and, 150–151
  HO-1 deficiency and, 207
  hyper-sensitivity, 155
  neuromodulatory actions, 151–153
  NOS inhibition and, 154–158
  renal function and, 159–160
  salt-induced hypertension, 157
  spontaneously hypertensive rat models, 234
    arachidonic acid metabolites and, 234, 243, 251–252
    heme effects, 236–237
    HO-1 gene transfer and, 233–234, 240–243
    methods, 235–236
    stannous chloride effects on renal function, 234, 239–243
  vasorelaxant activity, 153–154
Bone marrow histology, HO-1 deficiency case, 189
Bone marrow transplantation, 207
Bradykinin, 128, 223
Brain
  cerebral vasculature, 13–14, 26, 69–70
  CO concentration, 290
  HO expression, developmental patterns, 126
  human HO-1 deficiency histopathology, 191
Breath analysis, 284, 296–297
8-Bromoguanosine-3',5'-cyclic monophosphate (8-Br cGMP), 69

C

Cadmium ion (Cd^{2+}), 37
Calcium, CO effects on intracellular levels, 36–37, 75, 85–86, 168, 175, *See also* Calcium-activated K^+ channels; Calcium channels
Calcium, diabetes and intracellular levels, 222, 224–228

309